Musculoskeletal Medicine

Series Editors
Grant Cooper • Joseph E. Herrera

For further volumes:
http://www.springer.com/series/7656

David A. Spinner • Jonathan S. Kirschner
Joseph E. Herrera
Editors

Atlas of Ultrasound Guided Musculoskeletal Injections

Springer

Editors
David A. Spinner, DO, RMSK
Department of Anesthesiology - Pain Medicine
Beth Israel Deaconess Medical Center
Arnold Pain Management Center
Harvard Medical School
Brookline, MA
USA

Joseph E. Herrera, DO, FAAPMR
Interventional Spine and Sports Medicine Division
Department of Rehabilitation Medicine
Icahn School of Medicine at Mount Sinai
New York, NY
USA

Jonathan S. Kirschner, MD, FAAPMR, RMSK
Interventional Spine and Sports Medicine Division
Department of Rehabilitation Medicine
Icahn School of Medicine at Mount Sinai
New York, NY
USA

Series Editors
Grant Cooper, MD
Princeton Spine and Joint Center
Princeton, NJ
USA

Joseph E. Herrera, DO, FAAPMR
Icahn School of Medicine at Mount Sinai
New York, NY
USA

ISBN 978-1-4614-8935-1 ISBN 978-1-4614-8936-8 (eBook)
DOI 10.1007/978-1-4614-8936-8
Springer New York Heidelberg Dordrecht London

Library of Congress Control Number: 2013954547

Printed on acid-free paper

Springer is part of Springer Science+Business Media (www.springer.com)

Grant me an opportunity to improve and extend my training, since there is no limit to knowledge. Help me to correct and supplement my educational defects as the scope of science and its horizon widen day by day.

Moses ben Maimon (Maimonides)
Mishneh Torah. IV, 19

Dedicated to my wife, Jessica, and daughter, Shirley, who spent nights and weekends without me so that I could bring this book to completion.
To my sister, Randi, and mother, Ricki, for a lifetime of setting the bar high and leading by example.
And to my father, Charles, who had an unequivocal belief in me to succeed. When I scored a 93 on a test, he asked what happened to the other 7 points, ensuring whatever the score on a test, I understood the material for it would make a difference. No matter the cost or family adversity, my education would never be sacrificed. He believed that one day I would help people in their suffering. I hope this helps.

David A. Spinner, DO, RMSK

To those who I have learned so much from, my parents, Bruce and Gwenn; my sisters, Greta and Kaye; my brother, Eli; my wonderful friends; my mentors; and my students.

Jonathan S. Kirschner, MD, FAAPMR, RMSK

This book is dedicated to my wife, Sandra, and children, Alex, Mikhayla, and Andrew, for their love and encouragement. To my parents, Eduardo and Rosario, and my sister, Sacha, for their sacrifice and unconditional support.

Joseph E. Herrera, DO, FAAPMR

Foreword

I am very fortunate to have had the opportunity to write the foreword for this excellent piece of work, *Atlas of Ultrasound Guided Musculoskeletal Injections,* inspired and created by Drs. Spinner, Kirschner, and Herrera.

The use of ultrasound to diagnose and treat musculoskeletal conditions is an evolving and incredible medical skill. We now have the ability to go beyond palpation and physical examination maneuvers and truly visualize neuromusculoskeletal structures and their spatial relationships and dynamic interactions. We can do focused visual evaluations seeing structures and specific tissue planes and dynamically visualize obvious and subtle defects.

Structures such as nerves and tendon sheathes can now be clearly visualized while we direct our treatments more precisely adjacent to them while avoiding injecting within their substance. Equally, if not more importantly, we can visualize vascular and other structures we want to avoid. This leads to improved, safer, and more comfortable treatments.

Ultrasound is also an evolving supplemental tool in the interventional spine field. For the last several decades, our spinal treatments have improved in efficacy and safety due to fluoroscopic techniques. They have improved even further with contrast installation and more recently with digital subtraction usage. I anticipate that these spinal ultrasound techniques will not replace, but *supplement*, fluoroscopy in the evolving spinal intervention treatment field. As the ultrasound technology and resolution improve, we will get improved visualization of the nerves we want to treat and the vessels we want to avoid, along with the landmarks we know from fluoroscopically performed spinal procedures.

This Atlas is an enormous and distinctive contribution to the evolving ultrasound field. It comprises *essential musculoskeletal ultrasound topics* important to physiatrists, sports medicine physicians, orthopedists, rheumatologists, and others devoted to the treatment of musculoskeletal disorders. The Atlas is unique since it also presents evolving understanding of spinal ultrasound options and controversial subjects including ultrasound-guided spasticity, myofascial pain syndrome, and biologic treatments.

This Atlas will be sure to have a profound impact on the education of musculoskeletal specialists, residents, and fellows. This Atlas is a representation of the commitment Drs. Spinner, Kirschner, and Herrera have as passionate teachers and educators. They have gone to great length and detail to present a plethora of appropriate *musculoskeletal references and evidence-based medicine* relevant to each procedure.

This Atlas is truly a work of art based on what now would seem simple premises. This is a *succinct visual reference* with figures, pictures, and diagrams to facilitate an easy understanding of the core concepts on patient presentation, relevant anatomy, and sonoanatomy. Common colors, symbols, and photographs are closely incorporated throughout the book to underscore a clear, consistent visual presentation. There is *emphasis on safety* and avoiding relevant structures while performing these ultrasound-guided procedures. This approach makes some very complex procedures easier, more efficient, and safer to perform.

As a result, you will have a better understanding of how to interpret and perform the procedures presented in this Atlas in a more efficient and safer way than you ever did before. We owe a great deal of gratitude to Drs. Spinner, Kirschner, and Herrera for this significant contribution.

With great appreciation and respect,

Michael B. Furman, MD, MS
Director,
Sports Medicine and Interventional Spine Fellowship Program,
OSS Health, York, PA, USA
Special Consultant,
Department of Rehabilitation Medicine,
Sinai Hospital, Baltimore, MD, USA
Assistant Clinical Professor,
Department of Physical Medicine and Rehabilitation,
Temple University School of Medicine, Philadelphia, PA, USA
Associate, OSS Health, York, PA, USA

Preface

Atlas of Ultrasound Guided Musculoskeletal Injections is intended to be a comprehensive source of ultrasound-guided techniques to help physicians in their practice to heal, decrease pain, and increase their patients' quality of life. Advances in ultrasound technology have created an environment where the ultrasound probe has become our stethoscope. It helps both diagnostically and therapeutically by guiding a needle and its contents to a pain generator to provide relief. The book is not intended to support the use of corticosteroids or other injectates or to abuse overutilization of ultrasonography. The proper use of musculoskeletal ultrasound in properly trained hands can provide diagnostic and therapeutic benefits to patients. Never before in medicine has an office-based technology allowed us to visualize anatomic structures in a dynamic way.

There are currently other books that provide a comprehensive approach to musculoskeletal scanning/sonography. This book is designed to provide the most up-to-date evidence where available for performing the related musculoskeletal injections. It is intended for neuromuscular physicians in Physiatry, Orthopedics, Neurology, Pain, and Rheumatology. We encourage further technical advances and techniques on how to perform injections as well as research and cost-effective analysis on using musculoskeletal ultrasound.

The book does not replace the time required to practice scanning and injecting. The editors of this book spend time each year practicing new and different injection techniques on cadavers with follow-up dissections to continually improve our skills, as well as lecturing and taking ultrasound courses ourselves.

Users of this book should be looking for ways to enhance and improve patient care by providing the safest injection techniques, whether anatomical (blind), ultrasound, fluoroscopy, or CT guided. We support the use of whichever technique provides the best and safest outcomes.

Musculoskeletal medicine is an exciting and growing specialty. We are encouraged by the many ways ultrasound enhances our current abilities to practice and treat patients, and we are excited for whatever the future and its research and technology have in store.

Basic ultrasound pictures are provided to enhance the terms, concepts, and procedures described. No other book provides in one place the breadth or detail of musculoskeletal specific injections as may be found in this 1st edition of *Atlas of Ultrasound Guided Musculoskeletal Injections*.

Brookline, MA, USA David A. Spinner, DO, RMSK

Acknowledgements

Although many individuals have offered help and participated in the preparation of this book, several deserve special mention. We are very grateful to Dr. Kristjan Ragnarsson, Chairman, Rehabilitation Medicine, Icahn School of Medicine at Mount Sinai, for his interest and support of our academic endeavors at this institution. A special thank you to Dr. Dallas Kingsbury, Rehabilitation Medicine Resident, Icahn School of Medicine at Mount Sinai, for providing valuable assistance in preparing the images for this book.

The editors wish to acknowledge and thank the many contributors of this book who have devoted countless hours bringing this project to fruition.

David A. Spinner, DO, RMSK
Jonathan S. Kirschner, MD, FAAPMR, RMSK
Joseph E. Herrera, DO, FAAPMR

I especially want to thank my two mentors and coeditors, Dr. Jonathan Kirschner and Dr. Joseph Herrera, for not only sharing the vision of the vast applications of musculoskeletal ultrasonography but for also being enthusiastic and dedicated mentors.

They created an academic environment that strives to further enhance medical knowledge.

David A. Spinner, DO, RMSK

Contents

1 **Introduction** 1
Jonathan S. Kirschner

2 **Shoulder** 7
Naimish Baxi and David A. Spinner

3 **Elbow** 17
Emerald Lin, Kathy Aligene, and Jonathan S. Kirschner

4 **Wrist and Hand** 29
David A. Spinner and Melissa I. Rosado

5 **Hip** 43
Mahmud M. Ibrahim, Yolanda Scott, David A. Spinner, and Joseph E. Herrera

6 **Knee** 57
David A. Spinner, Houman Danesh, and Waheed S. Baksh

7 **Foot and Ankle** 69
Kiran Vadada, Richard G. Chang, Christopher Sahler, and Jonathan S. Kirschner

8 **Trigger Point Injections** 89
Stephen Nickl and Lauren M. Terranova

9 **Neuromuscular/Chemodenervation** 101
Sarah Khan, Emerald Lin, and Jonathan S. Kirschner

10 **Spine** 123
David A. Spinner

Appendix 139

Index 145

Contributors

Kathy Aligene, MD Department of Rehabilitation Medicine, Icahn School of Medicine at Mount Sinai, New York, NY, USA

Waheed S. Baksh, MD, DPT Advanced Pain Relief Center, Winchester Medical Center, Winchester, VA, USA

Naimish Baxi, MD OSS Health, York, PA, USA

Richard G. Chang, MD Interventional Spine and Sports Medicine Division, Department of Rehabilitation Medicine, Icahn School of Medicine at Mount Sinai, New York, NY, USA

Houman Danesh, MD Department of Anesthesiology – Pain Medicine, Icahn School of Medicine at Mount Sinai, New York, NY, USA

Joseph E. Herrera, DO, FAAPMR Interventional Spine and Sports Medicine Division, Department of Rehabilitation Medicine, Icahn School of Medicine at Mount Sinai, New York, NY, USA

Mahmud M. Ibrahim, MD Performance Spine and Sports Medicine, Lawrenceville, NJ, USA

Sarah Khan, DO Brain Injury Unit, Department of Rehabilitation Medicine, Hofstra Medical School, North Shore Long Island Jewish Glen Cove Hospital, Glen Cove, NY, USA

Jonathan S. Kirschner, MD, FAAPMR, RMSK Interventional Spine and Sports Medicine Division, Department of Rehabilitation Medicine, Icahn School of Medicine at Mount Sinai, New York, NY, USA

Emerald Lin, MD Kessler Institute for Rehabilitation, West Orange, NJ, USA

Stephen Nickl, DO Department of Rehabilitation Medicine, Icahn School of Medicine at Mount Sinai, New York, NY, USA

Melissa I. Rosado, MD Maxwell Medical, New York, NY, USA

Christopher Sahler, MD Interventional Spine and Sports Medicine Division, Department of Rehabilitation Medicine, Icahn School of Medicine at Mount Sinai, New York, NY, USA

Yolanda Scott, MD Department of Rehabilitation Medicine, Icahn School of Medicine at Mount Sinai, New York, NY, USA

David A. Spinner, DO, RMSK Department of Anesthesiology – Pain Medicine, Arnold Pain Management Center, Beth Israel Deaconess Medical Center, Harvard Medical School, Brookline, MA, USA

Lauren M. Terranova, DO Department of Rehabilitation Medicine, Icahn School of Medicine at Mount Sinai, New York, NY, USA

Kiran Vadada, MD Interventional Spine and Sports Medicine Division, Department of Rehabilitation Medicine, Icahn School of Medicine at Mount Sinai, New York, NY, USA

Introduction

1

Jonathan S. Kirschner

Background

Physical medicine was initially named not based on the treatment of musculoskeletal conditions but the use of physical modalities, including electrical stimulation, diathermy, heat, cold, and ultrasound. The American Institute of Ultrasound Medicine, broadly recognized as the premier association for medical ultrasound, was originally founded in the 1950s by 24 physical medicine and rehabilitation physicians with a common interest in ultrasonic energy as a medical tool [1]. The use of ultrasound in obstetrics, cardiology, and emergency medicine grew exponentially from the 1960s onward. As ultrasound technology improved, the ability and the way physical medicine and rehabilitation is practiced transformed as well. Whether a specialist in spinal cord injury, traumatic brain injury, sports medicine, pain management, or pediatrics, ultrasound can play a role in the diagnosis and treatment of your patients.

If you are reading this book, then you already understand the benefits that ultrasound guidance can provide. Ultrasound has excellent soft tissue resolution (better than MRI), has no radiation, has no known contraindications (anyone can have one), and it is portable, hands-on, interactive, and dynamic. Patients can provide their own control (contralateral side); you can image around hardware, sutures, and screws; and you can perform an immediate therapeutic intervention.

You can also understand its pitfalls. It is operator dependent (but isn't life?) and can be time intensive. There is increased cost, but perhaps cost savings in the long run from more accurate placement of medications and the avoidance of further diagnostic and therapeutic procedures, earlier return to work or sports, and improved well-being and function. There is a limited field of view, decreased resolution at high depth, and an inability to image through or inside of bone.

This book is designed to describe comprehensive injection techniques for targets encountered in a typical physiatric, orthopedic, rheumatologic, and pain or sports medicine practice. Common injections for spasticity, sports medicine, and pain management will be reviewed including joint, tendon, ligament, bursa, muscle, biologics, trigger points, and botulinum toxin. This book is a reference but not a substitute for hands-on training and practice with experienced mentors in a supervised setting.

Each section will discuss the relevant local anatomy, structures to target or to watch out for. Recommended equipment, injection setups, and sample injectates will be provided. Pearls and safety considerations will be discussed. The choice of injectate is up to the individual provider and may include any combination of local anesthetic, corticosteroid, hyaluronic acid, platelet-rich plasma, prolotherapy, and possibly stem cells in the future. *Injectates provided are suggestions only; this is always patient and operator dependent.*

For each type of injection, relevant evidence on the accuracy of different approaches will be included. Multiple methods may be presented to accommodate different patient or practitioner preferences.

Ultrasound Terms

Ultrasound works using a reverse piezoelectric effect [2]. Electrical energy is transmitted through a crystal that vibrates to create sound waves. "Ultra" sound is >20 kHz; we are operating in the MHz range.

Ultrasound waves become *attenuated* as they pass through tissue, losing some of their energy. This increases at higher frequencies. Some waves are absorbed and turned into heat. Others diverge when waves are emitted from the transducer at an angle and do not return back to be processed. *Deflection*

J.S. Kirschner, MD, FAAPMR, RMSK
Interventional Spine and Sports Medicine Division,
Department of Rehabilitation Medicine,
Icahn School of Medicine at Mount Sinai, New York, NY, USA
e-mail: jonathan.kirschner@mountsinai.org

D.A. Spinner et al. (eds.), *Atlas of Ultrasound Guided Musculoskeletal Injections*, Musculoskeletal Medicine,
DOI 10.1007/978-1-4614-8936-8_1, © Springer Science+Business Media, LLC 2014

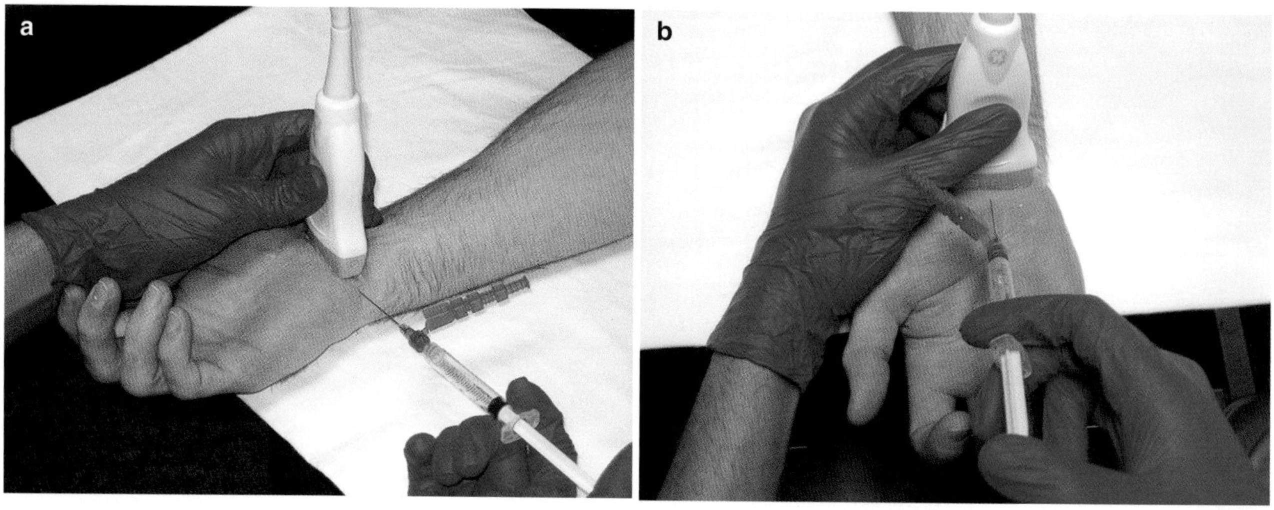

Fig. 1.1 (**a**) Example of short-axis (to the nerve) in-plane (to the needle) injection. (**b**) Example of short-axis (to the nerve) out-of-plane (to the needle) injection

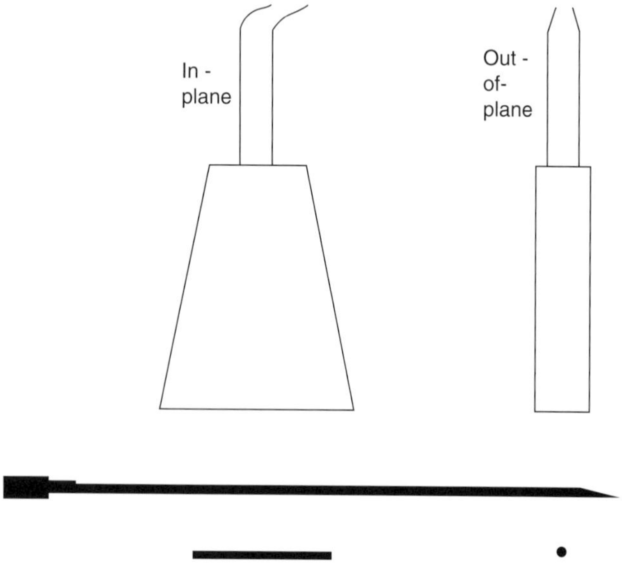

Fig. 1.2 When the needle is inserted in-plane it can be seen in its entirety, tip always in view. When the needle is inserted out-of-plane, only a cross section of the needle can be visualized and you cannot tell how deep it has advanced

includes reflection, refraction, and scattering. *Refraction* occurs when there are two fluid interfaces, changing direction of the wave as it passes from one another. *Reflection* occurs when some of the propagating sound energy strikes a boundary between two media and returns to the transducer. *Scatter* is reflection and refraction of waves away from the transducer [3].

The probe position may be described in anatomical terms or relative to the direction the structure is traveling. For example, the probe may be placed in the coronal, sagittal, or axial plane. It also may be "short axis," obtaining a cross-sectional view of a given structure, such as an axial view of the median nerve at the wrist. It may be "long axis" to the structure, which in the same example would be a sagittal view of the median nerve at the wrist [4, 5].

Injections, on the other hand, can be "in-plane" or "out-of-plane." In-plane means the needle is inserted parallel to the transducer, and the entire needle shaft (and tip) is visualized along its course. Out-of-plane means the needle is inserted perpendicular to the transducer (Figs. 1.1, 1.2).

Setting Up an Exam

First and foremost, the practitioner must be in a comfortable and ergonomic position to perform an injection. Next the patient must be comfortable. Injections can be done with the patient seated, supine, side-lying or prone. For patients prone to vasovagal responses or with poor balance or trunk control, seated is not recommended. For anxious patients, oral anxiolytics may be needed on occasion. For cervical procedures, an intravenous line may be placed. Risks, benefits, and alternatives of all procedures should be discussed with the patient and their family, and informed consent obtained. Common risks to all injections include bleeding, infection, worsening pain, allergic reaction, nerve damage, tendon, or ligament rupture. Risks specific to corticosteroids include local atrophy or skin depigmentation, increased blood pressure or sugar, mood swings, insomnia, rash, and flushing, but these are rare at the doses most commonly used.

The appropriate type of machine and transducer should then be selected. High-frequency linear array transducers (usually 10 MHz+) have higher resolution and have allowed the growth in musculoskeletal ultrasound (MSK-US) to be possible [6]. They are usually preferred for injections and come in wide,

Table 1.1 Transducers and frequency

Type of transducer		Frequency	
Linear	More accurate, less anisotropy	High frequency (10 MHz+)	Better resolution, less depth
Curvilinear	May help with needle visualization Larger footprint	Low frequency (5–2 MHz)	Poorer resolution, better depth
Hockey stick	Smaller footprint for interventions	High frequency (10 MHz+)	Better resolution, less depth

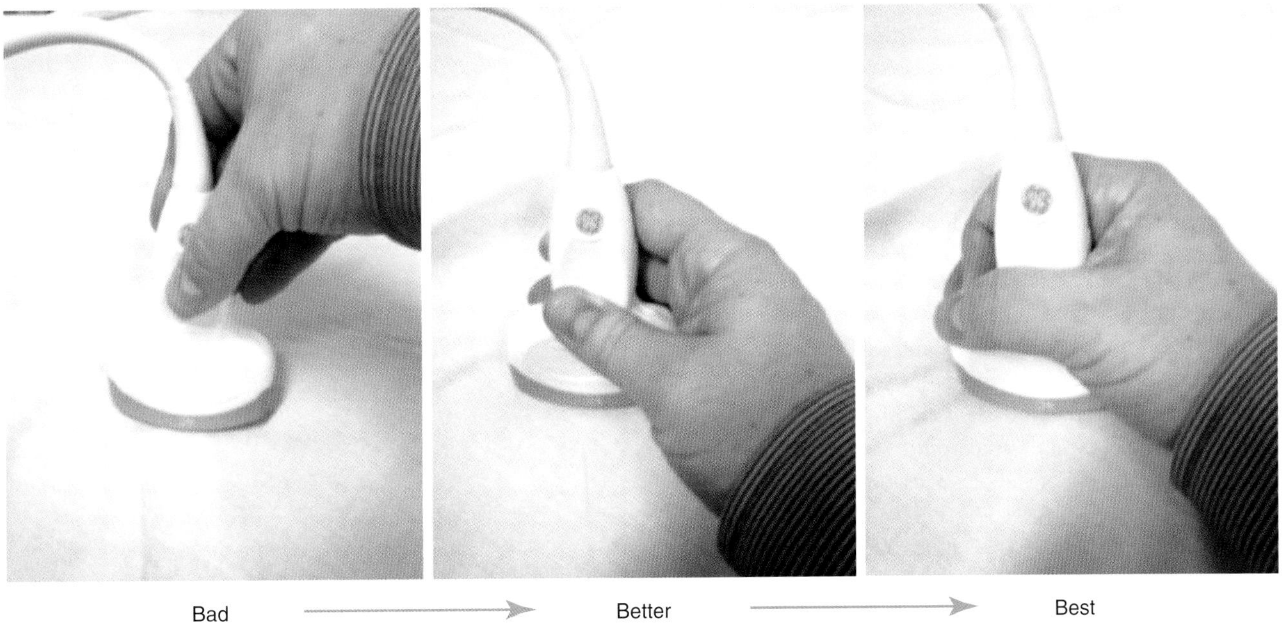

Fig. 1.3 Hold the transducer firmly while bracing the pinky or ulnar side of the hand on the patient for added control

medium, or small footprint "hockey-stick" sizes. Certain structures are more easily injected with small footprint probes (finger, toe joints), but usually the larger the footprint, the better because greater areas of tissue can be scanned at a time.

Low-frequency (curvilinear) transducers are helpful for imaging deeper structures, have large footprints, but have poorer resolution. They usually run in the 2–6 MHz range. It is easier to localize a needle at the beginning of an injection because the ultrasound beams are directed perpendicularly at the obliquely oriented needle; as the needle is advanced, the center of the transducer now emits beams 90° to the skin but oblique to the advancing needle. The transducer must be "heel-toed" or "rocked" to promote a more perpendicular beam orientation (Table 1.1).

Once the appropriate machine and transducer are selected, input the patient's demographics and adjust the presets (small parts, MSK, superficial, etc.). Many machines also come with needle enhancement software, which directs the beam more perpendicular to the needle rather than the skin. While helpful in some cases, these software tools are in no way as helpful as proper technique in maximizing needle visualization.

Place gel and a probe cover, followed by additional gel, then apply the probe. Grab the probe firmly and always brace the hand scanning against the skin. Once an image is obtained, identify a bony landmark and work off of that. Optimize the image by adjusting the depth, then focal zone. The number and width of focal zones can often be adjusted. The time gain compensation (TGC) can also be tuned to optimize visualization of structures at specific depths by selectively directing the sound beams, reducing attenuation and absorption. The last thing to adjust is the gain, which changes the overall brightness of the screen (Fig. 1.3).

Doppler mode can be used to identify flow. This is helpful in identifying blood vessels but can also be used to detect needle movements or small amounts of injectate, improving needle localization in difficult cases. Color Doppler shows directional flow, but Power Doppler is more sensitive for picking up movement.

Tissue Characteristics

Anisotropy occurs when sound beams exiting the transducer are not at 90° to the target. It must be adjusted for before declaring pathology. Correct it with "heel-toe," tilting or rocking the transducer (Table 1.2).

Table 1.2 General ultrasound terms

Echogenicity – the capacity of a structure in the path of an ultrasound beam to reflect back sound waves

Anechoic	*Isoechoic*	*Hypoechoic*	*Hyperechoic*
No internal echoes	Same echogenicity as the surrounding soft tissues	Low reflective pattern, manifesting as an area where the echoes are not as bright as the surrounding tissue	High reflective pattern appears brighter than the surrounding tissue
Examples:			
Blood vessels		Tendinosis	Calcifications
Fluid collections		Tears	Bone
Cartilage		Fluid collections	Ligaments, tendons
			Cartilage (uncovering sign)

Tendons appear as a fibrillar pattern of parallel hyperechoic lines in the longitudinal plane and hyperechoic round-to-ovoid shape (cut broom-end) in the transverse plane. They are very subject to anisotropy and so may appear hypoechoic if not visualized perpendicular to the transducer (i.e., biceps tendon). Follow tendons to their musculotendinous junction if you are not sure you are seeing tendon.

Ligaments appear similar to tendons with an intermediate echogenicity. They are structurally more dense, therefore more compact and fibrillar. They are also subject to anisotropy but less so.

Muscle appears as hypoechoic interstitial tissue interspersed with hyperechoic fascial planes. In the longitudinal plane, they have a pennate architecture. In the transverse plane, they have a "starry sky" appearance.

Nerves are less densely packed therefore less echogenic than tendons or ligaments but regular and fascicular. They have a train-track appearance in the longitudinal view and a honeycomb appearance in cross section [7]. They are less subject to anisotropy than tendons, which helps distinguish them in areas like the carpal tunnel. With nerve pathology you will see proximal hypoechoic swelling, an area of compression, then distal tapering. Indirect signs of nerve pathology are atrophy of the muscles innervated by that nerve (Fig. 1.4).

When examining joints, look for two articulating surfaces, fat pads, a capsule, and an intervening meniscus or synovial fold. Look for increased anechoic or hypoechoic fluid, fat pad displacement, or a "Geyser sign" to suggest effusion. Differentiate compressive effusions from non-compressible synovial hypertrophy, cartilage, or debris.

Hyaline cartilage lines articular surfaces of joints and appears as a thin hypoechoic rim paralleling the echogenic articular cortical surface. Because it is very hypoechoic, it may be confused for fluid. Due to the property of reflection, when there is a defect in the structure just superficial to the cartilage, increased sound waves can penetrate and bounce off of the cartilage, creating a hyperechoic line called the "cartilage uncovering sign." A large area of echogenic material lining the cartilaginous surface suggests pseudogout.

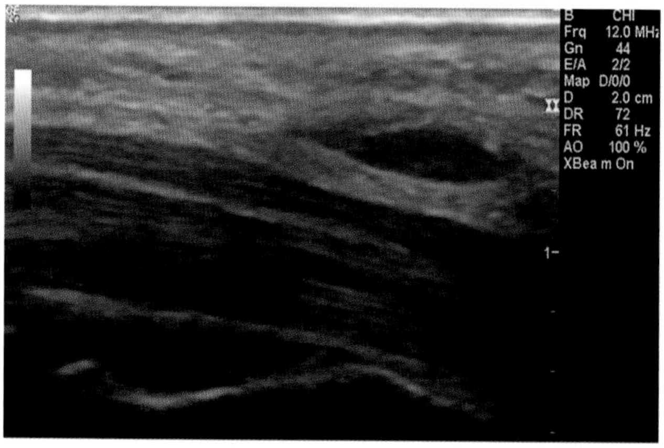

Fig. 1.4 Example of median nerve compression at the wrist, hypoechoic with proximal swelling

Bone cortex appears as an echogenic surface with posterior shadowing. Only the superficial surface of the bone can be consistently evaluated. Occult fractures may be seen as a "step-off" cortical disruption. Look for erosions or cortical irregularity in arthritis or tendinosis. Bony spurs at tendon or ligament insertion sites suggest enthesopathy.

Interventions

All potential injection sites should be scanned for relevant pathology, structures to avoid, and anomalous anatomy. It is a requirement, in fact, to document findings when billing for an ultrasound-guided procedure. Blood vessels, nerves, pleura, and other "safety" areas should be marked. Blood vessels can be seen with Doppler mode. Small nerves may not be well visualized, but many run with arteries so Doppler mode can identify the appropriate region or tissue plane to target (i.e., suprascapular nerve) even if the nerve is not directly seen. Constantly rock the transducer side to side ("toggling") or back and forth ("heel-toe") to improve image quality.

The preferred method of ultrasound-guided injection for most procedures is the in-plane approach, because the needle

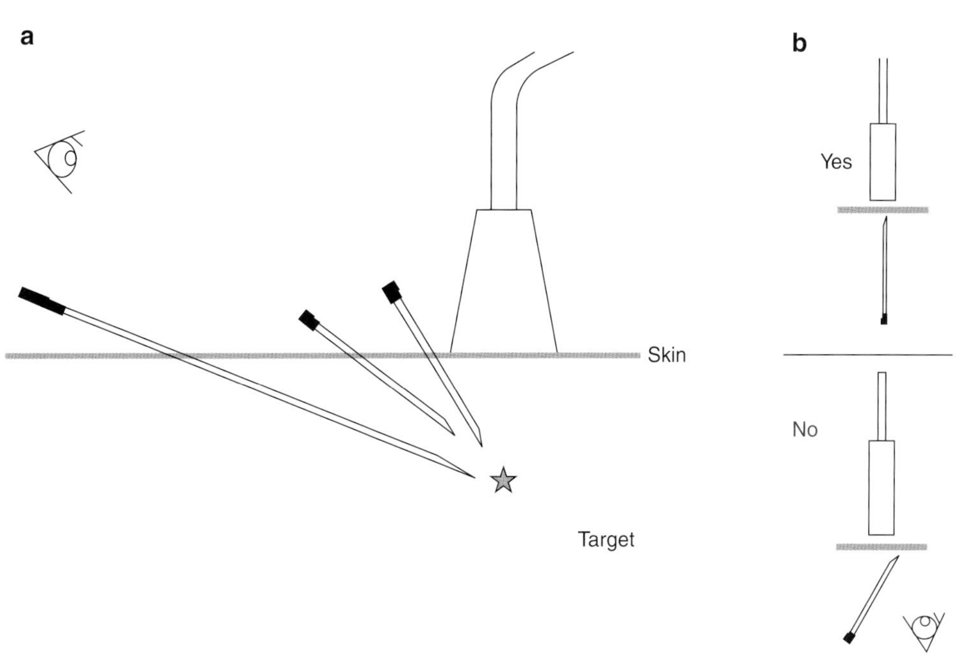

Fig. 1.5 Example of needle trajectory

and tip can be visualized along their entire course. Optimal imaging occurs when the needle is parallel to the transducer (sound beams perpendicular to the needle). The injectionist may have better visualization by starting further away from the transducer and using a longer needle at a flatter trajectory (Fig. 1.5).

Out-of-plane is less desirable because the needle is only seen as an echogenic dot, so once the needle passes under the transducer there is no way of knowing how far it is advancing. One way to correct for this is to advance the transducer after every needle advancement, so that the needle is never advanced beyond where it is seen directly under the transducer. Another method is the "walk-off" method, whereby the needle is inserted until it just appears under the transducer, then is retracted and redirected deep, then retracted, etc. until the correct depth is reached.

Tips and Tricks

Larger needles do not necessarily improve visualization, being parallel to the transducer and directly under the transducer at all times is much more helpful. There are echogenic needles on the market but these add cost and are of variable utility. A styletted spinal needle may be more helpful because the stylet can be rapidly inserted and removed or "jiggled" to increase sound reverberation and brighten the needle tip. Look for needle reverberation artifacts which occur when the needle is perfectly lined up.

Sometimes the target structure is so superficial or at such a steep angle that it is very difficult to advance a needle with adequate visualization. As mentioned above, *the steeper the needle insertion angle, the more difficult it is to see.* In these situations, a gel "standoff" may be used. With this technique, a mound of gel is placed under one end of the transducer while the other is anchored down on the skin. The needle is either introduced through this gel or just proximal to it. This allows the needle to be more parallel to the transducer for better imaging (Fig. 1.6).

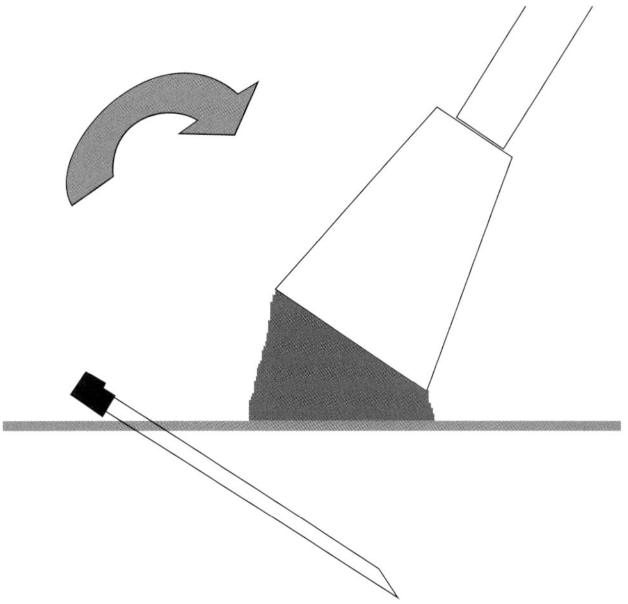

Fig. 1.6 Example of gel standoff positioning

Insert the needle quickly since breaking the skin is the most painful part of the injection. For local anesthesia, create a wheal of lidocaine or use ethyl chloride spray. Advance the needle just deep enough so that its leading edge is located directly under the transducer, optimizing the image to find the needle. Make sure the transducer is directly over the needle, the needle is parallel, and the angle is not too steep. Rotate the transducer clockwise or counterclockwise if you can see part of the shaft but not the whole needle or tip. Heel-toe (especially in obese patients) to get the needle more parallel to the transducer. Now advance the tip toward the intended target or retract and direct at a different angle. If you cannot see the tip, try rotating the needle and look for the sound beams reflecting off of the irregularly cut bevel.

Once at the intended target, inject some lidocaine or normal saline to confirm the correct location by watching the spread of the hypoechoic fluid. Injecting into a joint, the fluid will often seem to disappear (knee) or distend the joint capsule (acromioclavicular), whereas when in a fat pat or soft tissue, it will ball up. When perineural or peritendinous, you may see a "donut sign." When intratendinous or intraligamentous, there will be high pressure. If injecting corticosteroids or platelet-rich plasma (PRP), the injectate will be hyperechoic, especially at the end. Shaking up the medicine beforehand induces air bubbles which can act as a contrast medium. If you cannot see where the injectate is going, turn on Doppler to see a flash and help localize the needle tip.

For percutaneous needle tenotomies (aka barbitage, fenestration), a larger needle is often used after local anesthesia is given. The needle is retracted and redirected toward the more damaged (hypoechoic) or calcific (hyperechoic) areas. Infiltration of lidocaine or saline can help break up these calcifications. To cover a large area of tendinopathy, a "K or Kirschner turn" can be used. Analogous to parking terms, the needle is inserted in-plane, retracted, the transducer rotated clockwise or counter clockwise, and the needle reinserted in-plane. This process is repeated, allowing the injectionist to cover a large area of tendon with one skin insertion.

How to Use This Book

To remain consistent throughout the book, all injections contain a summary of clinical presentation, relevant local anatomy, and evidence-based treatments, if available. Each will have corresponding pictures that show the patient positioning and setup, normal ultrasound anatomy, and ultrasound anatomy with the needle in position. The needles will be denoted by white arrows, the needle tip by a white arrowhead. Needle reverberation artifact will be denoted by brackets. Black arrows and arrowheads refer to miscellaneous anatomy. Blood vessels will be shown as they appear on Doppler imaging or as an arrow with a line over it. Muscle and tendon are orange, purple, or occasionally magenta. Nerve is yellow. Ligaments, tendon sheathes, and aponeuroses are neon green.

We hope you find this book useful as a reference for commonly performed musculoskeletal injections. Keep it handy in the clinic. Residents or fellows can read up on a procedure they have not seen before, performing preliminary scanning and setting the patient up. Experienced practitioners can refresh their memory performing an injection they haven't done in a while. We hope others will use it to stimulate thought on different, better ways to perform injections accurately and safely. This is an evolving field and the techniques described here are expected to grow as well.

References

1. Valente C, Wagner S. History of the American Institute of Ultrasound in Medicine. J Ultrasound Med. 2005;24:131–42.
2. Smith J, Finnoff JT. Diagnostic and interventional ultrasound in contemporary musculoskeletal practice: part 1. Fundamentals. PM&R. 2009;1:6–75.
3. Kremkau F. Diagnostic ultrasound: principles and instruments. 6th ed. Philadelphia: WB Saunders; 2002. p. 428.
4. Lew HL, Chen CPC, Wang T-G, Chew KTL. Introduction to musculoskeletal diagnostic ultrasound: examination of the upper limb. Am J Phys Med Rehabil. 2007;86:310–21.
5. Smith J, et al. Sonographically guided carpal tunnel injections: the ulnar approach. J Ultrasound Med. 2008;27:1485–90.
6. Lin J, et al. An illustrated tutorial of musculoskeletal sonography. Part I. Introduction and general principles. Am J Roentgenol. 2000;175:637–45.
7. Sernik R, Abicalaf C, Pimentel B, Braga-Baiak A, Braga L, Cerri GG. Ultrasound features of carpal tunnel syndrome: a prospective case control study. Skeletal Radiol. 2008;37:49–53.

Shoulder

2

Naimish Baxi and David A. Spinner

The shoulder is an excellent region for the use of ultrasound-guided diagnosis and intervention due to its high injury prevalence and the superficial nature of commonly injured structures [1]. The shoulder girdle, composed of the scapula, clavicle, and proximal humerus, gives rise to the glenohumeral (GH), acromioclavicular (AC), and sternoclavicular joints. The deltoid, long head of the biceps brachii, and rotator cuff muscles (the supraspinatus, infraspinatus, teres minor, and subscapularis) facilitate shoulder movement in almost every plane [2]. The biceps tendon sheath, AC and GH joints, and subacromial/subdeltoid bursa (SASDB) are common sites for injection. There are also newer promising interventions, including prolotherapy, percutaneous needle tenotomy, and platelet-rich plasma, targeting rotator cuff tendons with ultrasound guidance.

Long Head of Biceps Brachii Tendon Sheath

Inflammation of the biceps tendon or sheath (tenosynovitis) from isolated injury or overuse is a common source of shoulder pain [3]. As the tendon passes through the bicipital groove of the humerus toward its insertion onto the superior labrum, it is exposed over the anterior region of the shoulder. The long head of the biceps contributes to humeral head stability, especially during abduction and external rotation [4]. Presenting symptoms may include anterior shoulder pain and discomfort. Injections to the biceps tendon sheath are historically performed blind.

N. Baxi, MD
OSS Health, York, PA, USA
e-mail: naimishb@gmail.com

D.A. Spinner, DO, RMSK (✉)
Department of Anesthesiology – Pain Medicine,
Arnold Pain Management Center,
Beth Israel Deaconess Medical Center,
Harvard Medical School, Brookline, MA, USA
e-mail: dspinnerny@gmail.com

A recent study by Hashiuchi et al. (Table 2.1) demonstrated that 86.7 % of ultrasound-guided injections achieved contrast within the tendon sheath compared to 26.7 % performed with the blind technique. Of those that were performed blind, another 33 % were completely outside the tendon sheath compared to 0 % when ultrasound was utilized [5]. Gazzillo et al. demonstrated that palpation-guided needle placement locating the long head of the biceps tendon was accurate only 5.3 % of the time without ultrasound verification [6].

Scanning Technique and Anatomy to Identify

For an optimal view of the biceps tendon, the patient's hand should be supinated with the elbow flexed, lying on the ipsilateral thigh. With the transducer placed in the axial plane over the proximal humerus, the hyperechoic tendon of the long head of the biceps brachii can be visualized within the bicipital groove. The transverse humeral ligament lies superficial to the tendon. The subscapularis tendon can be seen medially. Using Doppler imaging, the ascending branch of the circumflex humeral artery may be visualized laterally. Turn the transducer 90° to view the tendon longitudinally. Sweep medially to view the pyramid shape of the lesser tuberosity (Fig. 2.1) [7].

Injection Techniques: In-Plane Axial Approach

Patient positioning: Sit the patient with the hand supinated and elbow flexed.

Probe positioning: Place the transducer in the axial plane on the patient's proximal humerus, visualizing the greater and lesser tuberosities and the bicipital groove (Fig. 2.2a).

Markings: Identify the ascending branch of the circumflex humeral artery using power Doppler imaging. This vessel runs up the lateral side of the bicipital groove.

D.A. Spinner et al. (eds.), *Atlas of Ultrasound Guided Musculoskeletal Injections*, Musculoskeletal Medicine,
DOI 10.1007/978-1-4614-8936-8_2, © Springer Science+Business Media, LLC 2014

Table 2.1 Accuracy of blind vs. ultrasound-guided LHBT injection

		Type 1	Type 2	Type 3
Author	Location of injectate	Within tendon sheath	Inside tendon, tendon sheath, and surrounding area	Outside tendon sheath
Hashiuchi, 2011	Ultrasound-guided	86.7 %	13.3 %	0 %
	Unguided	26.7 %	40.0 %	33.3 %

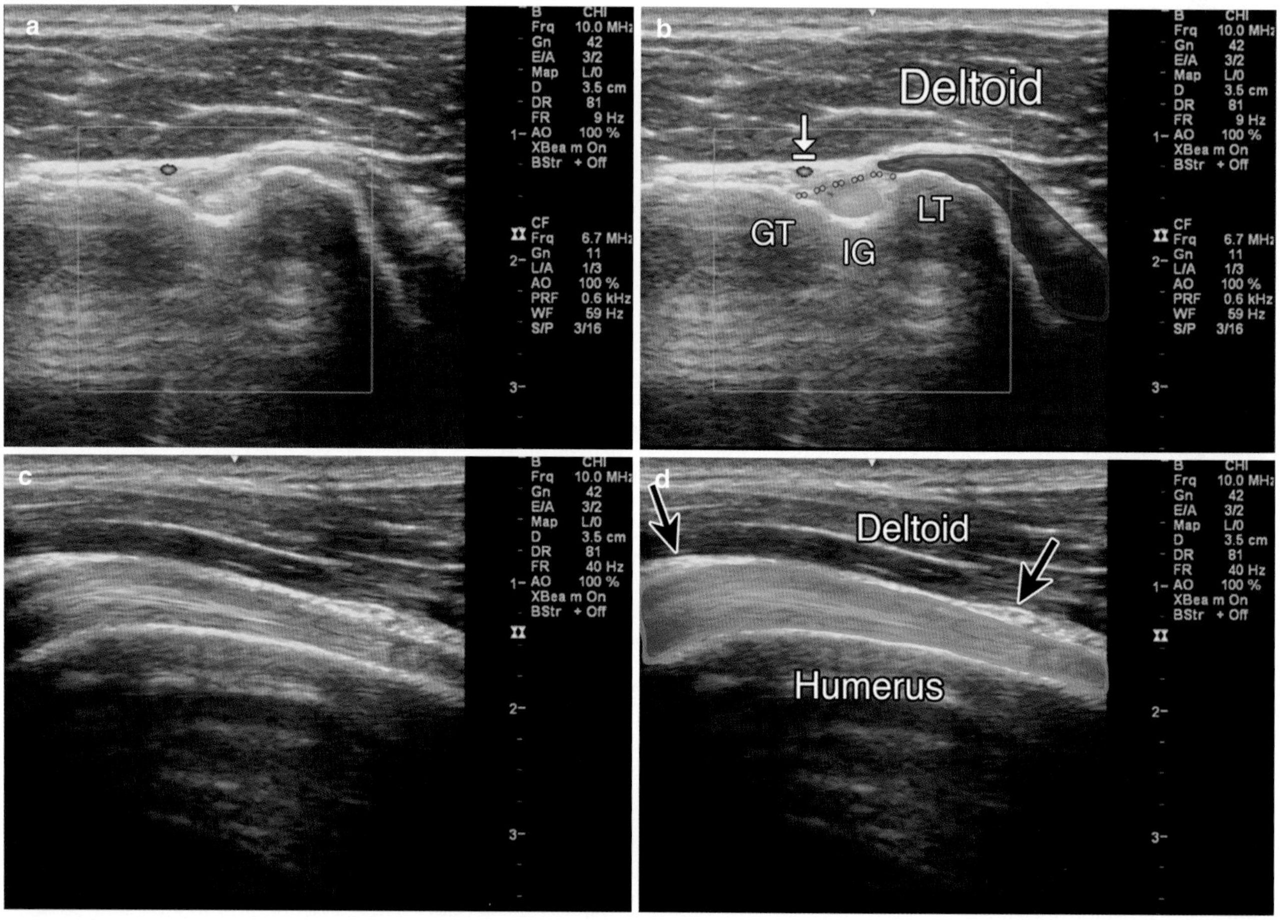

Fig. 2.1 (**a**) Short-axis view of the biceps tendon with circumflex humeral artery in *red*. (**b**) GT-greater tuberosity, *IG* intertubercular groove, *LT* lesser tuberosity, *arrow* with stop indicates circumflex humeral artery, deltoid labeled, *purple* subscapularis muscle, *orange circle* biceps tendon, *dotted green line* transverse humeral ligament. (**c**) Longitudinal view of biceps tendon. (**d**) Humerus deep to biceps tendon (*orange*) with thin bursa overlying it marked by *black arrows*, deltoid labeled

Needle position: Insert the needle from lateral to medial in-plane with the probe targeting the biceps tendon sheath situated between the biceps tendon and the transverse humeral ligament.

Safety considerations: Avoid directly injecting the tendon, as this may increase susceptibility to tendon rupture [8, 9]. Although the space between the tendon and the greater tuberosity can also be injected, the circumflex humeral artery should be properly visualized and avoided.

Pearls:

- The subacromial/subdeltoid bursa lies just superficial to the biceps tendon sheath and may be injected at the same time if so desired.
- Make sure injectate is seen flowing around the biceps tendon ("donut sign") and not in the bursa.

Injection Techniques: In-Plane Sagittal Approach

Patient positioning: Same as above

Probe positioning: Place the transducer sagittally to visualize the length of the biceps tendon within its groove and the pyramid shape of the lesser tuberosity (Fig. 2.3a).

Markings: The lesser tuberosity will appear medial to the bicipital groove. Fluid may be seen in the tendon sheath.

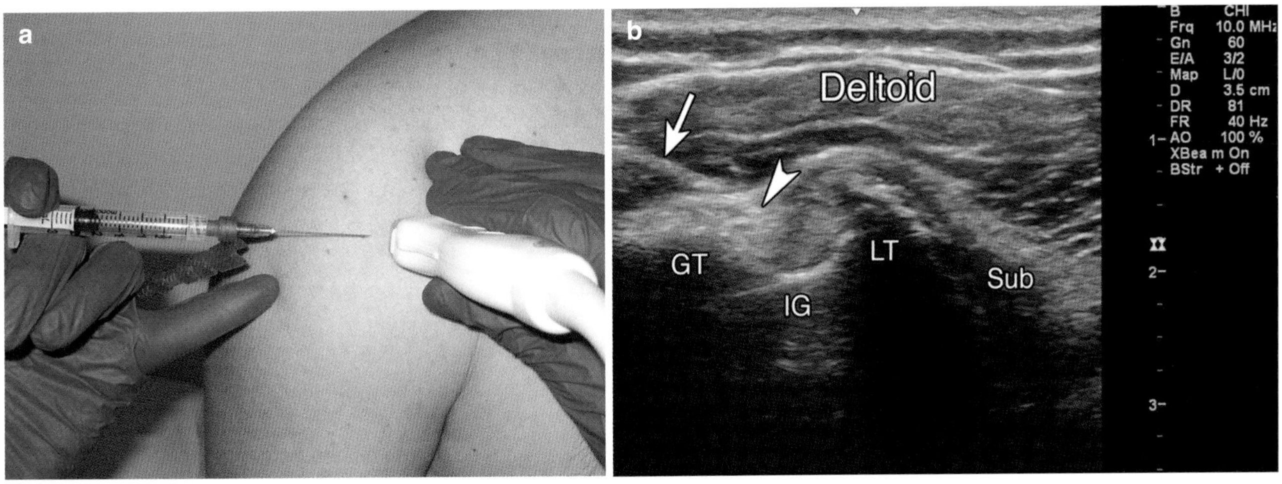

Fig. 2.2 (**a**) Example of axial probe position over biceps tendon with in-plane needle position. (**b**) Example of in-plane axial injection into the biceps tendon sheath, *GT* greater tuberosity, *IG* intertubercular groove, *LT* lesser tuberosity, *arrow* indicates needle, *arrowhead* indicates needle tip, sub-subscapularis muscle, deltoid labeled

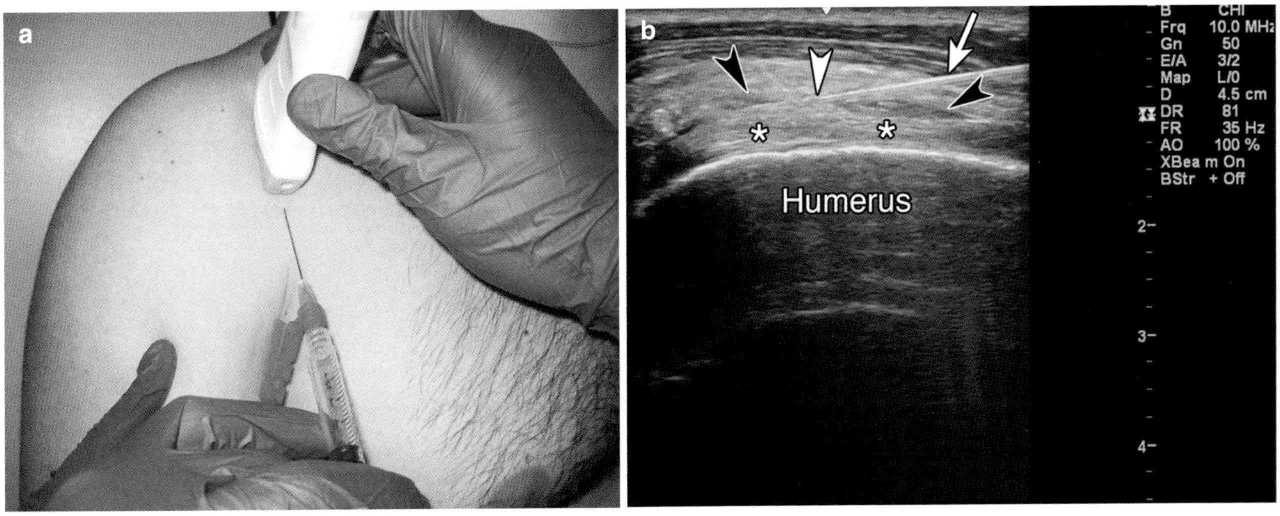

Fig. 2.3 (**a**) Example of longitudinal probe position over biceps tendon with in-plane injection technique. (**b**) Example of in-plane long axis approach, *asterisk* indicates biceps tendon, *black arrowheads* indicate tendon sheath filling with injectate, *white arrow* indicates needle, *white arrowhead* indicates needle tip

Needle position: Enter the skin from caudad to cephalad and in-plane with the probe.

Safety considerations: Same as above

Pearls:

- Supinate the hand to rotate the bicipital groove anteriorly.
- Angulate the transducer cephalad to eliminate anisotropy caused by the deep course of the biceps tendon.

Equipment needed:

- High-frequency linear array transducer (10 MHz+)
- 25 gauge, 1.5″ needle
- 0.5 ml of steroid preparation (typically 40 mg of triamcinolone or methylprednisolone)
- 1 ml of local anesthetic

Acromioclavicular (AC) Joint

The AC joint is formed by the articulation of the distal end of the clavicle and acromion process of the scapula, where a step-off can be palpated. Osteoarthritis of the AC joint is a frequent source of pain and occurs due to trauma or overuse from frequent rotational motion, shear stress, high compressive forces, or failure of the surrounding muscles [1, 10].

Ultrasound-guided AC joint injections can help diagnose AC joint mediated pain. Physical exam maneuvers such as the cross body arm abduction (scarf) sign and focal tenderness have low sensitivity [10]. Palpation-guided AC joint injections range in accuracy from 40 to 66 % (Table 2.2), while image-guided injections have been shown to have a much higher degree of accuracy [11–15].

Scanning Technique and Anatomy to Identify

The patient can be positioned supine or seated upright. The medial acromion or lateral clavicle can be palpated and the ultrasound probe placed in the anatomic coronal plane over the AC joint. Alternatively the joint can be found by scanning superiorly from the bicipital groove in the transverse plane [7]. With the probe directly over the AC joint, an anechoic joint space can be visualized separating the hyperechoic cortex of the acromion and clavicle (Fig. 2.4). The hyperechoic fibrocartilaginous disk interposing the joint may be visualized in younger patients [2].

Table 2.2 Accuracy of AC joint injections

Author	Specimen	Guidance	Accuracy	Verification
Partington, 1998	Cadaver	Blind	67 %	Dissection
Peck, 2010	Cadaver	Blind/US	Blind (40 %) US (100 %)	Dissection
Pichler, 2009	Cadaver	Blind	57 %	Dissection
Bisbinas, 2006	Clinical	Blind	39.4 %	Fluoroscopy
Sabeti-Aschraf, 2011	Cadaver	Blind/US	Blind (72 %) US (95 %)	US expert

Injection Techniques: In-Plane Coronal Approach

Patient positioning: Sit the patient with the arm in a neutral position, hanging at the side. This position is optimal as the weight of the shoulder and arm maximally opens the joint space. Downward traction on the arm can further accentuate this.

Probe position: Center the probe over the AC joint in the coronal plane (Fig. 2.5a).

Markings: No significant vascular or neural structures need to be marked.

Needle position: Insert the needle in-plane from lateral to medial aiming at the lateral margin of the clavicle. A gel standoff technique can be utilized.

Safety considerations: The subacromial space is approximately 4 mm below the capsule, so the needle should be carefully placed to avoid puncturing the deep capsule and entering the subacromial space.

Pearls:

- Direct the needle parallel to the probe, as the joint lies relatively superficial.
- Immediately after successful injection, the capsule may appear elevated and the joint space wider.
- A gel standoff technique may be used to allow more room for the needle approach.

Equipment needed:

- High-frequency linear array transducer (10 MHz+)
- 25 gauge, 1.5″ needle

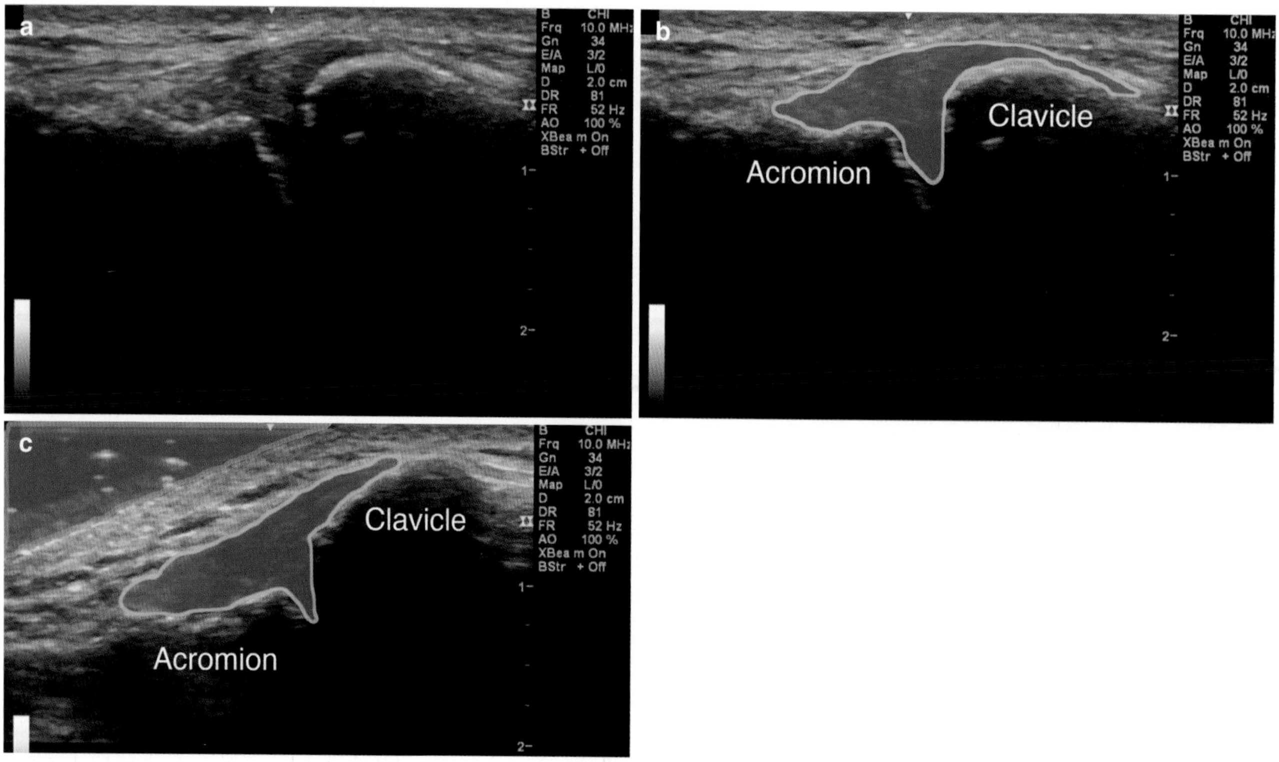

Fig. 2.4 (**a**) Coronal view of the acromioclavicular joint. (**b**) *Green* indicates AC joint fluid within the joint capsule, acromion and clavicle labeled. (**c**) Coronal view for a gel standoff approach, *light blue* indicating gel

- 0.5 ml of steroid preparation (typically 40 mg of triamcinolone or methylprednisolone)
- 1–2 ml of local anesthetic

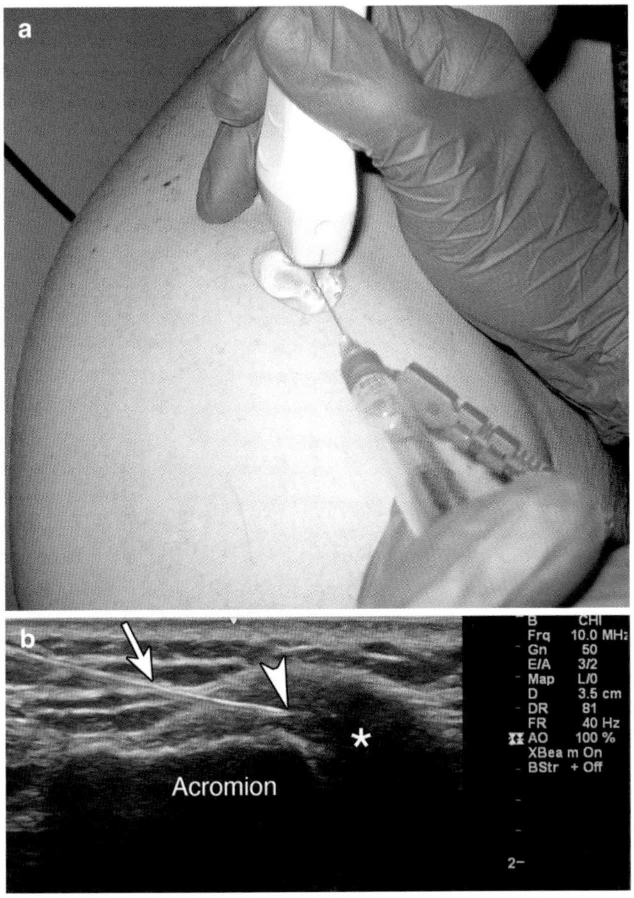

Fig. 2.5 (**a**) Example of coronal probe position over AC joint with gel standoff in-plane injection technique. (**b**) *Asterisk* indicates injectate in AC joint space, *arrow* points to needle, *arrowhead* points to needle tip, acromion labeled

Suprascapular Nerve Block

The suprascapular nerve innervates the supraspinatus and infraspinatus muscles and provides sensory branches to the posterior glenohumeral joint capsule, acromioclavicular joint, subacromial bursa, coracoclavicular, and coracoacromial ligaments [16]. A nerve block can be used to temporarily relieve pain or provide local anesthesia to any of these structures [17].

Scanning Technique and Anatomy to Identify

Place the ultrasound probe transversely over the superior medial border of the spine of the scapula, over the supraspinatus muscle. Follow the orientation of the superficial supraspinatus muscle and the deeper bony scapula; move the probe laterally along the axis of the supraspinatus muscle until the suprascapular notch appears (Fig. 2.6a) [18]. The suprascapular nerve will be visualized beneath the transverse scapular ligament in the suprascapular notch [19]. The nerve may be difficult to visualize but can be seen adjacent to the suprascapular artery, which can be identified with Doppler.

Injection Technique: In-Plane Coronal Approach

Patient positioning: Sit the patient with the arm in lap or with the hand of the side being blocked resting on the contralateral shoulder [19].

Probe positioning: The probe is placed parallel to the superior aspect of the scapular spine and then moved laterally and cephalad in a coronal plane to visualize the scapular floor and the suprascapular notch. Toggling the probe from

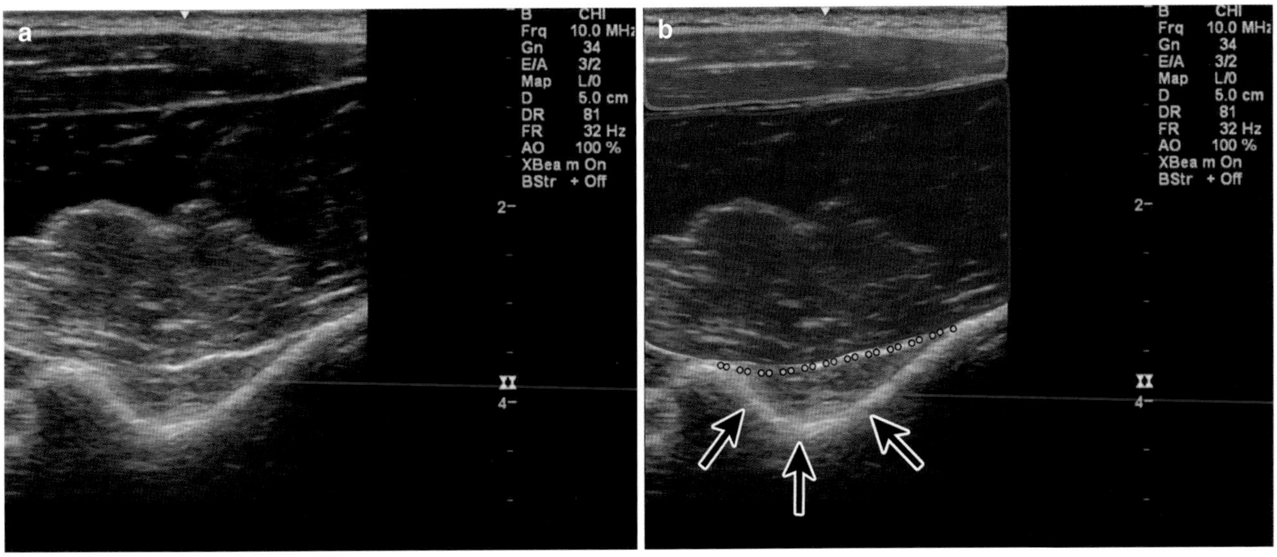

Fig. 2.6 (**a**) Coronal view of suprascapular notch. (**b**) *Orange* indicates trapezius muscle, *purple* indicates supraspinatus muscle, *black arrows* point to suprascapular notch, *green dotted line* indicates suprascapular ligament

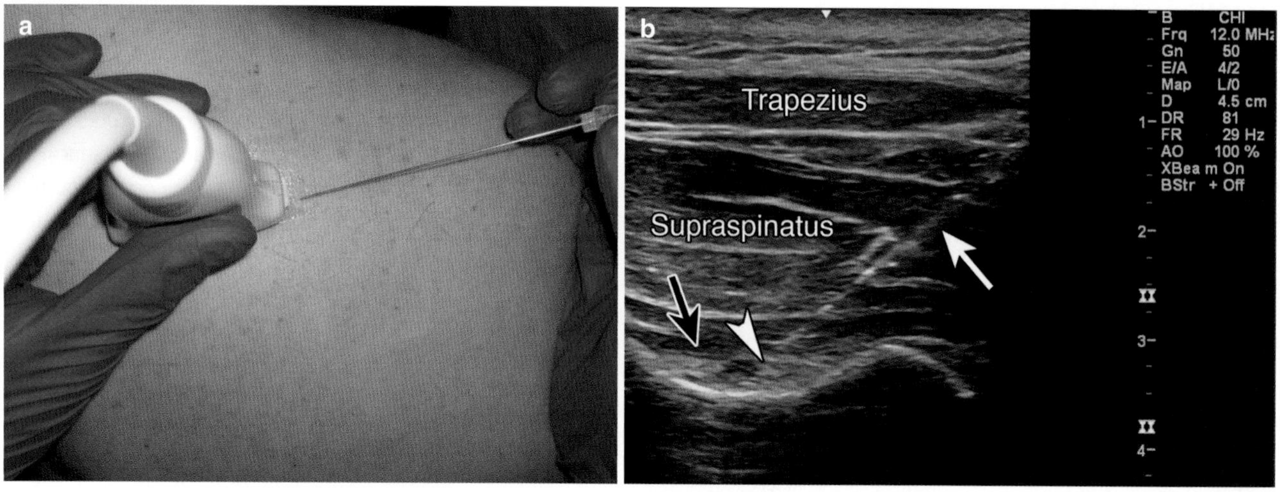

Fig. 2.7 (**a**) Example of coronal probe position over suprascapular notch. (**b**) Example of in-plane needle approach, *black arrow* point to suprascapular ligament, white arrow indicates needle, *white arrowhead* points to needle tip adjacent to suprascapular nerve, trapezius and supraspinatus muscles labeled

axial to coronal planes may help to visualize the suprascapular nerve and the transverse ligament (Fig. 2.7a).

Markings: The trapezius and supraspinatus will be clearly visualized deep to the subcutaneous tissue. The suprascapular artery can be confirmed with Doppler.

Needle position: The needle is directed from the lateral side of the probe in-plane toward the nerve sheath.

Safety considerations: The needle should be visualized at all times to avoid pneumothorax.

Pearls:

- Live ultrasound can demonstrate the spread of the injectate around the nerve and under the suprascapular ligament.

Equipment needed:

- High-frequency linear array transducer (10 MHz+)
- 22–25 gauge, 3″ or 3.5″ needle
- 0.5 ml of steroid preparation (typically 40 mg of triamcinolone or methylprednisolone)
- 4 ml of local anesthetic

Glenohumeral (GH) Joint

The GH joint is formed by the humeral head and glenoid cavity and is deepened and supported by the cartilaginous glenoid labrum. Its capsule is strengthened by three glenohumeral ligaments and extends down the bicipital tendon sheath in the intertubercular groove [16]. In patients with adhesive capsulitis or glenohumeral arthrosis, the shoulder can be an intense source of pain and limited mobility and function. Although primary osteoarthritis is uncommon in this region, rotator cuff failure, trauma, previous surgery, avascular necrosis, inflammatory arthropathies, osteochondritis dissecans, and iatrogenic injury can all lead to secondary osteoarthritis [1]. Adhesive capsulitis, commonly referred to as "frozen shoulder," initially presents as pain followed by progressively worsening range of motion. Although active or passive ranges of motion have been shown to improve function in adhesive capsulitis, GH joint injection expedites progress and symptom relief [20]. The accuracy of blind injections ranges from 27 to 72 % (Table 2.3) compared to ultrasound-guided injections which have been shown to be accurate 92–99 % of the time [21–29].

Scanning Technique and Anatomy to Identify

The glenohumeral joint can be visualized from either a posterior or an anterior approach. In a pathological joint, synovial hypertrophy and joint effusion can be visualized, most commonly in the posterior recess. Bone erosions of the humeral head can also be detected, often indicating a rotator cuff injury [30]. Posteriorly, the humeral head, bony glenoid, and labrum can be visualized deep to the infraspinatus and deltoid muscles (Fig. 2.8). Just medial, the spinoglenoid notch with the suprascapular neurovascular bundle can be seen [1].

Injection Techniques: In-Plane Axial Posterior Approach [1]

Patient positioning: Sit or place the patient in a semi-prone position with the hand of shoulder being injected crossing the chest (ipsilateral humerus adducted across thorax) or hanging at the side. The scapula should also remain protracted.

Probe position: Place the probe caudal and parallel to the lateral end of the scapular spine (Fig. 2.9a).

Table 2.3 Accuracy of GH joint injections

Author	Specimen	Guidance	Accuracy	Verification
Eustace, 1997	Clinical	Blind	42 %	Radiograph
Patel, 2012	Cadaver	Blind/US	72.5 %/92.5 %	Radiograph
Sethi, 2005	Cadaver	Blind	26.8 %	MR arthrography
Choudur, 2011	Clinical	US	99 %	MR arthrography
Gokalp, 2010	Clinical	US	96.7 %	MR arthrography
Koivikko, 2008	Clinical	US	Posterior 100 % Anterior 100 %	MR arthrography
Souza, 2010	Clinical	US	92 %	MR arthrography
Schaeffeler, 2010	Clinical	US/Fluoroscopy	US 100 % Fluoro 100 %	MR arthrography
Rutten, 2009	Clinical	US/Fluoroscopy	US 94 % Fluoro 72 %	MR arthrography

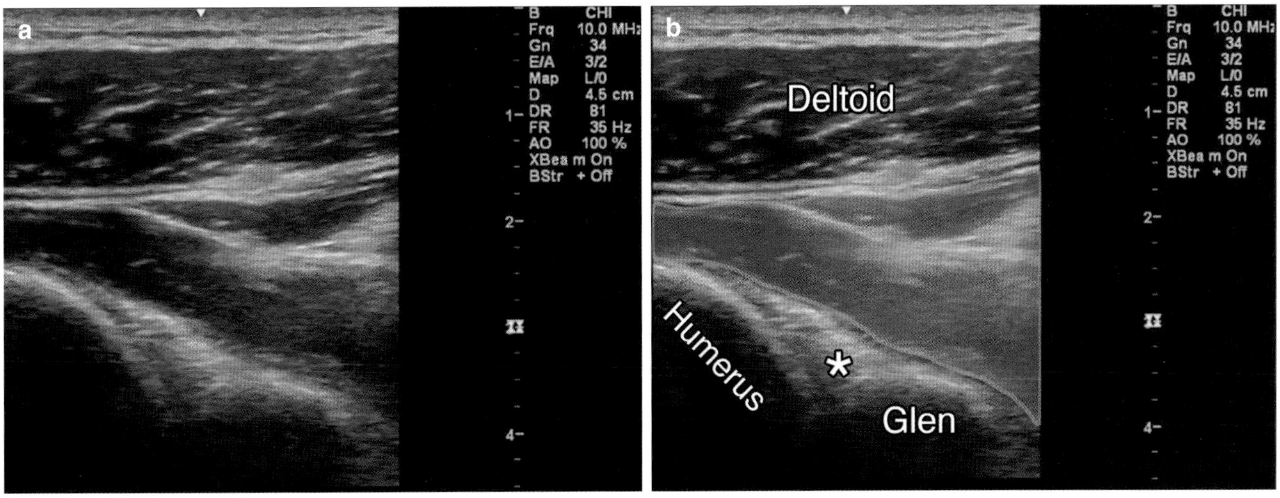

Fig. 2.8 (**a**) Posterior view of glenohumeral joint. (**b**) View of the posterior glenohumeral joint, deltoid and humerus labeled, *Glen* glenoid, *asterisk* indicates labrum, *orange* overlies infraspinatus muscle

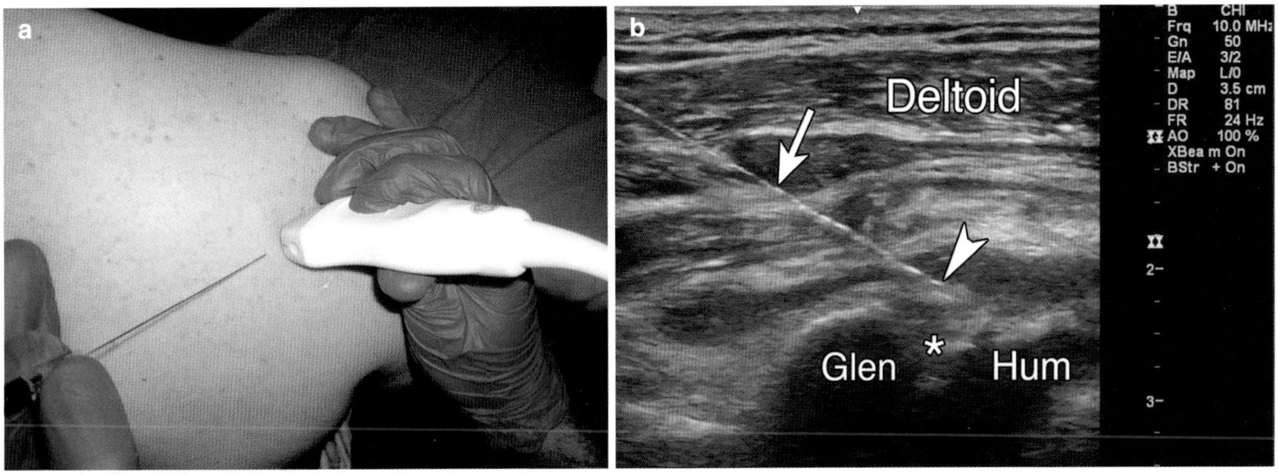

Fig. 2.9 (**a**) Example of probe position over posterior glenohumeral joint. (**b**) Example of in-plane needle approach, *white arrow* indicates needle, *white arrowhead* indicates needle tip, Hum-humerus, *Glen* glenoid, *asterisk* indicates labrum, deltoid labeled

Markings: The infraspinatus muscle, humeral head, posterior glenoid rim, and labrum can be visualized. Doppler can be checked to visualize the suprascapular artery in the spinoglenoid notch.

Needle position: The needle is directed, in-plane, from the medial or lateral side of the probe until it is subcapsular and contacts the humeral head.

Safety considerations: Avoid puncturing the glenoid labrum. Care must be taken to drive the needle directly toward the humeral head. For larger shoulders, a steeper approach may be necessary employing a walk-off technique of the needle off the posterior aspect of the humeral head.

Pearls:

- If resistance is encountered during injection, the needle may be embedded in the cartilage or capsule and may require slight manipulation to allow better flow of injectate into the joint.

Equipment needed:

- Linear array transducer (8 MHz+)
- 22–25 gauge, 3″ or 3.5″ needle
- 0.5–1.0 ml of steroid preparation (typically 40 mg of triamcinolone or methylprednisolone)
- 4 ml of local anesthetic

Subacromial/Subdeltoid Bursa (SASDB)

The SASDB is the most commonly injected shoulder structure and is helpful in diagnosing and treating impingement syndrome, rotator cuff tears, tendinosis, and other sources of bursitis. Impingement typically occurs from postural factors, rotator cuff deficits (partial tear, tendinosis, weakness), anatomic variations of the acromion or AC joint, thickening of the coracoacromial ligament, or repetitive overhead activities which then inflame the bursa. The mainstay of initial treatment is rest, nonsteroidal anti-inflammatory medication, and physical therapy, but patients with impingement may benefit from a SASDB corticosteroid injection to facilitate a more active therapy program when pain limited [1]. Blind SASDB injections are inconsistent, with studies demonstrating accuracy ranging from 60 to 100 % compared to near 100 % accuracy with ultrasound (Table 2.4) [31–37].

Scanning Technique and Anatomy to Identify

When viewing the SASDB, the acromion and deltoid muscles can be used as landmarks. The bursa will appear lateral to the acromion, below the relatively hypoechoic deltoid muscle and above the more hyperechoic supraspinatus tendon. When distended, a thin rim of hypoechoic fluid may be seen within the bursa (Fig. 2.10). When not distended, the location of the bursa can be estimated from the peribursal fat in between the deltoid muscle and supraspinatus tendon [1].

Injection Technique: In-Plane Coronal Approach

Patient position: Sit the patient with the ipsilateral arm hanging down.

Probe position: Place the probe in the coronal plane over the lateral end of the acromion perpendicular to the coracoacromial arch (Fig. 2.11a).

Marking: The acromion can be visualized on the medial most part of the ultrasound screen. The SASDB lies between the hyperechoic peribursal fat, below the hypoechoic deltoid muscle.

Needle position: Insert the needle in-plane directed toward the anechoic space between the peribursal fat, representing the SASDB [1].

Safety considerations: No significant structures are vulnerable to injury. Avoid spreading corticosteroid into the deltoid or supraspinatus tendon.

Table 2.4 Accuracy of SASDB injections

Author	Specimen	Guidance	Accuracy	Verification
Yamakado, 2002	Clinical	Blind	Anterolateral (70 %)	Radiographs
Henkus, 2006	Clinical	Blind	Posterior (76 %) Anteromedial (69 %)	MRI
Kang, 2008	Clinical	Blind	Posterior (75 %) Anterolateral (75 %) Lateral (60 %)	Radiographs
Park, 2010	Clinical	Blind	Anterolateral (49 %)	Radiographs
Rutten, 2007	Clinical	Blind/US	Posterior blind (100 %) Posterior US (100 %)	MRI
Hanchard, 2006	Cadaver	Blind	Posterior lateral (91 %)	Dissection
Mathews, 2005	Cadaver	Blind	Anterolateral (90 %) Posterior (80 %)	Dissection

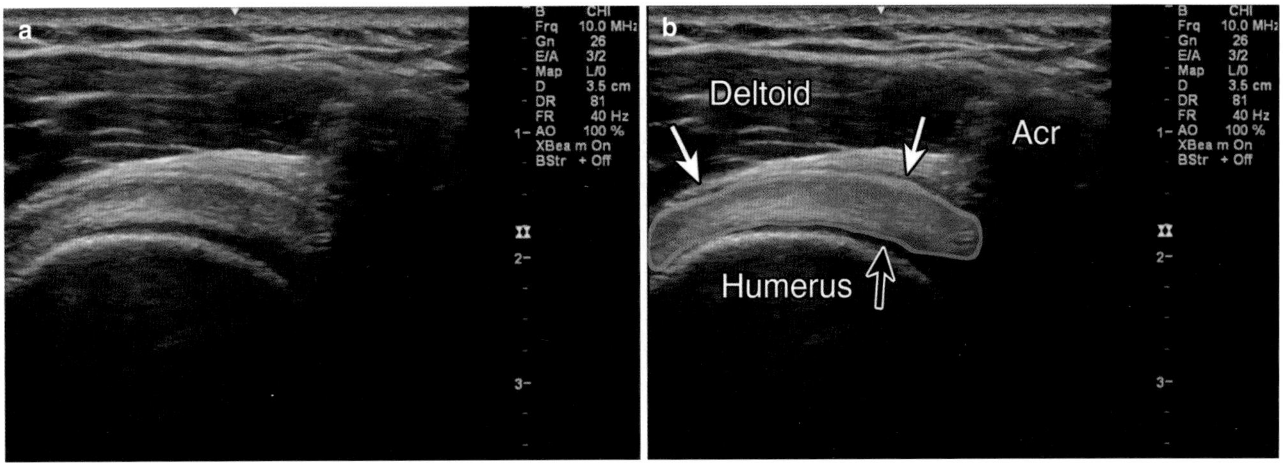

Fig. 2.10 (**a**) Coronal view of the SASDB. (**b**) Deltoid and humerus labeled, *Acr* acromion, *black arrow* indicates hyaline cartilage, *white arrows* indicate SASDB, *orange* indicates supraspinatus muscle

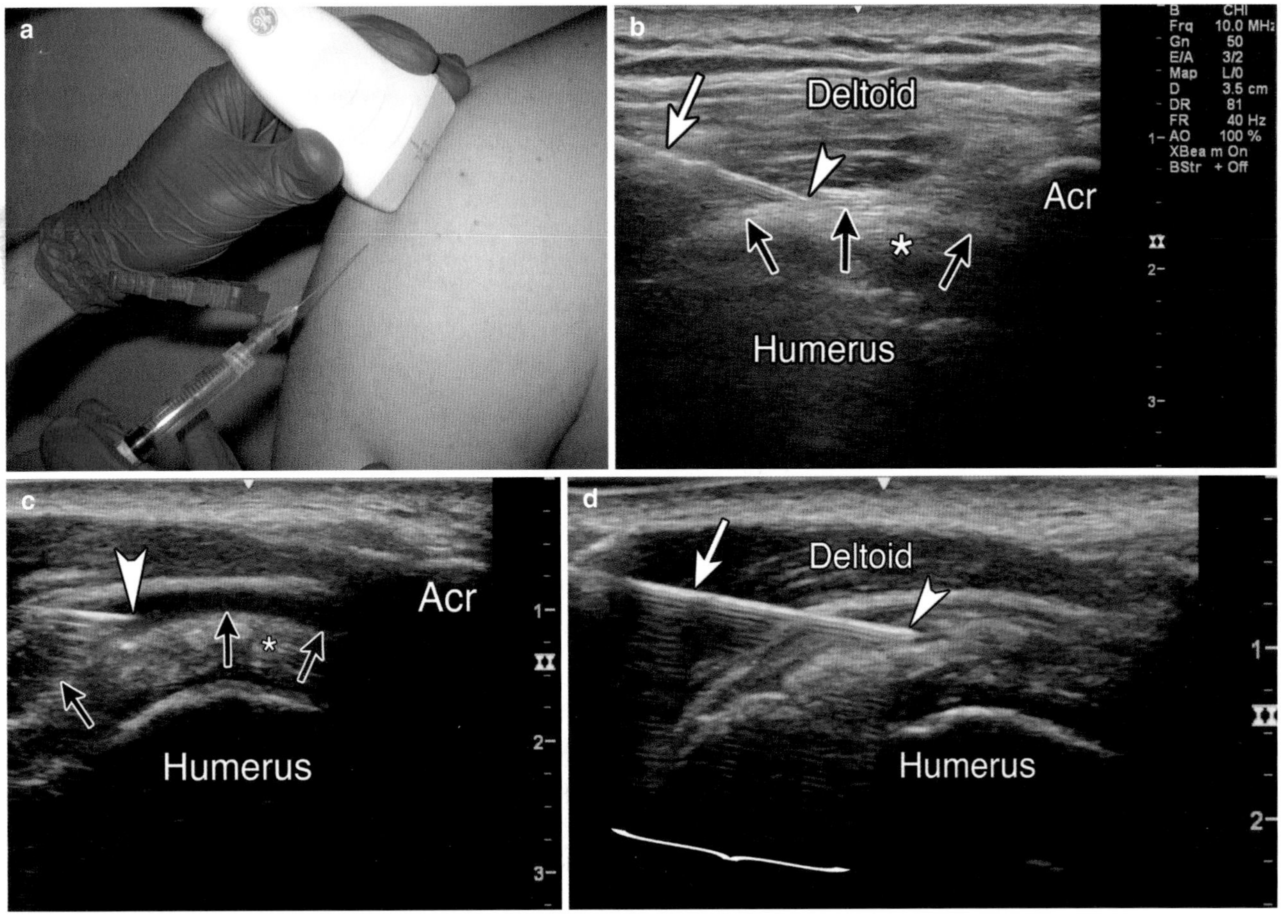

Fig. 2.11 (**a**) Example of probe position over SASDB with in-plane injection technique. (**b**) Example of in-plane needle approach, *white arrow* indicates needle, *white arrowhead* indicates needle tip, humerus and deltoid labeled, *Acr* acromion, *black arrows* indicate location of SASDB, *asterisk* indicates supraspinatus muscle with anisotropy. (**c**) *White arrowhead* indicates needle tip, *black arrows* indicate injectate filling bursa, *asterisk* indicates supraspinatus muscle with anisotropy, *Acr* acromion, humerus labeled. (**d**) Example of calcific tenotomy, *white arrow* indicates needle, *white arrowhead* indicates needle tip, *bracket* indicates needle reverberation, deltoid and humerus labeled

Pearls:

- Following injection, the separation between the supraspinatus and deltoid muscle can be seen under live ultrasound; make sure the fluid is seen diving underneath the acromion to confirm accurate placement.

Equipment needed:

- High-frequency linear transducer (10 MHz+)
- 25 gauge, 1.5″ needle
- 40 mg of triamcinolone or methylprednisolone
- 4–6 ml of local anesthetic

References

1. Peng P, Cheng P. A review of anatomy, sonoanatomy, and procedures. Part III: shoulder. Reg Anesth Pain Med. 2011;36:592–605.
2. Chiang YP, Feng CF, Lew HL. Ultrasound-guided examination and injection of the shoulder. Am J Phys Med Rehabil. 2011;90:616–7.
3. Ahrens P, Boileau P. The long head of biceps and associated tendinopathy. J Bone Joint Surg Br. 2007;89(8):1001–9.
4. Durham B. Emedicine [Online]. 8 February 2012. [Cited: 19 June 2012.] http://emedicine.medscape.com/article/96521-overview#a0106
5. Hashiuchi T, et al. Accuracy of the biceps tendon sheath injection: ultrasound-guided or unguided injection? A randomized controlled trial. J Shoulder Elbow Surg. 2011;20:1069–73.
6. Gazzillo GP, Finnoff JT, Hall MM, Sayeed YA, Smith J. Accuracy of palpating the long head of the biceps tendon: an ultrasonographic study. PM R. 2011;3:1035–40.
7. Jacobson JA. Fundamentals of musculoskeletal ultrasound. Philadelphia: Saunders/Elsevier; 2007.
8. Haraldsson BT, Langberg H, Aagaard P, Zuurmond AM, van El B, Degroot J, Kjaer M, Magnusson SP. Corticosteroids reduce the tensile strength of isolated collagen fascicles. Am J Sports Med. 2006;34:1992–7.
9. Carpenito G, Gutierrez M, Ravagnani V, Raffeiner B, Grassi W. Complete rupture of biceps tendons after corticosteroid injection in psoriatic arthritis "Popeye sign": role of ultrasound 2. J Clin Rheumatol. 2011;17:108.
10. Renfree KJ, Wright TW. Anatomy and biomechanics of the acromioclavicular and sternoclavicular joints. Clin Sports Med. 2003;22:219–38.
11. Pichler W, Weinberg AM, Grechenig S, Tesch NP, Heidari N, Grechenig W. Intra-articular injection of the acromioclavicular joint. J Bone Joint Surg Br. 2009;91:1638–40.
12. Partington PF, Broome GH. Diagnostic injection around the shoulder: hit and miss? A cadaveric study of injection accuracy. J Shoulder Elbow Surg. 1998;7:147–50.
13. Peck E, Lai JK, Pawlina W, Smith J. Accuracy of ultrasound-guided versus palpation-guided acromioclavicular joint injections: a cadaveric study. PM R. 2010;9:817–21.
14. Bisbinas I, Belthur M, Said H, Green M. Learmonth. Accuracy of needle placement in ACJ injections. Knee Surg Sports Traumatol Arthrosc. 2006;14:762–5.
15. Sabeti-Aschraf M, Lemmerhofer B, Lang S. Ultrasound guidance improves the accuracy of the acromioclavicular joint infiltration: a prospective randomized study. Knee Surg Sports Traumatol Arthrosc. 2011;19:292–5.
16. Drake R, Wayne A, Mitchell A. Gray's anatomy for students. Philadelphia: Elsevier; 2010.
17. Sigenthaler A, et al. Ultrasound-guided suprascapular nerve block; description of a novel supraclavicular approach. Reg Anesth Pain Med. 2012;37:325–8.
18. Taskaynatan MA, Ozgul A, Aydemir K, Koroglu OO, Tan AK. Accuracy of ultrasound-guided suprascapular nerve block measured with neurostimulation. Rheumatol Int. 2012;32:2125–8.
19. Harmon D, Hearty C. Ultrasound-guided suprascapular nerve block technique. Pain Physician. 2007;10(6):743–6.
20. Marx RG, Malizia RW, Kenter K. Intra-articular corticosteroid injection for the treatment. HSS J. 2007;3(2):202–7.
21. Patel DN, Nayyar S, Hasan S, Khatib O, Sidash S, Jazrawi LM. Comparison of ultrasound-guided versus blind glenohumeral injections: a cadaveric study. J Shoulder Elbow Surg. 2012;21(12):1664–8.
22. Sethi PM, Kingston S, Elattrache N. Accuracy of anterior intra-articular injection of the glenohumeral joint. Arthroscopy. 2005;21:77–80.
23. Eustace JA, Brophy DP, Gibney RP, Bresnihan B, FitzGerald O. Comparison of the accuracy of steroid placement with clinical outcome in patients with shoulder symptoms. Ann Rheumatol Dis. 1997;56:59–63.
24. Choudur HN, Ellins ML. Ultrasound-guided gadolinium joint injections for magnetic resonance arthrography. J Clin Ultrasound. 2011;39:6–11.
25. Gokalp G, Dusak A, Yazici Z. Efficacy of ultrasonography-guided shoulder MR arthrography using a posterior approach. Skeletal Radiol. 2010;39:575–9.
26. Koivikko MP, Mustonen AO. Shoulder magnetic resonance arthrography: a prospective randomized study of anterior and posterior ultrasonography-guided contrast injection. Acta Radiol. 2008;49:912–7.
27. Souza PM, Aguiar RO, Marchiori E, Bardoe SA. Arthrography of the shoulder: a modified ultrasound-guided technique of joint injection at the rotator interval. Eur J Radiol. 2010;74:29–32.
28. Rutten MJ, Collins JM, Maresch BJ. Glenohumeral joint injection: a comparative study of ultrasound and fluoroscopically guided techniques before MR arthrography. Eur Radiol. 2009;19:722–30.
29. Schaeffeler C, Brügel M, Waldt S, Rummeny EJ, Wörtler K. Ultrasound-guided intraarticular injection for MR arthrography of the shoulder. Rofo. 2010;182:267–73.
30. Petranova T, et al. Ultrasound of the shoulder. Med Ultrason. 2012;14(2):133–40.
31. Rutten MJ, Maresch BJ, Jager GJ, de Waal Malefijt MC. Injection of the subacromial-subdeltoid bursa: blind or ultrasound-guided? Acta Orthop. 2007;78:24–257.
32. Henkus HE, Cobben LP, Coerkamp EG, Nelissen RG, van Arkel ER. The accuracy of subacromial injections: a prospective randomized magnetic resonance imaging study. Arthroscopy. 2006;22: 227–82.
33. Yamakado K. The targeting accuracy of subacromial injection to the shoulder: an arthrographic evaluation. Arthroscopy. 2002; 18:887–91.
34. Kang MN, Rizio L, Prybicien M, Middlemas DA, Blacksin MF. The accuracy of subacromial corticosteroid injections: a comparison of multiple methods. J Shoulder Elbow Surg. 2008;17:61–6.
35. Park JY, Siti HT, O KS, Chung KT, Lee JY, Oh JH. Blind subacromial injection. J Shoulder Elbow Surg. 2010;19:1070–5.
36. Hanchard N, Shanahan D, Howe T, Thompson J, Goodchild L. Accuracy and dispersal of subacromial and glenohumeral injections in cadavers. J Rheumatol. 2006;33:1143–6.
37. Mathews PV, Glousman R. Accuracy of subacromial injection: anterolateral versus posterior approach. J Shoulder Elbow Surg. 2005;14:145–8.

3 Elbow

Emerald Lin, Kathy Aligene, and Jonathan S. Kirschner

Ultrasound can play an important role in differentiating the etiology of elbow pain since most pathology is extra-articular and superficial, including tendinosis and tears, ligamentous injury, nerve injury or entrapment, and bursitis [1–4]. Elbow arthritis, fractures, and other intra-articular pathologies can also be diagnosed indirectly by visualizing effusions which are easily seen. Due to the prevalence of tendinopathies, the elbow is a good region for some of the more emerging interventional procedures including prolotherapy, percutaneous needle tenotomy, and platelet-rich plasma injection [5].

Medial Epicondylosis (ME): Common Flexor Tendon (CFT)

The two most common pathologies involving the CFT are medial epicondylosis and tendon tear. Clinically distinguishing between these two diagnoses can be challenging [6]. However, with ultrasound guidance, diagnosis of degenerative changes versus tendon tear can be readily made. This information helps guide the early management of medial elbow pain. In addition, serial scanning with ultrasound can help assess response to intervention. Medial epicondylosis, known as "golfer's elbow," is characterized as an overuse syndrome or degenerative tendinosis caused by repetitive motion, especially during pronation and flexion of the wrist, involving the attachment at the CFT origin [3]. Medial epicondylosis is also frequently reported in baseball pitchers due to intense valgus force, and in athletes participating in tennis, bowling, racquetball, and javelin [4].

Clinically, the patient presents with localized tenderness at the medial epicondyle that is exacerbated by pronation and often associated with decreased grip strength [5]. One provocative test, called the medial epicondylitis test ("reverse Cozen's test"), reproduces medial elbow pain with resisted wrist flexion while the elbow is in full extension and the forearm is supinated [7]. Treatments vary from oral anti-inflammatory medications, rest, ice, physical therapy, and a variety of injections including ultrasound-guided corticosteroids and newer alternative minimally invasive procedures such as percutaneous needle tenotomy (PNT), autologous blood injection (ABI), and platelet-rich plasma (PRP) [5, 8]. Combined approach of PNT and autologous blood (AB) with ultrasound guidance has been shown as an effective treatment for refractory medial epicondylosis [8].

Scanning Technique and Anatomy to Identify

With the patient's hand in supination, the ultrasound probe is placed in a longitudinal orientation over the medial epicondyle [1]. In this view, the medial epicondyle is seen proximally with the trochlea and ulna. The anterior band of the ulnar collateral ligament is seen overlying the ulna and trochlea and ultimately inserts onto the epicondyle. The common flexor tendon appears fibrillar and overlies these structures inserting on the ridge of the epicondyle [2].

Ultrasound assessment usually reveals a normal hyperechoic triangular tendon interspersed with focally thickened or hypoechoic areas. As these changes may appear quite subtle it is critical to compare with the contralateral side [2]. In the presence of more progressive changes, hypoechogenicity, loss of normal fibrillar pattern, and even hyperemia from neovascularization can be visualized with color or power Doppler mode [3]. In chronic medial epicondylosis, calcifications may be observed that can lead to increased risk of partial or complete tendon rupture. Acute medial tendon

E. Lin, MD (✉)
Kessler Institute for Rehabilitation, West Orange, NJ, USA
e-mail: lin.emerald@gmail.com

K. Aligene, MD
Department of Rehabilitation Medicine,
Icahn School of Medicine at Mount Sinai, New York, NY, USA
e-mail: kaligene@gmail.com

J.S. Kirschner, MD, FAAPMR, RMSK
Interventional Spine and Sports Medicine Division,
Department of Rehabilitation Medicine,
Icahn School of Medicine at Mount Sinai, New York, NY, USA
e-mail: jonathan.kirschner@mountsinai.org

D.A. Spinner et al. (eds.), *Atlas of Ultrasound Guided Musculoskeletal Injections*, Musculoskeletal Medicine,
DOI 10.1007/978-1-4614-8936-8_3, © Springer Science+Business Media, LLC 2014

ruptures can be diagnosed quickly and effectively by scanning in both the longitudinal and transverse plane. Typically, there is a loss or replacement of the regular hyperechoic fibrillar tendon pattern with irregular hypoechoic fluid and debris. If this is visualized, confirm clinically by palpating the identified location. One may feel a subtle step-off defect [9]. In this case, surgical intervention is often indicated (Fig. 3.1).

Injection Technique: In-Plane Coronal Approach

Patient positioning: The patient should be seated or lay supine with 90° of elbow flexion and the shoulder externally rotated. Place a towel underneath the lateral epicondyle for comfort.

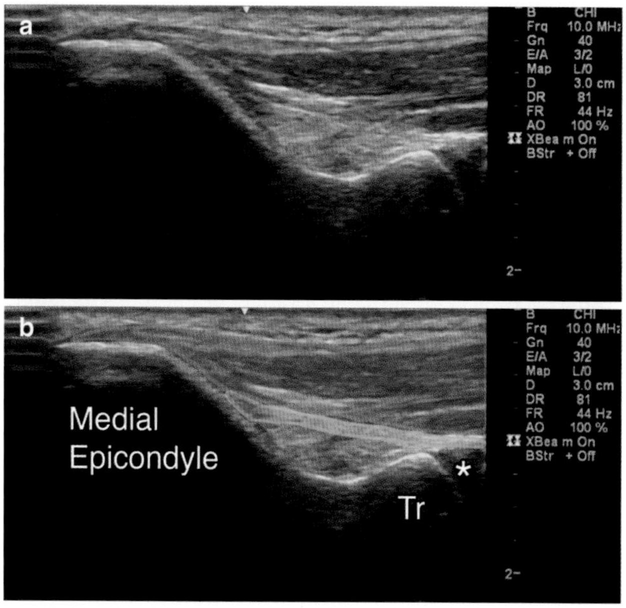

Fig. 3.1 (**a**) Coronal view of the common flexor tendons. (**b**) Tr-trochlea, *asterisk* indicates joint space, *orange* indicates common flexor tendons, and *green* indicates ulnar collateral ligament

Probe position: Place the probe longitudinally (coronal) with the proximal end of the transducer over the medial epicondyle to visualize the common flexor tendon. Scan proximally and distally until the medial epicondyle and the proximal attachments of the CFT are clearly identified (Fig. 3.2a).

Markings: Mark any obvious vessel or tendon prior to injection. Mark the medial epicondyle and the olecranon process.

Needle position: The needle should be inserted parallel to the transducer from either proximal to distal or distal to proximal. Due to the superficial nature of the tendon, a gel standoff may be helpful. For PNT, insert the needle into the tendon itself. For a peritendinous injection, keep the needle above or below the tendon.

Safety considerations: For corticosteroid injections, be careful when injecting superficial to the tendon since this can cause subcutaneous atrophy or depigmentation. PNT may cause local bleeding and post-procedure pain. Be careful to not inject too posterior, as this is where the ulnar nerve may lie.

Pearls:

- If performing PNT, intermittently switch to an out-of-plane/short-axis view in order to determine the anterior-posterior/radial-ulnar position of the needle within the region of tendinosis [4]. Repetitively fenestrate the entire region of tendinosis while injecting local anesthetic, PRP, or AB. Resistance should decrease with increased passes. Calcifications and enthesophytes should be mechanically broken up [11–13].

Equipment needed:

- High-frequency linear array transducer (10 MHz+).
- 25 gauge, 1.5″ needle.
- 0.5 mL of steroid preparation.
- 1–3 mL of local anesthetic.
- For PNT, use a larger (18–20 gauge) needle.
- May include 0.5–1 mL of steroid preparation with 1–3 mL of local anesthetic or 2–3 mL of PRP or autologous whole blood [11, 12].

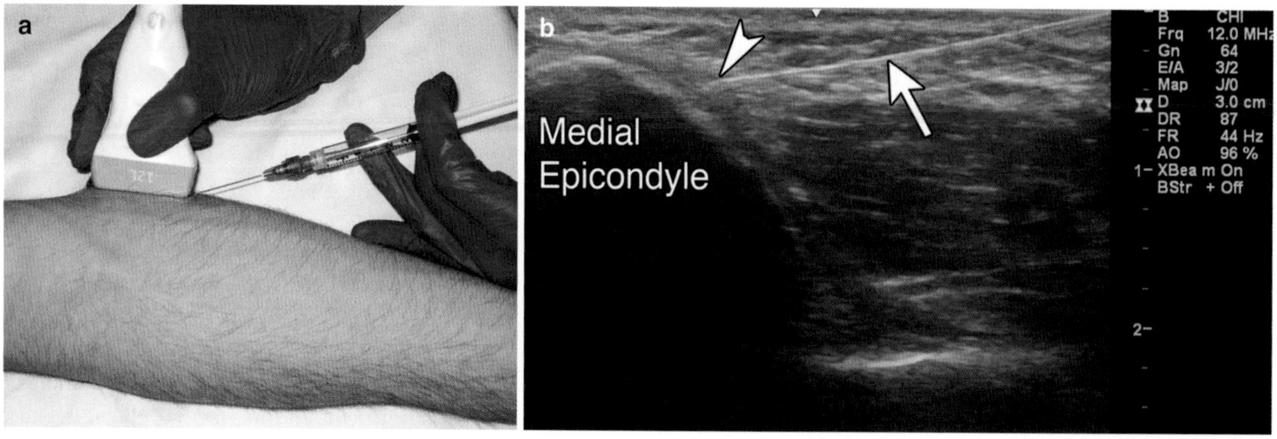

Fig. 3.2 (**a**) Example of probe position over medial epicondyle with in-plane injection technique. (**b**) Example of in-plane long-axis approach, *white arrow* indicates needle, *arrowhead* indicates needle tip, medial epicondyle labeled

Ulnar Collateral Ligament (UCL)

Ultrasound is very useful for distinguishing UCL pathology, including partial or complete tears, avulsion fractures, and chronic UCL injury and thickening. The UCL is a short and broad-based ligament divided into three components: an anterior, posterior, and transverse segment [5]. The anterior bundle provides the primary stabilization of the medial elbow, playing a critical role during valgus stress of the joint [10]. In injuries from sports requiring overhead throwing, prompt diagnosis is critical in determining appropriate management, whether it is surgical intervention for a complete tear versus conservative care for a partial tear or sprain [10]. For a professional athlete, delayed diagnosis of a torn ligament that ultimately requires surgery will have a significant adverse impact and may lead to the abrupt end of a professional sports career.

Clinically, a patient will present with medial elbow pain, tenderness to palpation along the ligament, and increased laxity with valgus stress at 30–90° [6]. Treatment with corticosteroid injection or PRP shows variable to promising improvement [5, 11]. In acute UCL injury, avoid using steroids for symptomatic relief, as there is an increased risk of ligamentous laxity and potential rupture [7]. In these cases, lidocaine injection may be used for temporary pain relief. After a corticosteroid injection, the patient should undergo a rehabilitation program focusing on proximal muscle strength, trunk rotation, core and gluteal strength, and the entire kinetic chain. A formal physical therapy program may be helpful [12].

Scanning Technique and Anatomy to Identify

The UCL is best visualized with the elbow positioned at 30° of flexion and the forearm supinated [4, 6]. Sprains include stretch injury with continuity of the ligament (Grade 1), partial tears (Grade 2), or complete rupture (Grade 3). With grade 1 sprains, the UCL may appear mildly thickened and hypoechoic [2]. Partial tears of the UCL appear as abnormal ligament thickening with internal hypoechoic disruption; the presence of hypoechoic fluid is variable [2, 9]. Complete tears or full thickness rupture appear as focal discontinuity of the ligament with surrounding hypoechoic edema or inability to visualize the ligament at all [13]. Increased gapping with valgus stress implies partial or full thickness tear. The anterior bundle extends from the anterior-inferior aspect of the medial epicondyle to the medial edge of the coronoid process [2, 3]. UCL avulsion, more commonly seen in the adolescent population, appears as a hyperechoic bony fragment adjacent to the medial epicondyle [2]. Chronic UCL injury from repetitive microtrauma causes progressive thickening, hypoechoic foci and calcifications that can lead to ligamentous instability (Fig. 3.3) [2, 5].

Injection Technique: In-Plane Coronal Approach

Patient positioning: The patient should be seated or lay supine with 30° of elbow flexion and the shoulder externally rotated. Place a towel underneath the lateral epicondyle for comfort.

Probe position: Place the probe longitudinally (coronal) with the proximal end of the transducer over the medial epicondyle to visualize the CFT. Scan proximally and distally until the medial epicondyle and the proximal attachments of the CFT are clearly identified. The UCL appears deep to the CFT (Fig. 3.4a). A normal UCL appears compact, fibrillar, and hyperechoic compared to an abnormal UCL, which appears as a thin hypoechoic band [3].

Markings: Mark the length of the anterior band of the UCL to plan the needle approach.

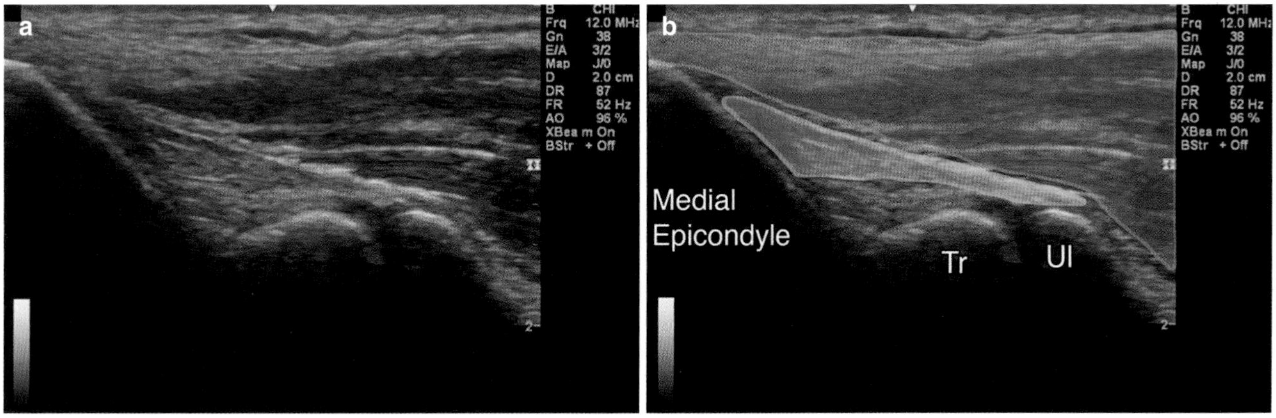

Fig. 3.3 (**a**) Coronal view of ulnar collateral ligament. (**b**) *Green* indicates ulnar collateral ligament, *orange* indicates common flexor tendons, *Tr* trochlea, *Ul* ulna, medial epicondyle labeled

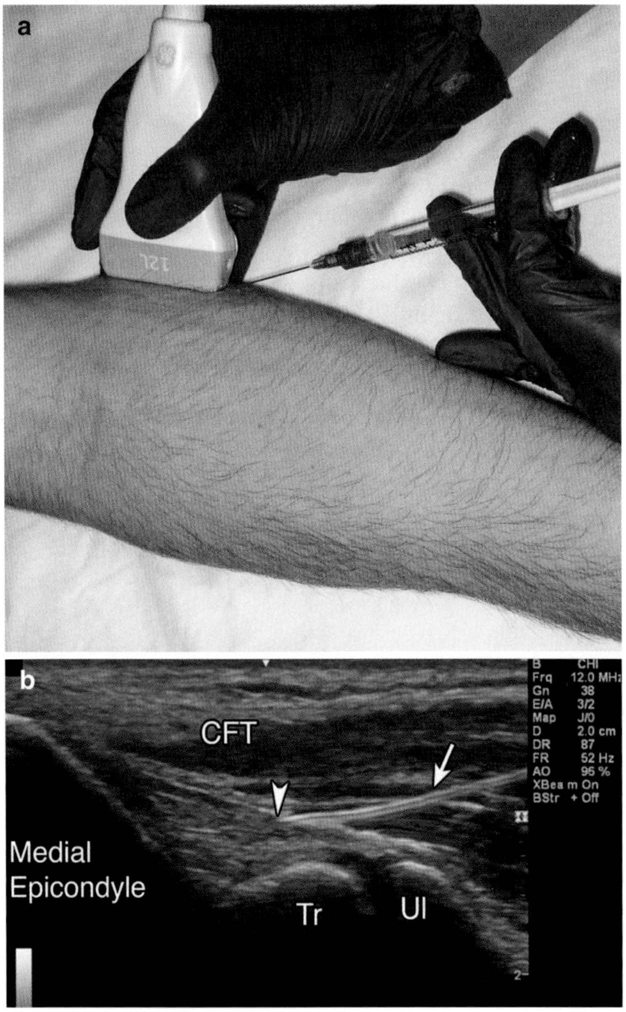

Fig. 3.4 (**a**) Example of probe position over ulnar collateral ligament. (**b**) Example of in-plane long-axis approach, white arrow indicates needle, arrowhead indicates needle tip, *Tr* trochlea, *Ul* ulnar, CFT-common flexor tendon, medial epicondyle labeled

Needle position: The needle should be inserted in-plane to the transducer. Inject into the hypoechoic region of the pathologic ligament with a single injection directed from distal to proximal [5].

Safety considerations: There is a risk of fatty atrophy and local depigmentation with corticosteroid injection. Be careful to not inject too posterior, where the ulnar nerve may lie.

Pearls:

- Valgus stress on the elbow will help to identify laxity of the UCL.
- An abnormal UCL appears hypoechoic with discontinuous fibers.

Equipment needed:

- High-frequency linear array transducer (10 MHz+)
- 25G 1.5″ needle
- 22G needle for PRP or autologous whole blood
- 0.5–1 mL of steroid preparation or 2–3 mL of PRP or autologous whole blood [11, 12]
- 1–3 mL local anesthetic

Ulnar Nerve at the Elbow

The ability of ultrasound to evaluate structures dynamically is particularly useful when evaluating the ulnar nerve at the elbow for ulnar subluxation or other causes of neuropathy [14]. At the level of the elbow, the ulnar nerve lies in the retroepicondylar groove and has a variable amount of slack in extension. This predisposes it to subluxation over the medial epicondyle during flexion, which can occur in roughly 20 % of individuals, although many may be asymptomatic. This movement predisposes the patient to ulnar neuritis [9]. Ulnar nerve subluxation also occurs in "snapping triceps syndrome." This can occur when the distal medial head of the triceps muscle subluxes from a lateral direction during elbow flexion, causing displacement of the ulnar nerve from its groove over the medial epicondyle [9]. As a result, ulnar nerve compression and neuropathy can occur at the retroepicondylar groove and the edge of the flexor carpi ulnaris muscle aponeurosis.

Clinically, patients commonly present with upper extremity weakness, hand pain, and numbness in the ulnar distribution [15]. It may be difficult to determine if the ulnar nerve is involved and the level of involvement. Ultrasound guided diagnostic ulnar nerve blockade is an effective and efficient method to determine ulnar nerve involvement [16]. This method is often used prior to a peripheral nerve stimulator in cases of refractory ulnar neuropathy. In addition, regional anesthesia of the ulnar nerve using ultrasound guidance is an effective technique. This is often used to potentiate distal anesthesia in incomplete brachial plexus blocks and in post-operative anesthesia of forearm and hand procedures to help minimize the need for pain medication.

Scanning Technique and Anatomy to Identify

Begin by scanning proximal to distal in the transverse plane at the level of the medial epicondyle. Proximally, the nerve appears oval or triangular in shape with internal punctate hyperechoic areas [16]. The ulnar nerve has a characteristic honeycomb pattern in the transverse plane, which is the typical appearance of a peripheral nerve [17]. This pattern describes the arrangement of the hypoechoic nerve fascicles with the hyperechoic perineurium and endoneurium. Identify the medial epicondyle and triceps muscle. Distally, the nerve becomes

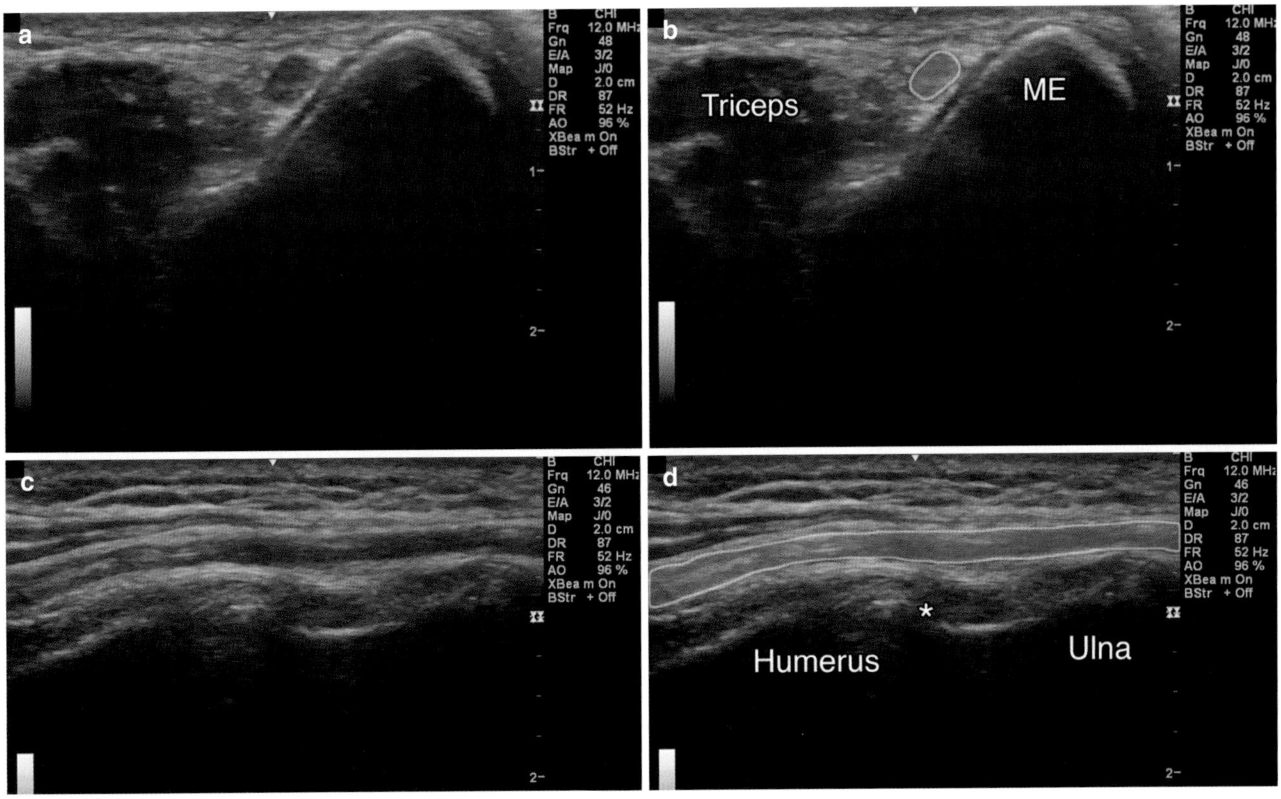

Fig. 3.5 (**a**) Transverse (axial) view of the ulnar nerve. (**b**) *Yellow* indicates ulnar nerve, *ME* medial epicondyle, triceps labeled. (**c**) Longitudinal view of the ulnar nerve. (**d**) *Yellow* indicates ulnar nerve, *asterisk* indicates joint space, humerus and ulna labeled

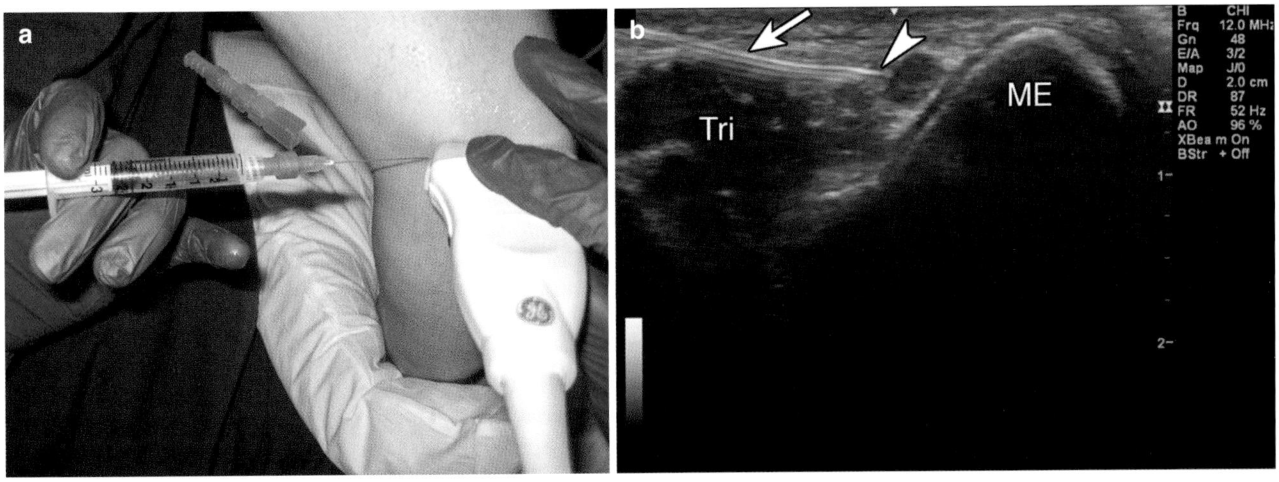

Fig. 3.6 (**a**) Example of probe position over ulnar nerve at the elbow. (**b**) Example of in-plane short-axis approach, *white arrow* indicates needle, *arrowhead* indicates needle tip, *Tri* triceps, *ME* medial epicondyle

thinner and difficult to differentiate from tendon. This is because the nerve contains smaller amounts of myelinated axons and thus can mimic the appearance of tendons. In the longitudinal plane, the ulnar nerve appears as a thin hyperechoic tubular structure. In an entrapment, the ulnar nerve becomes enlarged and edematous with an increase in hypoechoic appearance with loss of fascicular pattern (Fig. 3.5) [17].

Injection Technique: In-Plane Axial Approach

Patient positioning: The patient should lay supine, shoulder abducted 90° and elbow flexed approximately 90°, or be seated with the elbow flexed 90° with the hand on the table [15].

Probe positioning: Place the transducer transverse relative to the ulnar nerve at the elbow (Fig. 3.6a).

Markings: Mark any blood vessels prior to injection.

Needle position: Start from the ulnar (medial) aspect of the transducer. An in-plane approach is advised, as this provides continuous visualization of the needle tip. Identify the ulnar nerve and then guide the needle adjacent to the nerve and inject medication to create a "target sign." Look for spread around the circumference of the nerve and reposition as needed.

Safety considerations: Identify and avoid intravascular injection into the superior ulnar recurrent artery. Injections at this site should be limited to 3–5 mL in volume to minimize the risk of a compartment syndrome.

Pearls:

- Unlike blood vessels, nerves are not compressible structures.
- Injecting small amounts of anesthetic can help localize the needle tip.

Equipment needed:

- High-frequency linear array transducer (10 MHz+)
- 25G 1.5″ needle
- 3–5 mL local anesthetic

Injection Technique: In-Plane Longitudinal Approach

Patient positioning: Lay the patient supine, shoulder abducted 90° and elbow flexed approximately 90°, or with the patient sitting and the elbow flexed 90° with the hand on the table [15].

Probe positioning: Place the transducer longitudinal relative to the ulnar nerve at the elbow (Fig. 3.7a).

Markings: Mark any blood vessels prior to injection.

Needle position: Start from the ulnar (medial) aspect of the transducer. An in-plane approach is advised, as this provides continuous visualization of the needle tip. Identify the ulnar nerve and then guide the needle adjacent to the nerve. Look for spread around the superficial aspect of the nerve.

Safety considerations: Identify and avoid intravascular injection into the superior ulnar recurrent artery. Injections at this site should be limited to 3–5 mL in volume to minimize the risk of a compartment syndrome.

Pearls:

- Unlike blood vessels, nerves are not compressible structures.
- Injecting small amounts of anesthetic can help localize the needle tip.

Equipment needed:

- High-frequency linear array transducer (10 MHz+)
- 25G 1.5″ needle
- 3–5 mL local anesthetic

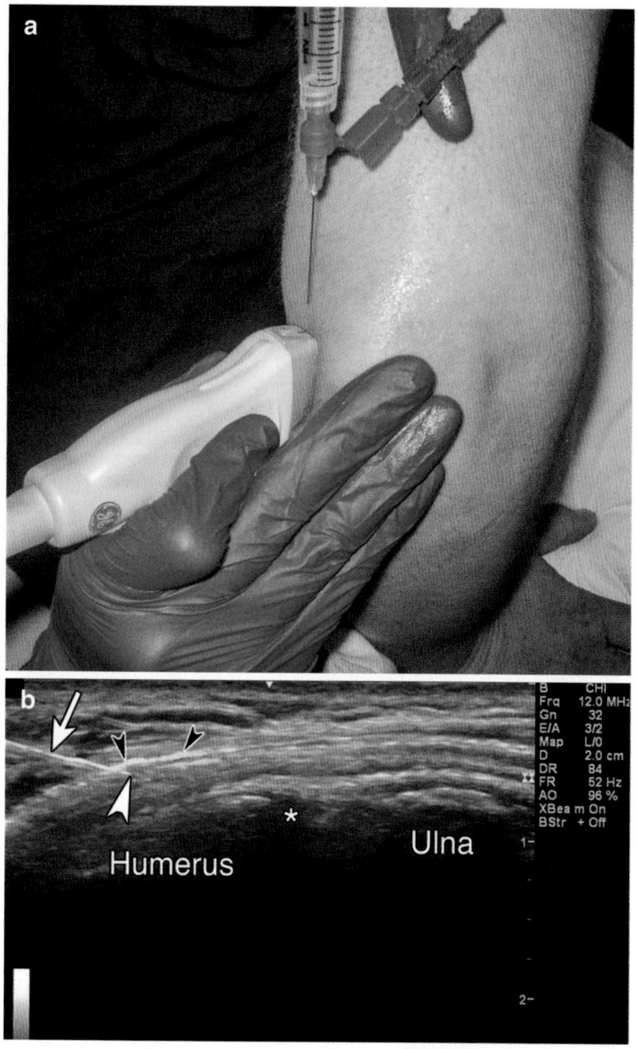

Fig. 3.7 (**a**) Example of probe position over ulnar nerve at the elbow. (**b**) Example of in-plane longitudinal approach, *white arrow* indicates needle, *white arrowhead* indicates needle tip, *black arrowheads* indicate injectate over nerve sheath, *asterisk* indicates joint space, humerus and ulna labeled

Lateral Epicondylosis (LE)

Lateral epicondylosis, also known as tennis elbow, is a common tendinopathy in the upper extremity. LE consists of pain at the proximal attachment of the common extensor tendon, usually arising from repetitive use and microtrauma. Patients often complain of pain in the region of the proximal wrist extensor attachments, especially with resisted wrist extension, twisting motions as the wrist, and grasping objects. Physical examination may reveal tenderness to palpation over the lateral epicondyle and reduced strength with resisted grip, supination, and wrist extension [18]. Provocative tests such as Cozen's and Mill's can reproduce the symptoms. Ultrasound may assist in identifying enthesophytes, tendon

Table 3.1 Outcomes of USG percutaneous needle tenotomy in the treatment of common extensor tendinosis in the elbow, $N=52$ [11]

Excellent	Good	Fair	Poor
30 (57.7 %)	18 (34.6 %)	1 (1.9 %)	3 (5.8 %)

Excellent – very happy with the procedure and had no room for improvement
Good – happy with the procedure and had only mild room for improvement
Fair – slight dissatisfaction with the outcome of the procedure and had room for considerable improvement
Poor – dissatisfied with the outcome of the procedure and had little or no improvement

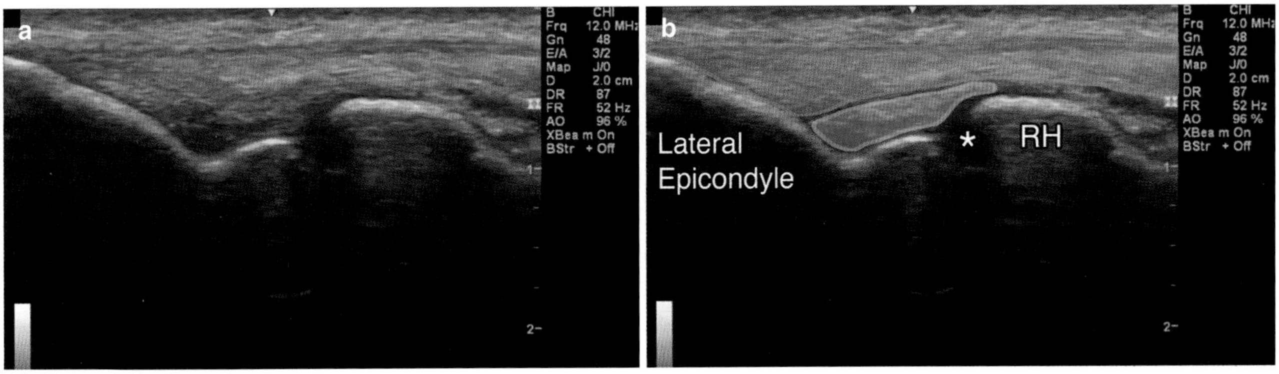

Fig. 3.8 (**a**) Coronal view of common extensor tendon. (**b**) *Green* indicates radial collateral ligament, *orange* indicates common extensor tendons, *RH* radial head, *asterisk* indicates joint space, lateral epicondyle labeled

thickening, and calcifications [17, 18]. PNT, PRP, and corticosteroid injection into or around the involved tendon have all shown varying efficacy in treating lateral epicondylosis (Table 3.1) [19–21].

Scanning Technique and Anatomy to Identify

The patient should lay supine with the forearm rested across the abdomen or be seated with the arm on a table. Place the transducer longitudinally, in line with the forearm, over the common extensor tendon (CET). This allows evaluation of the lateral epicondyle and the proximal attachments of the CET [22]. The CET can be seen here at its origin on the lateral epicondyle traversing distally over the radial head. The radial collateral ligament can be seen deep to the CET between the lateral epicondyle and the radial head. The CET may show tendon thickening at its origin, degenerative changes, and tears, which appear as linear focal or complex hypoechoic areas within the normal tendon matrix [9, 23]. Other findings may include calcification, adjacent cortical irregularity, and diffuse tendon heterogeneity [18]. The lateral collateral ligament complex (LCL) of the elbow is a Y-shaped complex composed of three components: the radial collateral ligament (RCL), the lateral ulnar collateral ligament (LUCL), and the annular ligament. The RCL extends from the lateral epicondyle to the annular ligament. The LUCL spans from the lateral epicondyle to the supinator crest of the ulna. The annular ligament courses from the ulnar anterior margin at the sigmoid notch to the supinator crest at the posterior margin of this bone, forming a ring encompassing the radial head and neck [24]. Part of the elbow joint between the radial head and the lateral epicondyle can also be appreciated deep to the CET (Fig. 3.8).

Injection Technique: In-Plane Long-Axis Approach

Patient positioning: The patient should lay supine with the arm internally rotated and elbow flexed. The patient can also be seated with the affected arm resting comfortably on a table with the elbow in 20–40° of flexion and forearm pronated. Place a towel underneath the medial epicondyle for comfort.

Probe positioning: Place the probe longitudinally (coronal) with the proximal end of the transducer over the lateral epicondyle to visualize the CET. Scan proximally and distally until the lateral epicondyle and the origin of the CET are clearly identified. The radial collateral ligament appears deep to the CET. If performing PNT, alternate changing to an out-of-plane/short-axis view to identify and confirm the position of the needle within the region of tendinosis (Fig. 3.9a).

Markings: None

Needle position: The needle should be inserted parallel to the transducer from either proximal to distal or distal to proximal. Due to the superficial nature of the tendon, a gel

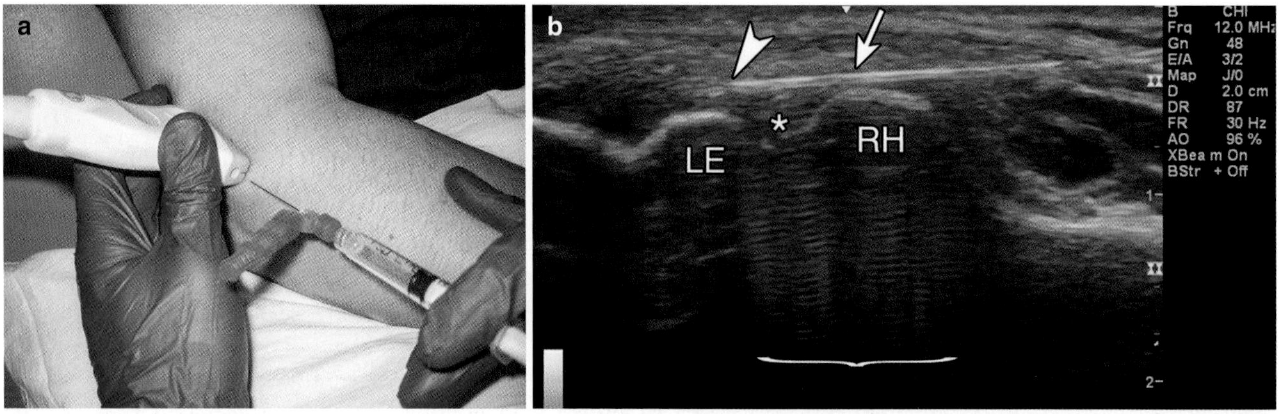

Fig. 3.9 (**a**) Example of probe position over common extensor tendon. (**b**) Example of in-plane long-axis approach, *arrow* indicates needle, *arrowhead* indicates needle tip, *asterisk* indicates joint space, *bracket* indicates needle reverberation, *LE* lateral epicondyle, *RH* radial head

standoff may be helpful. For PNT, insert the needle into the tendon itself and repetitively fenestrate the entire region of tendinosis. For a peritendinous injection, keep the needle above or below the tendon. The elbow joint can also be accessed using the same approach directed towards the space between the radial head and lateral epicondyle.

Safety considerations: For corticosteroid injections, be careful when injecting superficial to the tendon since this can cause subcutaneous atrophy or depigmentation. PNT may cause local bleeding and post-procedure pain. Avoid the lateral collateral ligament complex and the radial and posterior interosseous nerves.

Pearls:

- Doppler may help to identify hyperemia and chronic tendinosis.
- If performing PNT, intermittently switch to an out-of-plane/short-axis view in order to determine the anterior-posterior/radial-ulnar position of the needle within the region of tendinosis [4].
- For PNT, repetitively fenestrate the entire region of tendinosis while injecting local anesthetic, PRP, or AB. Resistance should decrease with increased passes. Calcifications and enthesophytes should be mechanically broken up.
- The elbow joint, between the radial head and lateral epicondyle, can be accessed using this approach by angling the needle deeper through the common extensor tendon.

Equipment needed:

- High-frequency linear array transducer (10 MHz+).
- 25 gauge, 1.5″ needle.
- 0.5 mL of steroid preparation.
- 1–3 mL of local anesthetic.
- For PNT, use a larger (18–20 gauge) needle.
- May include 0.5–1 mL of steroid preparation with 1–3 mL of local anesthetic or 2–3 mL of PRP or autologous whole blood [19–21].

Radial and Posterior Interosseous Nerve

Compression neuropathy of the posterior interosseous nerve (PIN) near or below the supinator muscle is known as supinator syndrome, posterior interosseous syndrome, or radial tunnel syndrome [25]. The PIN is the terminal motor branch of the radial nerve [26]. Entrapment may be due to hypertrophy of the supinator muscle, which acts in synergy with the biceps to supinate the forearm when the elbow is extended. Furthermore, the PIN may be bound and entrapped by fibrous bands or recurrent radial vessels at the arcade of Fröhse. Soft-tissue masses, such as periosteal lipomas and deep ganglia may also compress the nerve [27–29]. Radial head and neck fractures, including Monteggia fracture-dislocations, may displace and compress the PIN as it courses through the radial tunnel [30]. The PIN is a purely motor nerve, but patients usually complain of a dull ache and burning pain around the lateral epicondyle, very similar to lateral epicondylosis. Diagnosis is usually made clinically or with a diagnostic block. The radial nerve innervates the extensor carpi radialis longus, the extensor carpi radialis brevis, and the brachioradialis, while the PIN branch innervates the supinator, extensor digitorum communis, extensor digiti minimi, extensor carpi ulnaris, abductor polices longus, extensor polices brevis and longus, and extensor indicis proprius. Therefore, radial wrist extension should be preserved, and the patient has more of a "finger drop" than the characteristic radial "wrist drop" [30]. Provocation of the symptoms is performed by passive supination or active pronation of the forearm. There may also be a positive Tinel's sign [26].

Scanning Technique and Anatomy to Identify

Place the transducer in an axial plane over the elbow. The radial nerve courses between the brachioradialis and the brachialis muscles then bifurcates into the superficial sensory branch and

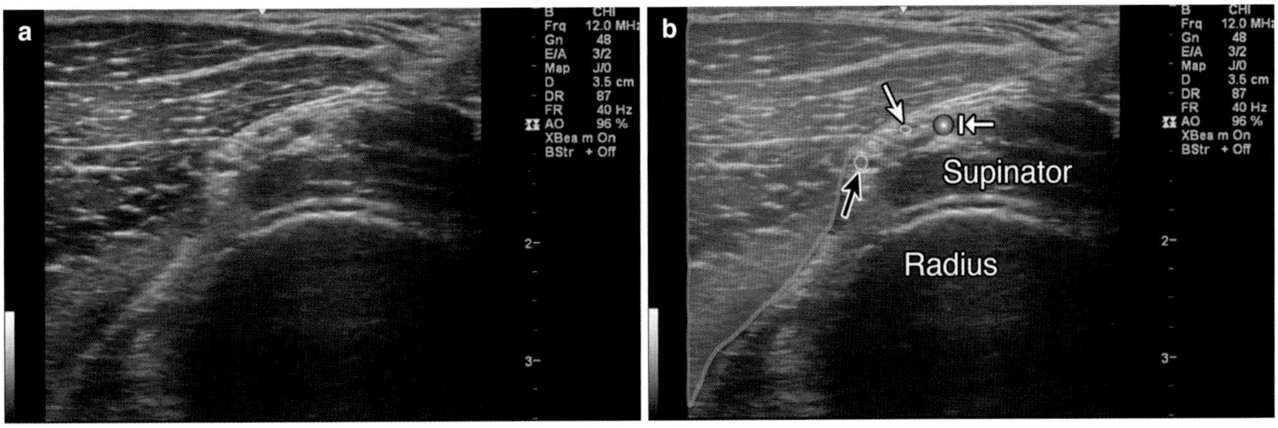

Fig. 3.10 (**a**) Transverse (axial) view of branching radial nerve. (**b**) *White arrow* indicates superficial radial nerve, *black arrow* indicates posterior interosseous nerve, *orange* indicates brachioradialis, *arrow with stop* indicates vessel, supinator and radius labeled

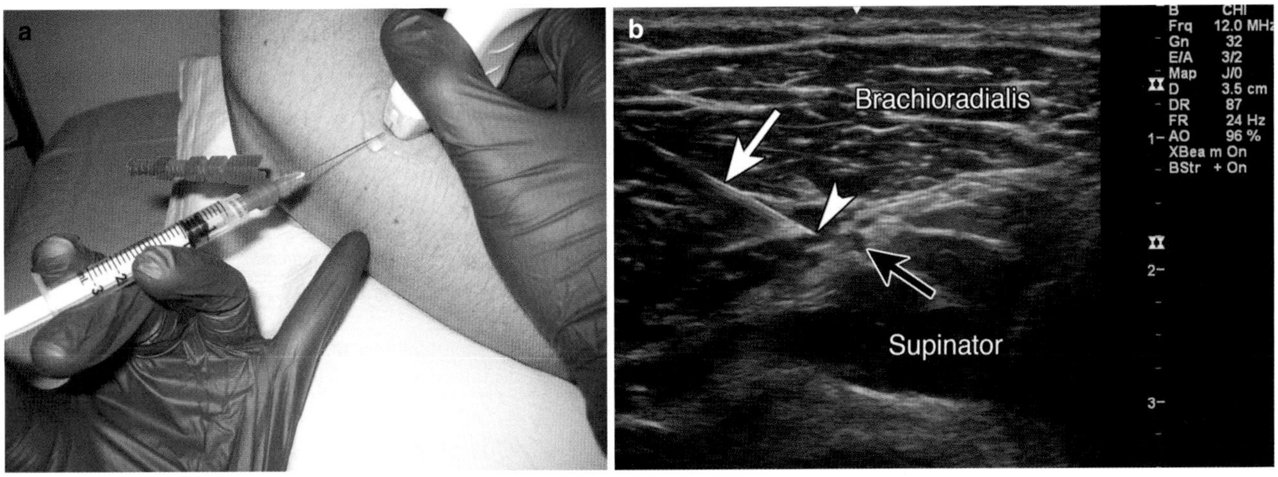

Fig. 3.11 (**a**) Example of probe position over branching radial nerve. (**b**) *White arrow* indicates needle, *arrowhead* indicates needle tip, *black arrow* indicates posterior interosseous nerve, brachioradialis and supinator labeled

the deep branch (PIN) just anterior to the lateral epicondyle. Scan these branches transversely to their termination. Almost immediately, the PIN can be seen entering the "radial tunnel," piercing between the superficial and deep parts of the supinator. The roof of this tunnel is known as the arcade of Fröhse. The PIN may also be assessed by pronating and supinating the forearm while passing the probe over the supinator in an axial plane [25, 26]. A compressed nerve typically appears enlarged and hypoechoic proximal to or inside the site of compression, in this case the supinator muscle [26]. After a radial fracture, the nerve may be surrounded by hypoechoic scar tissue (Fig. 3.10) [30].

Injection Techniques: In-Plane Short-Axis Approach

Patient positioning: The patient should be seated with the affected arm resting on the table, with elbow flexed, and forearm neutral or pronated.

Probe position: Place the transducer transverse relative to the PIN at the level of the distal humerus and locate the radial nerve laterally. Follow the nerve distally until it bifurcates into the superficial sensory branch and PIN (Fig. 3.11a).

Markings: Mark any obvious vessels prior to injection.

Needle position: Insert the needle in-plane from the ulnar (lateral) to radial (medial) aspect of the transducer, transverse to the PIN. Identify the PIN as it enters the arcade of Fröhse by following it distally from the radial bifurcation. Guide the needle tip adjacent to the nerve and then inject medication to produce a "target sign."

Safety considerations: Identify the superficial radial nerve and the recurrent radial artery and avoid intravascular injection.

Pearls:

- Injecting small amounts of anesthetic can help localize the needle tip.
- Adjust the forearm pronation/supination for optimal imaging of the PIN.

Equipment needed:

- High-frequency linear array transducer (10 MHz+)
- 22–25G 1.5″ needle
- 1–3 mL local anesthetic [31]

Olecranon Bursitis

Olecranon bursitis is the most common superficial bursitis [32]. Causes include inflammation from repetitive mechanical stress, trauma, infection, or systemic inflammatory diseases such as gout, pseudogout, and rheumatoid arthritis [33]. Ultrasound assesses olecranon bursa location, depth, and size while providing guidance for aspiration and therapeutic injection [5]. Olecranon bursitis typically presents as unilateral swelling over the posterior elbow, with or without pain. Aseptic bursitis is commonly painless; septic bursitis is more often painful with associated cellulitic changes [5, 33].

Scanning Technique and Anatomy to Identify

The olecranon bursa is an anatomical potential space, located between the proximal aspect of the olecranon process and the subcutaneous tissue on the extensor surface. Normally, the bursa appears as a thin hypoechoic area surrounded by a hyperechoic synovial lining. Fluid collection in this potential space displaces the posterior fat pad and creates a distended fluid-filled collection that appears anechoic or hypoechoic [34]. In the transverse view, fluid in the joint is evidenced by fat pad displacement, and frequently epicondylar injury can be detected [35]. Hypoechoic fluid can be distinguished from hypoechoic cartilage by its compressibility and altered fluid distribution with dynamic movement [34].The olecranon recess is accessible with the elbow flexed at 90°, either medial or lateral to the triceps tendon. Diagnostic sonography is more sensitive with the elbow in the flexed position; 1–3 mL of joint fluid can be identified on ultrasound, compared with the 5–10 mL

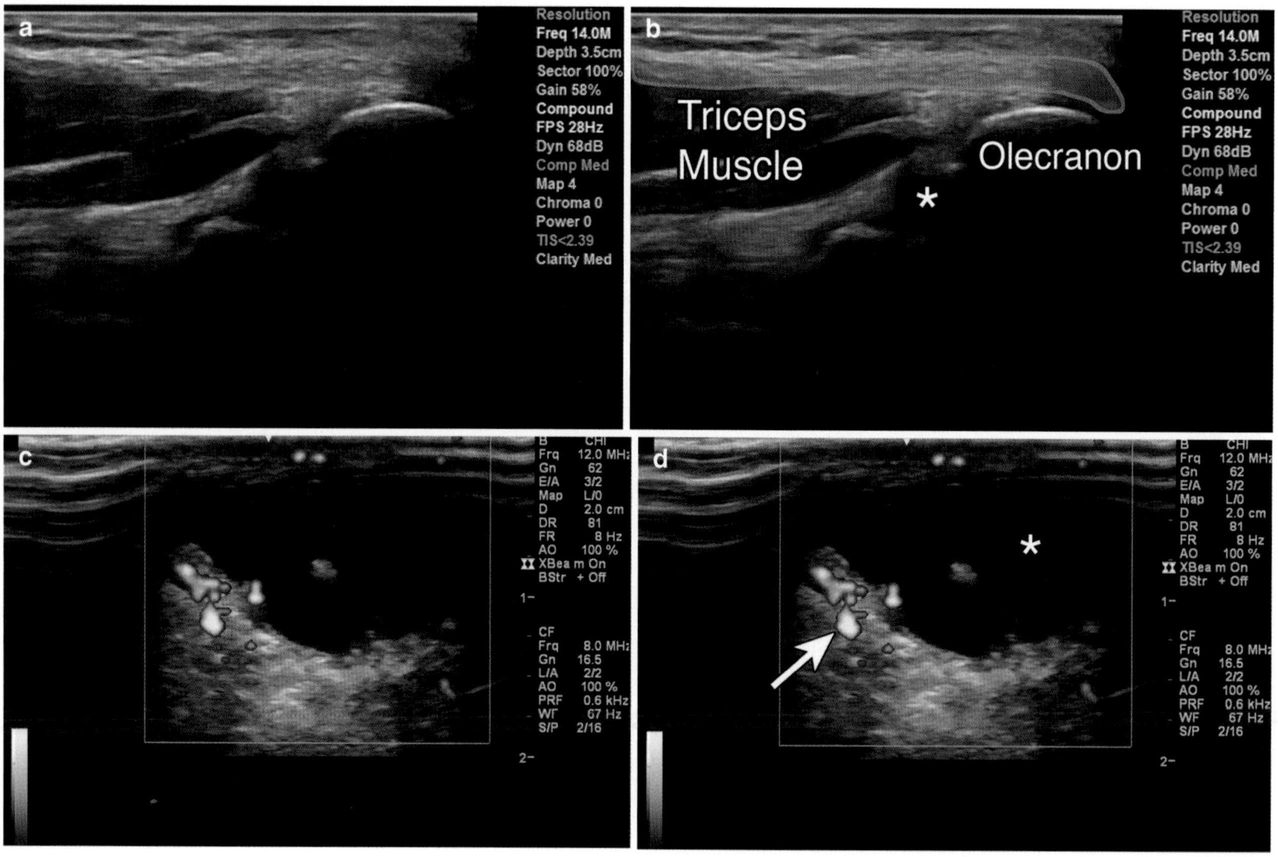

Fig. 3.12 (**a**) Example of sagittal view over posterior elbow. (**b**) Triceps muscle labeled, *orange* indicates tendinous portion of triceps muscle, *asterisk* indicates joint space between olecranon and trochlea, *magenta* indicates fat pad, olecranon labeled. (**c**) Example of transverse (axial) view over olecranon bursitis. (**d**) *White arrow* indicates hyperemia, *asterisk* indicates hypoechoic fluid-filled bursa

required for identification of a posterior fat pad on plain films [34]. Aspiration is used to decompress the bursa especially when it is painful, interferes with daily activity or causes a cosmetic concern, and it provides diagnostic analysis when infectious or crystal arthropathies are suspected [33].

Start by placing the transducer parallel to the triceps muscle and tendon and identify the olecranon joint recess, olecranon fossa, and posterior fat pad. Move the transducer inferiorly and the olecranon bursa will come into view. Rotate the transducer to the axial plane and identify the ulnar nerve in the retroepicondylar groove. Doppler may identify active inflammation in the bursa with local hypervascularity [3, 36]. Olecranon bursitis will have local hypervascularity along with bursal wall distention [37]. In chronic bursitis, the synovial wall of the bursae becomes thickened and appears hyperechoic (Fig. 3.12).

Injection Techniques: In-Plane Axial Approach

Patient positioning: Place the affected arm on a table with the elbow flexed to 90°.

Probe positioning: Place the probe transversely over the bursa (Fig. 3.13a).

Markings: It may be helpful to identify the cubital tunnel and ulnar nerve. Mark the border of the triceps tendon.

Needle position: The needle should be inserted in-plane from radial to ulnar, distal to proximal, or proximal to distal. A posterior intra-articular elbow injection can be performed in this position as well targeting the space between the olecranon and trochlea [38].

Safety considerations: There is a risk of reoccurrence of swelling or fistula formation from aspirating the olecranon bursa through the extensor compartment [39, 40]. If septic or infection suspected, steroid injections should not be used, until diagnostic confirmation.

Pearls:

- Aspirate from a lateral approach; needle is inserted at an angle into the bursa; use the "zigzag" needle method to prevent the formation of fistula or direct sinus with the skin or subcutaneous tissue.
- Posterolateral approach is used to help avoid the ulnar nerve.
- Doppler mode may help identify hyperemia.
- Compression with the ultrasound probe will compress the olecranon bursa.
- Avoid intratendinous injection and neurovascular structures.
- Hyperechoic particles within the fluid suggest a hemorrhagic, an inflammatory, or septic etiology [41].

Equipment needed:

- High-frequency linear array transducer (10 MHz+)
- 18 or 20 gauge needle 1.5″ needle
- 0.5 mL of steroid preparation
- 3–5 mL local anesthetic

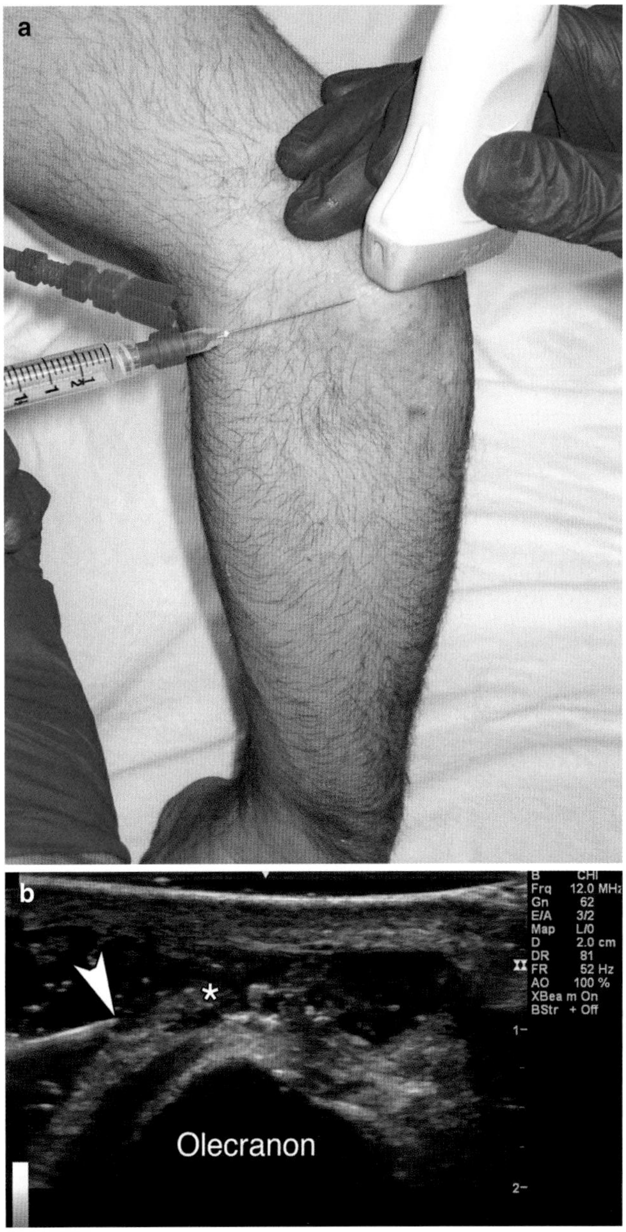

Fig. 3.13 (**a**) Example of probe position over olecranon with in-plane injection technique. (**b**) Example of in-plane axial approach, *arrowhead* indicates needle tip, *asterisk* indicates fluid-filled bursa, olecranon labeled

References

1. AIUM practice guideline for the performance of a musculoskeletal ultrasound examination. Journal of ultrasound in medicine. 2012;31(9):1473–88.
2. Tran N, Chow K. Ultrasonography of the elbow. Semin Musculoskelet Radiol. 2007;11(2):105–16.

3. Martinoli C, Bianchi S, Giovagnorio F, Pugliese F. Ultrasound of the elbow. Skeletal Radiol. 2001;30(11):605–14.
4. Lee KS, Rosas HG, Craig JG. Musculoskeletal ultrasound: elbow imaging and procedures. Semin Musculoskelet Radiol. 2010;14(4): 449–60.
5. Banffy MB, ElAttrache NS. Injection therapy in the management of musculoskeletal injuries: the elbow. Oper Tech Sports Med. 2012;20(2):124–31.
6. Ciccotti MC, Schwartz MA, Ciccotti MG. Diagnosis and treatment of medial epicondylitis of the elbow. Clin Sports Med. 2004;23(4): 693–705.
7. Piligian G, Herbert R, Hearns M, Dropkin J, Landsbergis P, Cherniack M. Evaluation and management of chronic work-related musculoskeletal disorders of the distal upper extremity. Am J Ind Med. 2000;37(1):75–93.
8. Suresh SP, Ali KE, Jones H, Connell DA. Medial epicondylitis: is ultrasound guided autologous blood injection an effective treatment? Br J Sports Med. N2006;40(11):935–9.
9. Bodor M, Fullerton B. Ultrasonography of the hand, wrist, and elbow. Phys Med Rehabil Clin N Am. 2010;21(3):509–31.
10. Callaway GH, Field LD, Deng XH, et al. Biomechanical evaluation of the medial collateral ligament of the elbow. J Bone Joint Surg Am. 1997;79(8):1223–31.
11. Podesta L, Crow SA, Volkmer D, et al. Treatment of partial ulnar collateral ligament tears in the elbow with platelet-rich plasma. Am J Sports Med. 2013;41(7):1689–94 [Epub ahead of print].
12. Van Hofwegen C, Baker 3rd CL, Baker Jr CL. Epicondylitis in the athlete's elbow. Clin Sports Med. 2010;29(4):577–97.
13. Jacobson JA, Propeck T, Jamadar DA, Jebson PJ, Hayes CW. US of the anterior bundle of the ulnar collateral ligament: findings in five cadaver elbows with MR arthrographic and anatomic comparison–initial observations. Radiology. 2003;227(2):561–6.
14. Beekman R, Schoemaker MC, Van Der Plas JP, et al. Diagnostic value of high-resolution sonography in ulnar neuropathy at the elbow. Neurology. 2004;62(5):767–73.
15. Beekman R, Visser LH, Verhagen WI. Ultrasonography in ulnar neuropathy at the elbow: a critical review. Muscle Nerve. 2011;43(5):627–35.
16. Gray AT. Ultrasound-guided regional anesthesia: current state of the art. Anesthesiology. 2006;104(2):368–73.
17. Smith J, Finnoff JT. Diagnostic and interventional musculoskeletal ultrasound: part 2. Clinical applications. PM R. 2009;1(2):162–77.
18. Levin D, Nazarian LN, Miller TT, et al. Lateral epicondylitis of the elbow: US findings. Radiology. 2005;237(1):230–4.
19. McShane JM, Shah VN, Nazarian LN. Sonographically guided percutaneous needle tenotomy for treatment of common extensor tendinosis in the elbow. J Ultrasound Med. 2008;27(8):1137–44.
20. McShane JM, Nazarian LN, Harwood MI. Sonographically guided percutaneous needle tenotomy for treatment of common extensor tendinosis in the elbow. J Ultrasound Med. 2006;25(10):1281–9.
21. Mishra A, Pavelko T. Treatment of chronic elbow tendinosis with buffered platelet-rich plasma. Am J Sports Med. 2006;34(11):1774–8.
22. AIUM practice guideline for the performance of the musculoskeletal ultrasound examination. Laurel: American Institute of Ultrasound in Medicine. http://www.acr.org/SecondaryMainMenuCategories/quality_safety/guidelines/us/us_msculoskeleta.aspx. Accessed 20 Feb 2012. (In other publications this is cited as originally cited: AIUM practice guideline for the performance of the musculoskeletal ultrasound examination. October 1, 2007. Laurel: American Institute of Ultrasound in Medicine.)
23. van Holsbeeck MT, Introcaso JH. Musculoskeletal ultrasound. 2nd ed. St. Louis: Mosby; 2001.
24. Augusto P, Teixeira G, et al. Ultrasound assessment of the lateral collateral ligamentous complex of the elbow: imaging aspects in cadavers and normal volunteers. Eur Radiol. 2011;21(7):1492–8.
25. Beggs I, Bianchi S, Bueno A and M Cohen. Elbow. In: ESSR Ultrasound Group Protocols. Musculoskeletal ultrasound technical guidelines. European Society of Musculoskeletal Radiology, Vienna, Austria. p. 1–6. http://www.essr.org/html/img/pool/elbow.pdf. Accessed Feb 20, 2012.
26. Bodner G, Harpf C, Meirer R, Gardetto A, Kovacs P, Gruber H. Ultrasonographic appearance of supinator syndrome. J Ultrasound Med. 2002;21(11):1289–93.
27. Dang AC, Rodner CM. Unusual compression neuropathies of the forearm. Part I: radial nerve. J Hand Surg Am. 2009;34(10): 1906–14.
28. Hamdi MF, Aloui I, Allagui M, Abid A. Letter to Editor: Paralysis of posterior interosseous nerve caused by parosteal lipoma. Neurol India. 2010;58(2):319–20.
29. Lubahn J, Cermak M. Uncommon nerve compression syndromes of the upper extremity. J Am Acad Orthop Surg. 1998;6: 378–86.
30. Bianchi S, Martinoli C. Elbow. In: Bianchi S, Martinoli C, editors. Ultrasound of the musculoskeletal system, Medical radiology. Berlin/Heidelberg: Springer; 2007. p. 349–407.
31. Frenkel O, Herring AA, Fischer J, Carnell J, Nagdev A. Supracondylar radial nerve block for treatment of distal radius fractures in the emergency department. J Emerg Med. 2011;41(4): 386–8.
32. Pien FD, Ching D, Kim E. Septic bursitis: experience in a community practice. Orthopedics. 1991;14(9):981–4.
33. Aaron DL, Patel A, Kayiaros S, Calfee R. Four common types of bursitis: diagnosis and management. J Am Acad Orthop Surg. 2011;19(6):359–67.
34. De Maeseneer M, Jacobson JA, Jaovisidha S, et al. Elbow effusions: distribution of joint fluid with flexion and extension and imaging implications. Invest Radiol. 1998;33(2):117–25.
35. Barr LL, Babcock DS. Sonography of the normal elbow. AJR Am J Roentgenol. 1991;157(4):793–8.
36. Koski JM. Ultrasonography of the elbow joint. Rheumatol Int. 1990;10(3):91–4.
37. Radunovic G, Vlad V, Micu MC, et al. Ultrasound assessment of the elbow. Med Ultrason. 2012;14(2):141–6.
38. Louis LJ. Musculoskeletal ultrasound intervention: principles and advances. Radiol Clin North Am. 2008;46(3):515–33.
39. Del Buono A, Franceschi F, Palumbo A, Denaro V, Maffulli N. Diagnosis and management of olecranon bursitis. Surgeon. 2012;10(5):297–300.
40. Stell IM. Septic and non-septic olecranon bursitis in the accident and emergency department – an approach to management. J Accid Emerg Med. 1996;13(5):351–3.
41. Finlay K, Ferri M, Friedman L. Ultrasound of the elbow. Skeletal Radiol. 2004;33(2):63–79.

4 Wrist and Hand

David A. Spinner and Melissa I. Rosado

The wrist and hand is an excellent region for the use of musculoskeletal ultrasound due to the superficial structures and the ability to perform dynamic scans. Common pathologies in this area include tenosynovitis of the dorsal wrist compartments, tendon ruptures, cysts, compression neuropathies, and arthritides.

Carpal Tunnel Syndrome

The carpal tunnel is located on the volar aspect of the wrist and is the most common compression neuropathy site in the upper limb [1]. Carpal tunnel syndrome (CTS) is a constellation of symptoms consisting of pain, paresthesias, and eventually thenar atrophy, arising from increased pressure within the tunnel, edematous states, or direct nerve trauma. Patients often complain of nocturnal paresthesias in the volar aspect of the thumb, index finger, middle finger, and radial half of the ring finger. Provocative tests such as compression over the carpal tunnel or Tinel's and Phalen's signs can help to reproduce the symptoms. The diagnosis is based on history, physical exam, electrodiagnostic studies, or cross-sectional area on ultrasound [2]. Corticosteroid injection into the carpal tunnel has been shown to provide improvement in pain, paresthesias, and function [3–5].

Scanning Technique and Anatomy to Identify

The patient should sit with the elbow flexed to 90°, forearm supinated with the hand resting comfortably. A towel may be placed under the wrist to place it in slight extension. The carpal tunnel lies just distal to the distal wrist crease. The transducer is placed transversely (short axis) to the median nerve, at the distal wrist crease. The bony borders of the tunnel include the scaphoid and trapezium laterally and the hamate and pisiform medially. The transverse carpal ligament or flexor retinaculum forms the superficial roof of the tunnel. The carpal tunnel contains the tendons of the flexor digitorum profundus, flexor digitorum superficialis, and flexor pollicis longus, and the median nerve. Identify the honeycomb-appearing median nerve in cross section. It generally appears relatively hypoechoic to the adjacent hyperechoic tendons in cross section. You can tilt the probe to adjust anisotropy; the nerve will remain present, but the flexor tendons may disappear at off angles. Have the patient move their flexor tendons to assess for adhesions which may be amenable to hydrodissection. Be sure to scan on the ulnar side of the canal to view the ulnar artery and nerve and radially to identify the radial artery (Fig. 4.1) [6, 7].

Injection Techniques: In-Plane Axial Ulnar-Sided Approach [8]

Patient positioning: Sit the patient with the affected arm resting comfortably on the table. A towel can be placed underneath the wrist to create mild extension.

Probe position: The transducer is placed short axis (transverse) to the median nerve at the wrist. Scan proximally and distally until the nerve is clearly identified under the transverse carpal ligament, at approximately the level of the pisiform (Fig. 4.2a).

Markings: Because of the shallow needle plane angle, make sure to identify and mark off the ulnar nerve and artery and insert the needle just radial or deep to these structures.

Needle position: The needle should be inserted on the ulnar side of the wrist crease parallel to the transducer for optimal needle visualization. Some practitioners attempt to get as close to the nerve as possible, while others argue that because the carpal tunnel is a confined space, placing the injectate anywhere in the tunnel may be effective. There are no studies comparing these approaches. Some practitioners

D.A. Spinner, DO, RMSK (✉)
Department of Anesthesiology – Pain Medicine,
Arnold Pain Management Center, Beth Israel Deaconess Medical Center, Harvard Medical School, Brookline, MA, USA
e-mail: dspinnerny@gmail.com

M.I. Rosado, MD
Maxwell Medical, New York, NY, USA

D.A. Spinner et al. (eds.), *Atlas of Ultrasound Guided Musculoskeletal Injections*, Musculoskeletal Medicine,
DOI 10.1007/978-1-4614-8936-8_4, © Springer Science+Business Media, LLC 2014

hydrodissect the nerve off of the flexor retinaculum or flexor tendons if adhesions are present.

Injection Techniques: Out-of-Plane Axial Approach [9]

Patient positioning: Sit the patient with the affected arm resting comfortably on the table. A towel can be placed underneath the wrist to create mild extension.

Probe positioning: The transducer is placed axially to the median nerve at the wrist. Center the probe over the median nerve (Fig. 4.3a).

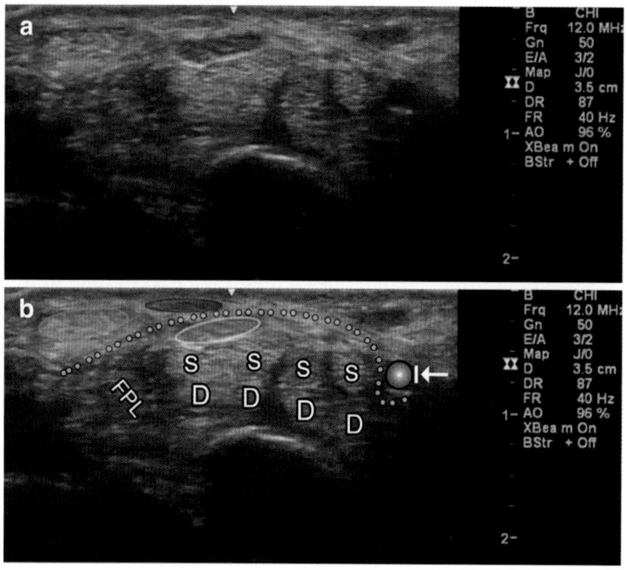

Fig. 4.1 (**a**) Axial view of the carpal tunnel. (**b**) *Orange oval*, flexor carpi radialis; *purple oval*, palmaris longus; *yellow oval*, median nerve; *FPL* flexor pollicis longus; *D* and *S* indicate the combined eight tendons of the flexor superficialis and digitorum muscles; *arrow with stop* indicates ulnar artery; and *dotted green line*, flexor retinaculum

Markings: Mark any obvious vessel or tendon prior to injection.

Needle position: The needle should be inserted at a steep angle at the center of the ultrasound probe, directed just adjacent to the median nerve. The needle tip is seen as a bright hyperechoic dot. The injectate is delivered next to the nerve. Hydrodissection is not performed with this technique since the whole needle path cannot be visualized.

Safety considerations: The palmar cutaneous branch of the median nerve arises just proximal to the flexor retinaculum and is a potential site for injury using a radial-sided approach; therefore, the ulnar approach is recommended. The palmar cutaneous branch of the ulnar nerve travels superficial to the flexor retinaculum and is a potential site for injury with the in-plane ulnar-sided approach [10]. The median nerve is very superficial therefore the in-plane approach is preferred to maximize visualization and avoid nerve injury. Patients may have hand numbness for the duration of the local anesthetic and should not plan on driving after the procedure.

Pearls:

- The median nerve is subject to anisotropy but not as much as the surrounding tendons. Nerve visualization can be improved by flexing and extending the fingers or wrist or by toggling the probe in the axial plane.
- Tracking the nerve proximally into the forearm may help differentiate it from the palmaris longus tendon.
- An oblique standoff technique may be helpful for small wrists.
- Doppler mode can help identify vascular structures such as a persistent median artery [11].

Equipment needed:

- High-frequency linear array transducer (10 MHz+)
- 25G 1.5″ needle
- 0.5 mL of steroid preparation
- 1–3 mL local anesthetic

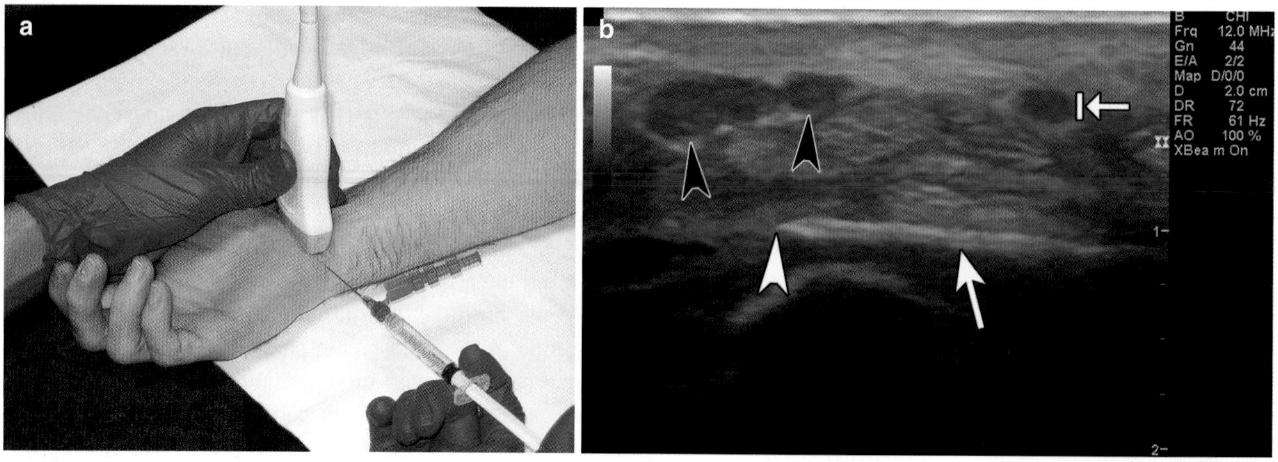

Fig. 4.2 (**a**) Example of probe position over carpal tunnel with ulnar-sided injection technique. (**b**) Example of in-plane approach. *Black arrowheads* point to bifid median nerve. *White arrowhead* points to needle tip. *White arrow* points to needle. *Arrow with stop* indicates ulnar artery

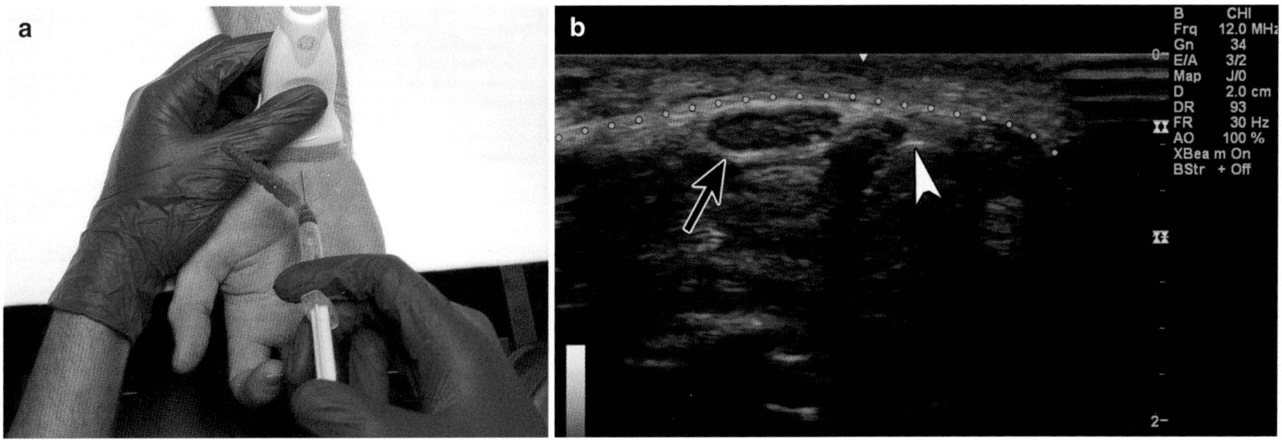

Fig. 4.3 (**a**) Example of probe position over carpal tunnel. (**b**) Example of out-of-plane approach. *White arrowhead* points to needle tip. *Black arrow* points to median nerve. *Green dotted line* represents flexor retinaculum

Table 4.1 Accuracy of ultrasound guided DRUJ injections

Study – DRUJ	Author	Accuracy (%)
Ultrasound guided	Smith et al. [35]	100

Distal Radioulnar Joint (DRUJ)

Although uncommon, the distal radioulnar joint (DRUJ) can be a source of ulnar-sided wrist pain [12]. The DRUJ allows for forearm supination and pronation and stabilizes the wrist. DRUJ pain typically comes from arthritis [13]. Presenting symptoms may include pain and weakness. Injections to confirm DRUJ pain were typically performed with fluoroscopy. Ultrasound guidance enables the effective placement of a needle into this small joint space with uneven anatomy (Table 4.1).

Scanning Technique and Anatomy to Identify

The patient should sit with the elbow in slight flexion and the forearm pronated so that the hand rests comfortably. The DRUJ lies deep to the fourth and fifth extensor compartments of the dorsal wrist. The transducer is placed transversely, short axis to the fourth and fifth extensor compartments over Lister's tubercle and the distal ulna. Identify the extensor digiti minimi (EDM) muscle which lies over the DRUJ (Fig. 4.4) [14, 15].

Injection Techniques: In-Plane Axial Approach [9]

Patient positioning: Sit the patient with the affected arm resting comfortably on a table with the wrist and hand in pronation, palm down.

Probe positioning: Place the transducer axially over the fourth and fifth extensor compartments at the wrist at the level of the ulnar styloid process and Lister's tubercle (Fig. 4.5a).

Markings: It may helpful to identify the ulnar styloid process and Lister's tubercle for bony anatomy and transducer placement and then the fifth extensor compartment to avoid needle placement into the EDM.

Needle position: The needle should be inserted on the ulnar side of the EDM parallel to the transducer for optimal needle visualization. The needle should be inserted deep to the EDM and aimed at the DRUJ recess between the ulna and radius.

Safety considerations: Prior to passing the needle below the extensor digiti minimi tendon, Doppler may help to identify the dorsal branch of the anterior interosseous artery which runs in a neurovascular bundle with transverse branches of the dorsal ulnar cutaneous nerve [12, 16].

Pearls:

- An oblique standoff technique may be used if the ulnar styloid process makes an appropriate needle angle difficult to attain.
- Doppler mode may help identify vascular structures.
- Extending the fingers may help improve identification of local anatomy.

Equipment needed:

- High-frequency linear array transducer (10 MHz+)
- 25G 1.5″ needle
- 0.5 mL of steroid preparation
- 1–3 mL local anesthetic

First Extensor Compartment

DeQuervain's disease is a painful tenosynovitis of the abductor pollicis longus (APL) and extensor pollicis brevis (EPB) tendons in the first dorsal extensor compartment of the wrist. DeQuervain's disease is thought to occur from overuse or trauma directly to the tendon sheath [17]. Symptoms include

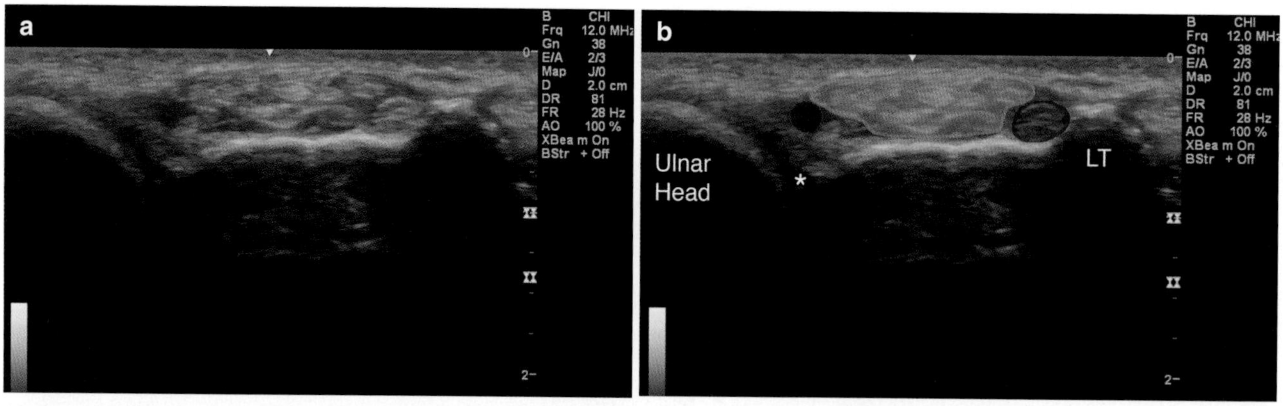

Fig. 4.4 (**a**) Axial view over dorsal distal radioulnar joint. (**b**) *Asterisk* indicates DRUJ; *purple circle*, third extensor compartment (extensor pollicis longus); *orange*, fourth extensor compartment (extensor digitorum and extensor indicis); *magenta circle*, fifth extensor compartment (extensor digiti minimi); *LT* Lister's tubercle; and ulnar head labeled

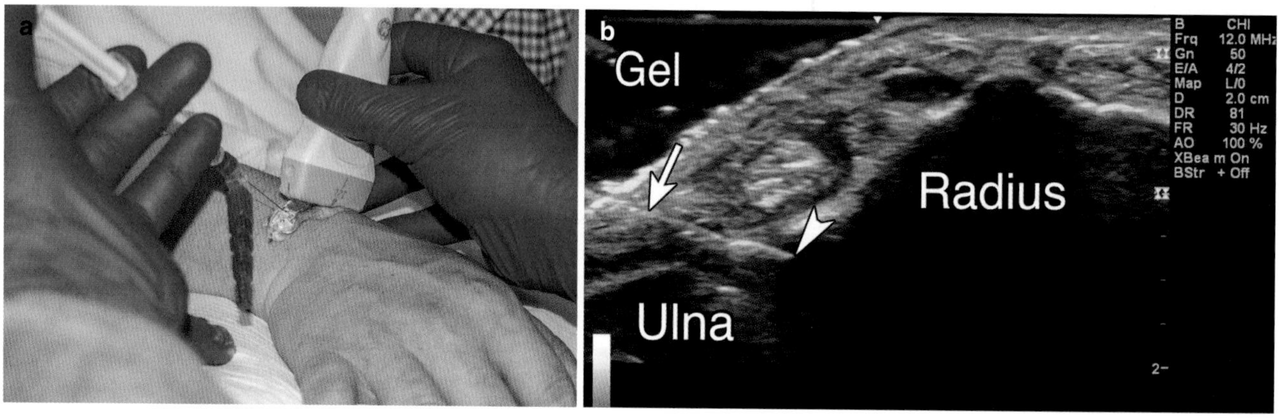

Fig. 4.5 (**a**) Example of probe position over DRUJ with gel standoff technique. (**b**) Example of in-plane approach. *White arrowhead* points to needle tip. *White arrow* points to needle. Gel-gel standoff, radius, and ulna labeled

Table 4.2 Relief following ultrasound guided 1st dorsal compartment injection

Study – 1st dorsal compartment	Author	Symptomatic relief at follow-up (%)
Ultrasound guided	Jeyapalan et al. [36]	94

hand, wrist, and thumb pain with activities that involve abduction and extension of the thumb. Provocative tests such as Finkelstein's maneuver may reproduce symptoms. The diagnosis is based on history and physical exam. Corticosteroid injection has been shown to provide improvement in pain and function (Table 4.2) [15, 18, 19].

Scanning Technique and Anatomy to Identify

The patient should sit with the elbow flexed and the wrist and hand in neutral position so that the radial styloid is facing up. The first extensor compartment is located directly over the radial styloid process. The transducer is placed transversely, short axis over the radial styloid. The APL and EPB tendons travel through this compartment and can be separated by a septum. The APL lies more volar than the EPB. Scanning further distally will show the two tendons diverging towards their insertions. Scanning proximally will show them side by side. The compartment is covered by an extensor retinaculum. Tendon sheath thickening may be apparent with transverse or longitudinal scanning; a "donut sign" may indicate synovitis (Fig. 4.6) [20, 21].

Injection Techniques: In-Plane Longitudinal Approach

Patient positioning: Sit the patient with the affected arm resting comfortably on a table. Place the hand in a neutral position with the radial styloid facing up.

Probe positioning: Place the probe longitudinal over the radial styloid and APL tendon (Fig. 4.7a).

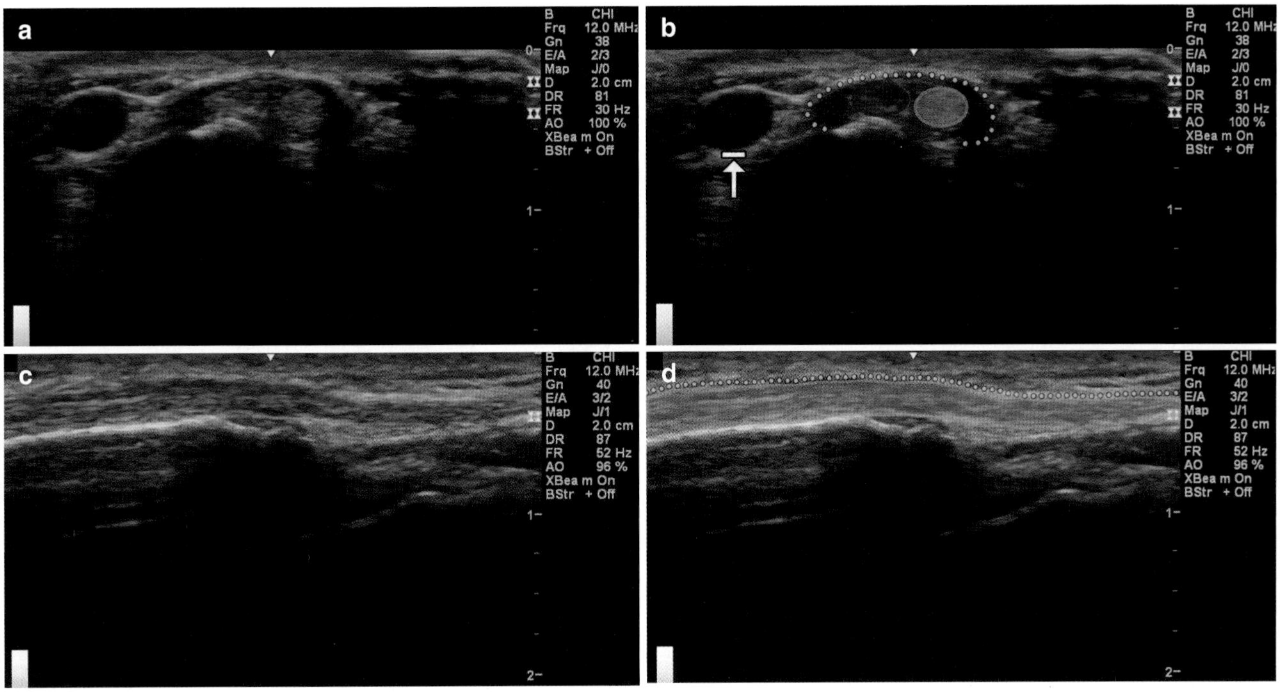

Fig. 4.6 (**a**) Axial view over first extensor compartment. (**b**) *Purple circle*, abductor pollicis longus; *orange circle*, extensor pollicis brevis; *dotted green line*, extensor retinaculum; *arrow with stop* indicates radial artery. (**c**) Longitudinal view over first extensor compartment. (**d**) *Orange* indicates abductor pollicis longus and extensor pollicis brevis; *dotted green line*, extensor retinaculum

Markings: Identify and mark any veins and the radial artery that lie volar to the 1st dorsal compartment.

Needle position: The needle should be inserted parallel to the transducer for optimal needle visualization. The needle tip target is the tendon sheath overlying the APL and EPB tendons.

Injection Techniques: Out-of-Plane Axial Approach

Patient positioning: The patient is seated with the affected arm resting comfortably on a table. Place the hand in a neutral position with the radial styloid facing up.

Probe positioning: Start by placing the transducer short axis (transverse) over the radial styloid and scan proximally and distally until the APL and EPB are clearly identified traveling in the same compartment (Fig. 4.8a).

Markings: Identify and mark any veins and the radial artery that lie volar to the 1st dorsal compartment.

Needle position: The needle should be inserted perpendicular to the transducer. Keep the needle tip superficial as the target site is the tendon sheath encasing the APL and EPB tendons.

Safety considerations: There is a risk of the following: prolonged bleeding, infection, tendon rupture, allergic reaction, increased pain, and decreased functional scores. If using corticosteroid, there is a risk of soft tissue (fat) atrophy and local depigmentation with corticosteroid injection.

Pearls:

- The superficial branch of the radial nerve can lie over the first dorsal compartment and may be temporarily blocked by the local anesthetic.
- The footprint of a standard probe is too large to fully cover a short axis view of the 1st dorsal compartment, and an oblique standoff technique may allow for better needle visualization.
- Doppler mode may help identify vascular structures.

Equipment needed:

- High-frequency linear array transducer (10 MHz+)
- 25G 1.5″ needle
- 0.5 mL of steroid preparation
- 1–3 mL local anesthetic

Scaphotrapeziotrapezoid (STT) Joint

The STT joint is located on the radial side of the wrist. STT joint pain is a common source of wrist pain; however, making an accurate diagnosis in this complex area of the wrist can be difficult [22]. The STT joint can produce pain on the dorsal or volar aspect of the wrist and mimic pain arising from the 1st carpometacarpal joint [23]. Patients often complain of deep achy arthritic-type pain. There are no specific provocative tests for STT joint pain; however, direct palpation of the volar STT joint should reproduce the pain [24, 25]. The diagnosis remains challenging with history and physical

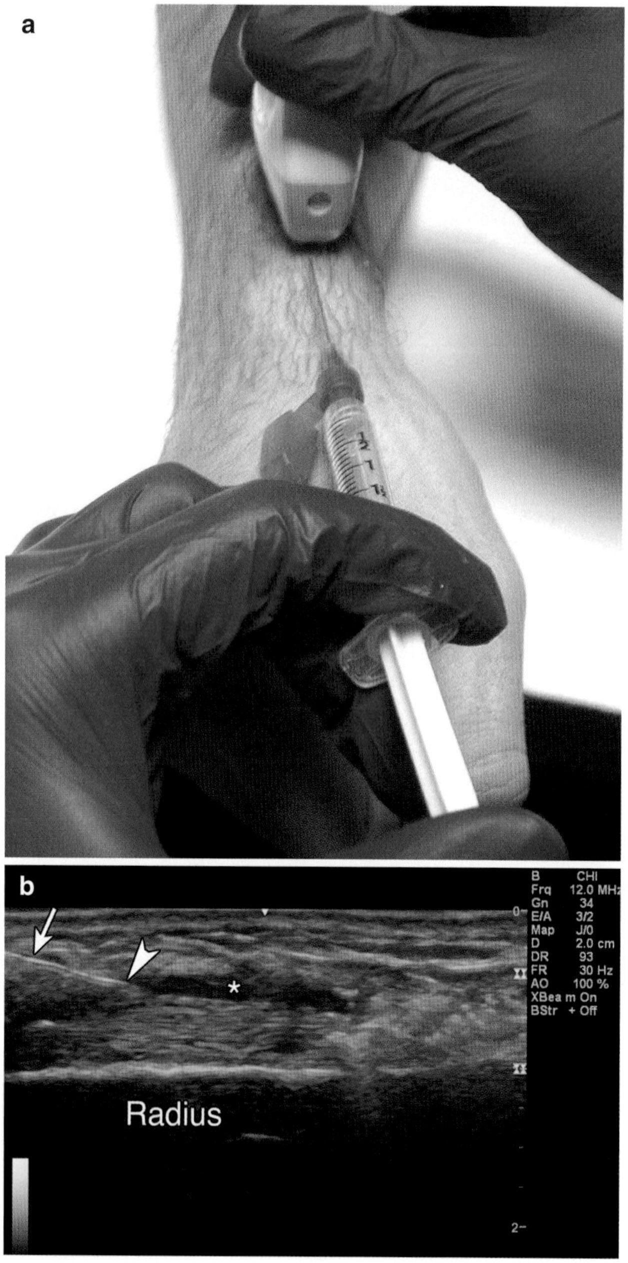

Fig. 4.7 (**a**) Example of longitudinal probe position over first extensor compartment. (**b**) Example of in-plane approach. *White arrowhead* points to needle tip. *White arrow* points to needle. *Asterisk* indicates injectate filling tendon sheath. Radius labeled

exam alone. Injection into the STT joint can provide symptomatic relief and serve as a diagnostic tool (Table 4.3).

Scanning Technique and Anatomy to Identify

The patient should sit with the elbow flexed and the hand lying comfortably in the supinated position. A high-frequency linear transducer is placed longitudinal to the distal radius. The hyperechoic bony radius is followed distally until the radioscaphoid articulation is identified. Continue scanning distally until the trapezium and carpometacarpal joint are identified. Moving the thumb can help to identify the CMC joint. The flexor carpi radialis tendon can be visualized superficial to the STT joint. Doppler can be used to help identify the superficial palmer branch of the radial artery (Fig. 4.9).

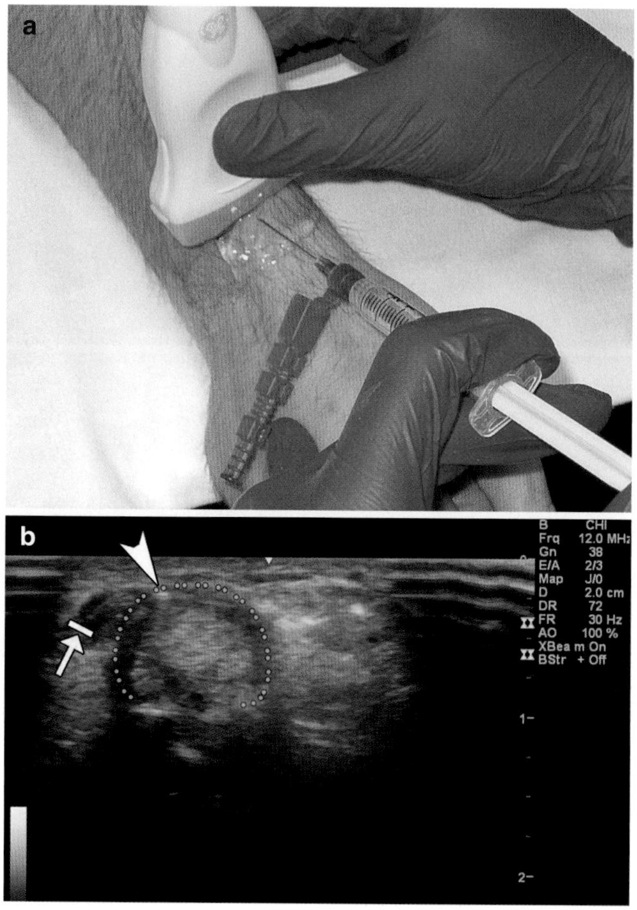

Fig. 4.8 (**a**) Example of transverse probe position over first extensor compartment. (**b**) Example of out-of-plane approach. *White arrowhead* points to needle tip. *Dotted green line* – tendon sheath. *Arrow with stop* indicates radial artery

Table 4.3 Accuracy of ultrasound guided versus palpation guided STT joint injections

Study – STT	Author	Accuracy (%)
Palpation guided	Smith et al. [37]	80
Ultrasound guided	Smith et al. [37]	100

Injection Technique: Out-of-Plane Longitudinal Approach

Patient positioning: Sit the patient with the affected arm resting comfortably on a table. Place the hand in a supinated position.

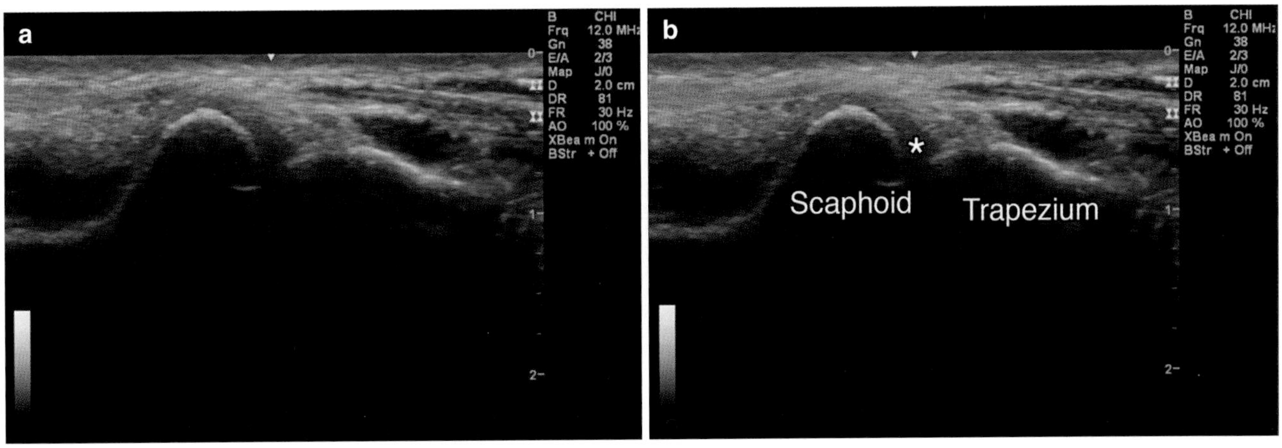

Fig. 4.9 (**a**) Sagittal view over volar aspect of STT Joint. (**b**) *Orange* – flexor carpi radialis traversing superficial to the scaphoid towards the second metacarpal bone, *asterisk* indicates STT joint, scaphoid and trapezium labeled

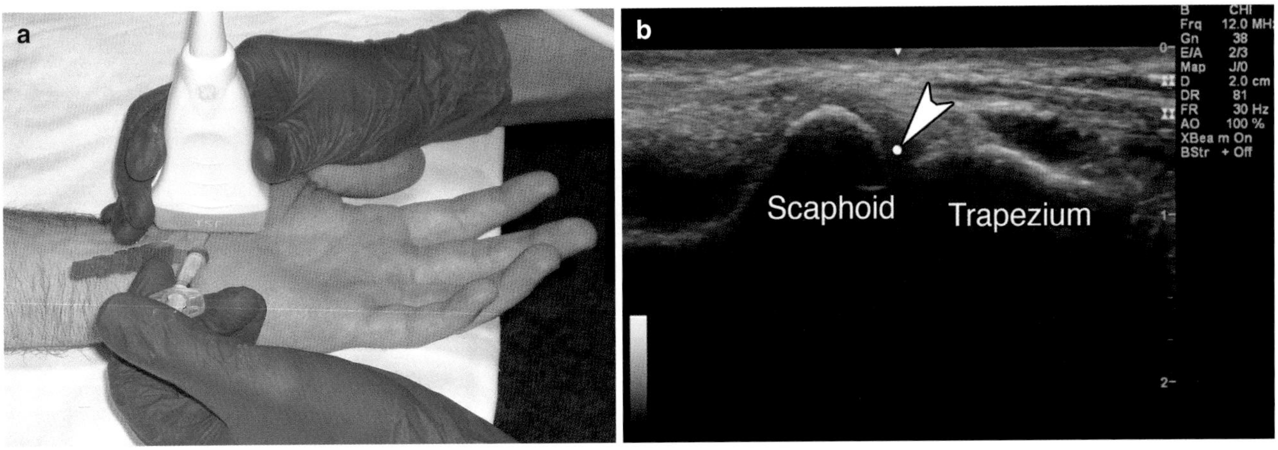

Fig. 4.10 (**a**) Example of longitudinal probe position over STT joint. (**b**) Example of out-of-plane approach. *White arrowhead* points to needle tip. Scaphoid and trapezium labeled

Probe positioning: Start by placing the transducer long axis (longitudinal) to the radius and scan distal until the scaphoid, trapezium, carpometacarpal joint, and the flexor carpi radialis tendon are clearly identified (Fig. 4.10a).

Markings: If the superficial palmar branch of the radial artery is identified, mark it so the probe and needle position can be adjusted to avoid puncture.

Needle position: The needle should be inserted on the radial side of the transducer, centered and perpendicular. The needle is advanced at a 45° angle until the needle tip is identified within the joint as a bright hyperechoic dot.

Safety considerations: Prior to advancing the needle, Doppler can be used to help identify the superficial palmer branch of the radial artery.

Pearls:

- Slightly extending the wrist and applying some radial or ulnar deviation may help to open up the joint space.

Equipment needed:

- High-frequency linear array transducer (10 MHz+)
- 25G 1.5″ needle
- 0.5 mL of steroid preparation
- 1–3 mL local anesthetic

Wrist Dorsal, Volar, and Flexor Tendon Sheath Ganglion Cyst

Ganglion cysts are soft tissue masses arising from the dorsal or volar aspects of the wrist. They are composed of mucoid material contained in randomly arranged sheets of collagen without a synovial lining and communicate with the joint via a pedicle [28]. Patients with ganglia can present with a painless mass, aching at the wrist, decreased ROM, decreased grip strength, or paresthesias if there is nerve compression. On exam, wrist ganglia are usually 1–2 cm cystic structures with limited mobility and rubbery feel. Often clinical presentation and exam can be enough to make the diagnosis [26]. Treatment consists of observation if asymptomatic or aspiration and

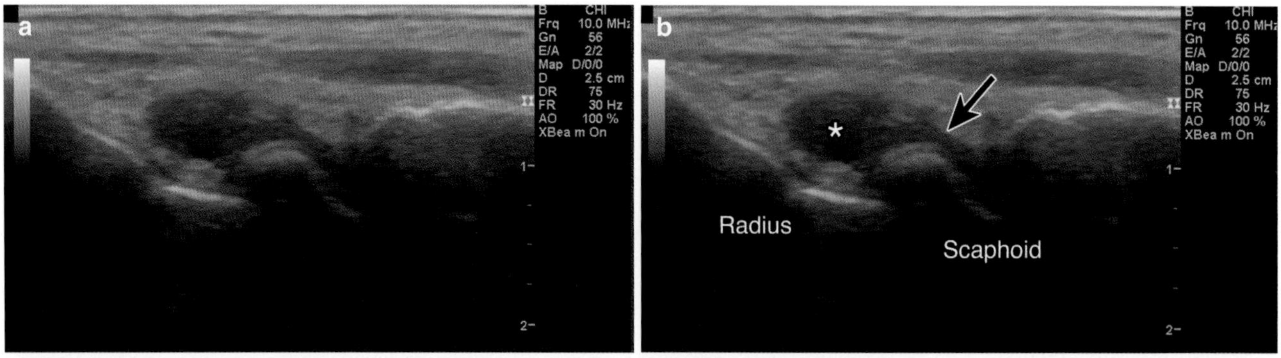

Fig. 4.11 (**a**) Longitudinal dorsal view over distal radius and scaphoid. (**b**) *Asterisk* indicates ganglion cyst. *Black arrow* shows (stalk) communication with the carpal joint. Radius and scaphoid labeled

surgical excision if symptomatic. Ultrasound-guided aspiration has been recommended especially for volar ganglia due to the risk of trauma to adjacent structures such as the radial artery and the recurrent branch of the median nerve [27].

Scanning Technique and Anatomy to Identify: Dorsal

The patient should sit with the elbow flexed to 90° and the forearm pronated so that the hand is resting comfortably. The most common site for ganglion cysts is the dorsal wrist as they arise from the scapholunate ligament 60–70 % of the time [28]. Begin with the probe longitudinally over the distal radius and scan distally until you identify the scaphoid bone. Once you identify the scaphoid, rotate the transducer to obtain an axial view of the scaphoid with the lunate located on the ulnar side. The majority of ganglia appear complex, look for well-defined margins, thick walls, posterior acoustic enhancement, and septations or locules [29].

Scanning Technique and Anatomy to Identify: Volar/Flexor Tendon Sheath

To evaluate the volar side of the wrist, have the patient supinate the forearm. A towel may be placed under the wrist to induce slight extension. Roughly 20 % of ganglia arise on the volar aspect of the wrist from the radiocarpal or scaphotrapezial joint [30]. In addition, 10 % can arise from the flexor tendon sheathes [26]. The transducer is placed longitudinally over the distal radius until the radiocarpal joint is identified. Note the proximity of the radial artery (Fig. 4.11).

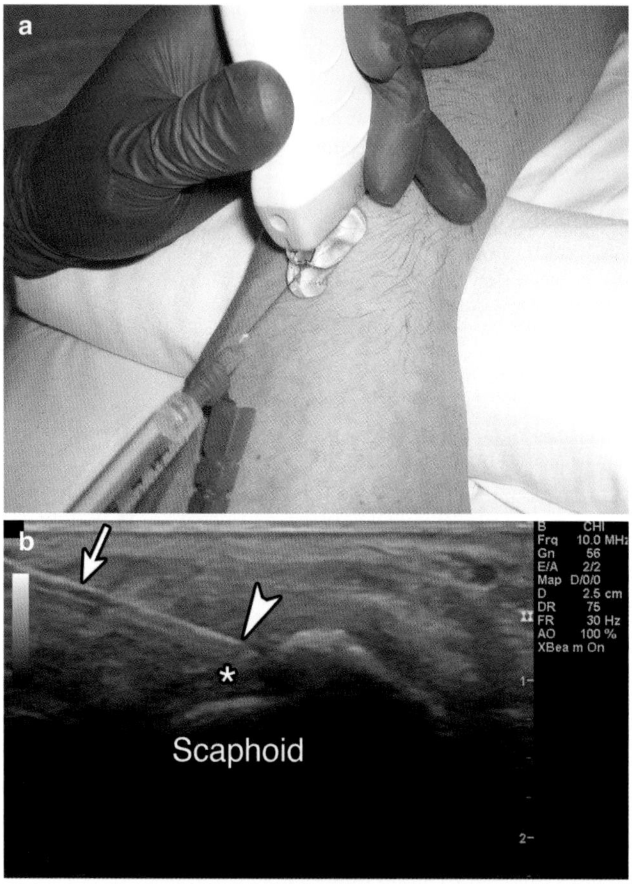

Fig. 4.12 (**a**) Example of longitudinal probe position over dorsal wrist with in-plane gel standoff technique. (**b**) Example of in-plane approach. *White arrowhead* points to needle tip. *White arrow* points to needle. *Asterisk* indicates ganglion cyst. Scaphoid labeled

Injection Techniques: In-Plane Sagittal Approach

Patient positioning: Sit the patient with the affected wrist resting comfortably on a table. The forearm is pronated for a dorsal cyst and supinated for a volar or flexor tendon sheath cyst.

Probe positioning: Place the transducer long axis over the ganglia until the ganglia is centered on the screen. Obtain short axis views to determine optimal needle placement (Fig. 4.12a).

Markings: Identify any neurovascular structures.

Needle position: The needle should be inserted in plane to the transducer for optimal needle visualization. Specific landmarks and direction of approach will vary based on the location of the cyst.

Safety considerations: Prior to injection, Doppler will help to identify adjacent vascular structures.

Pearls:

- An oblique standoff technique may be used if the ganglia are very superficial.
- Doppler mode may help identify vascular structures.
- Slightly flexing and extending the wrist may help improve visualization of the carpal bones.
- Flexing the fingers may help to identify structures surrounded ganglia opposed to flexor tendons.

Equipment needed:

- High-frequency linear array transducer (10 MHz+)
- 25G needle and 1–3 mL anesthetic for local anesthesia
- 16–18G 1.5″ needle for aspiration
- 0.5 mL of steroid preparation and 1 mL local anesthetic post-aspiration

Trigger Finger

Trigger finger is a stenosing tenosynovitis of the flexor digitorum and flexor pollicis longus tendons. Triggering or locking occurs at the first annular (A1) pulley which becomes thickened due to chronic repetitive friction. Diabetics have four times higher prevalence of triggering than the general population [31]. The diagnosis is based on history and physical exam. There may be pain at the A1 pulley, a palpable mass, or a tautness of the flexor tendons. The finger will get stuck when moving from active flexion to extension through the thickened A1 pulley (Tables 4.4 and 4.5).

Scanning Technique and Anatomy to Identify

The patient should sit with the hand resting comfortably and the fingers extended. The A1 pulley lies superficial and proximal to the metacarpophalangeal joint. The ultrasound probe is placed on the volar aspect of the hand just proximal to the MCP joint. Longitudinal scan shows the hyperechoic metacarpal head and the proximal phalanx deep with the tendons of the flexor digitorum profundus tendon and the flexor digitorum superficialis (FDS) tendon running over. The A1 pulley is seen here in cross section superficial to the tendon sheath. The probe is then rotated to give an axial image at the level of the A1 pulley. From superficial to deep, you should appreciate the FDS, flexor digitorum profundus (FDP), the volar plate (VP), and the metacarpal bone. The lumbricals can be seen laterally. Doppler can be utilized to identify the digital artery. Ultrasound diagnosis for trigger finger was described by Ebrahim et al., including hypoechoic thickening of the A1 pulley, visualization of a nodule in the FDS tendon, and dynamic visualization of triggering (Fig. 4.13) [32].

Table 4.4 Accuracy of blind versus ultrasound guided trigger point injections

Study – trigger finger		Accuracy tendon sheath (%)	Tendon proper injection (%)
Dae-Hee Lee et al. [38]	Blind	15	30
	Ultrasound guided	70	0

Table 4.5 Outcomes of blind versus ultrasound guided trigger finger injections

Study – trigger finger	Author	Success rate at 1 year (%)
Blind	Fleisch et al. [39]	57
Blind	Peters-Veluthamaningal et al. [40]	56
Ultrasound guided	Bodor et al. [41]	90

Injection Techniques: In-Plane Sagittal Approach

Patient positioning: Sit the patient with the affected hand resting palm up comfortably on a table.

Probe positioning: Obtain a long axis view of the affected flexor tendon at the level of the metacarpophalangeal joint. Identify the A1 pulley as a hyperechoic thickening of the volar aspect of the tendon sheath. A flexor tendon nodule or thickening may be noted. The A1 pulley synovial sheath may also demonstrate hypoechoic thickening or an effusion. The FDS, FDP, and VP should be centered on the screen. The A1 pulley wraps over these structures (Fig. 4.14a).

Markings: It may helpful to identify the digital arteries and nerves to avoid inadvertent needle puncture.

Needle position: The needle is inserted at a shallow angle from distal to proximal so that the tip of the needle is placed just distal to the A1 pulley and into the tendon sheath.

Injection Techniques: Out-of-Plane Axial Approach

Obtain a short axis view of the affected flexor tendon at the level of the metacarpophalangeal joint. Identify the A1 pulley overlying the FDS and FDP. The target is centered to the triangle formed by the FDS/FDP/VP, metacarpal bone, and the A1 pulley.

Patient positioning: Sit the patient with the affected hand resting palm up comfortably on table.

Probe positioning: Start by placing the transducer short axis (axial) over the A1 pulley at the level of the metacarpal

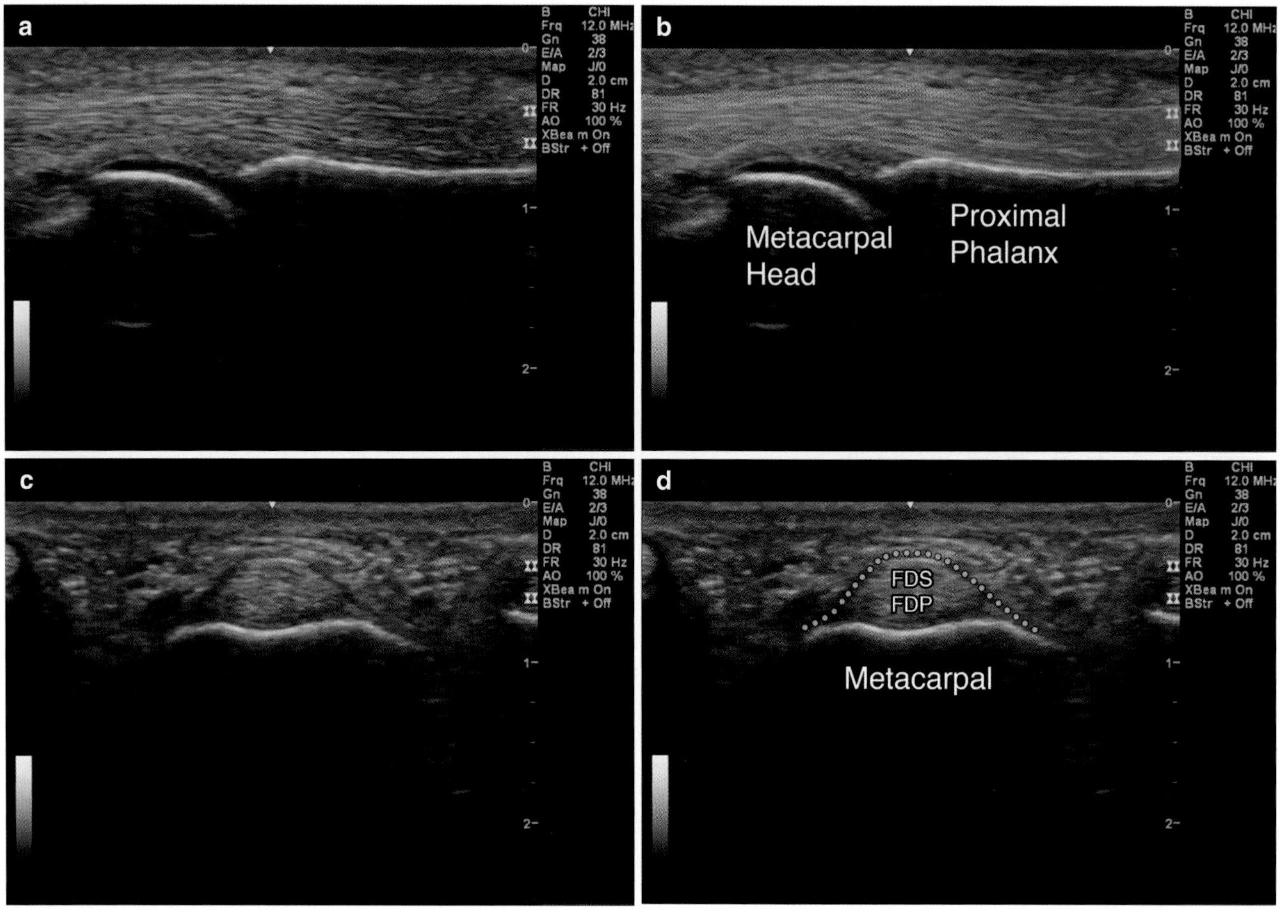

Fig. 4.13 (**a**) Sagittal view over FDS and FDP. (**b**) *Orange* – flexor digitorum superficialis and profundus tendons, metacarpal head and proximal phalanx labeled. (**c**) Axial view over A1 pulley at metacarpal head. (**d**) *Dotted green line* – tendon sheath, *FDS*, *FDP*, and metacarpal labeled

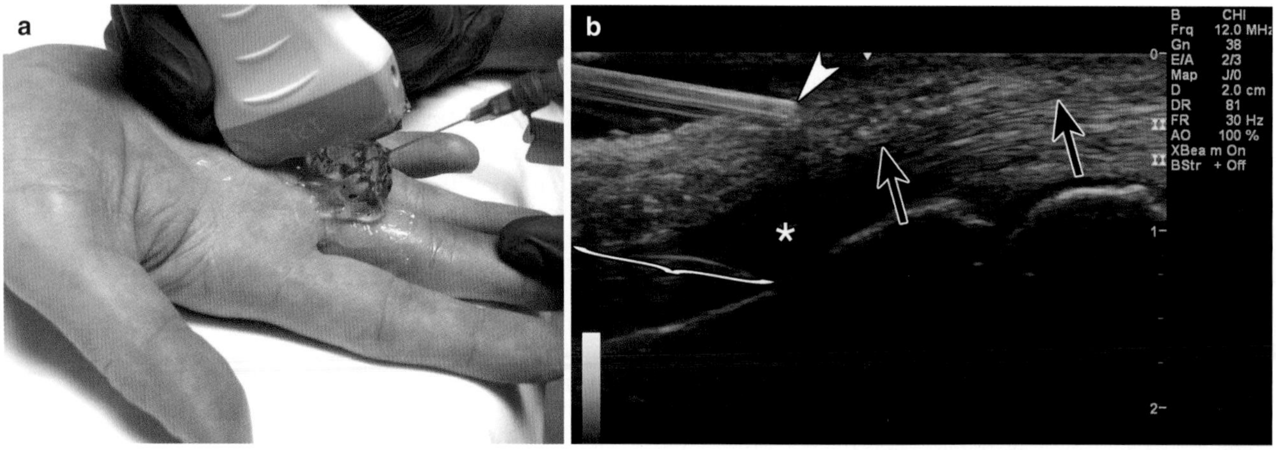

Fig. 4.14 (**a**) Example of sagittal probe position over trigger finger with gel standoff. (**b**) Example of in-plane approach. *Black arrows* point to tendon sheath. *White arrowhead* points to needle tip approaching target. *Asterisk* indicates anisotropy of FDS/FDP tendons. *Bracket* indicates needle reverberation

head. Make sure the pulley is located directly under the midpoint of the transducer (Fig. 4.15A).

Markings: It may helpful to identify the digital arteries and nerves to avoid inadvertent needle puncture.

Needle position: The needle is inserted at a steep angle, from either the proximal or distal end of the midpoint transducer so that the tip of the needle is seen within the target triangle. The needle tip is seen as a bright hyperechoic dot.

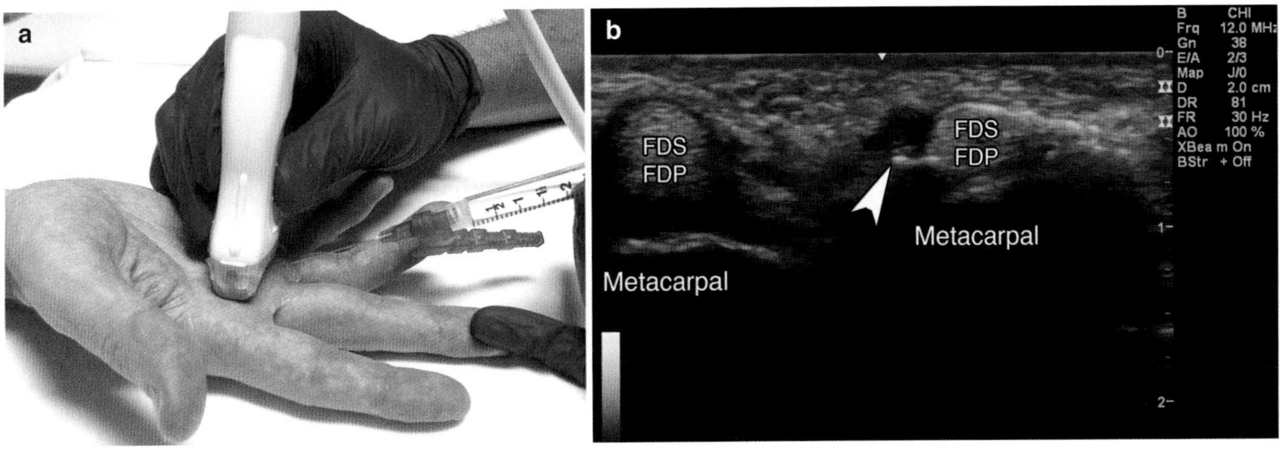

Fig. 4.15 (**a**) Example of axial probe position over trigger finger. (**b**) Example of out-of-plane approach. *White arrowhead* points to needle tip. *FDS*, *FDP*, and metacarpal labeled

Safety considerations: Do not inject the flexor tendons themselves. It may be helpful to retract the needle until loss of resistance is noted.

Avoid the digital arteries and nerves.

Pearls:

- A gel standoff technique may be used in the long axis injection.
- Doppler mode may help identify vascular structures.
- Slightly flexing and extending the fingers will help to identify a nodule if present within the tendon.

Equipment needed:

- High-frequency linear array transducer (10 MHz+)
- 25G 1.5″ needle for in-plane approach
- 25G 0.5″ needle for out-of-plane approach
- 0.5 mL of steroid preparation
- 1–3 mL local anesthetic

Hand: 1st Carpometacarpal (CMC) Joint

The thumb has three joints that can develop painful arthritis: the interphalangeal joint (IP), the metacarpophalangeal joint (MCP), and the carpometacarpal joint (CMC). CMC arthritis appears to be more frequent in women and is related to repetitive activity of the joint. Symptoms are typically thumb and wrist pain when pinching, grasping, and twisting the hand. Common physical exam findings include pain over the affected joint and a positive grind test [33, 34].

Scanning Technique and Anatomy to Identify

The patient should sit with the elbow flexed and the hand resting comfortably on a table. The hand position will move from pronated to neutral so that much of the joint can be circumferentially scanned. The transducer is placed in plane with the axis of the thumb so that the joint between the first metacarpal bone and base of the trapezium is identified. The APL and EPB tendons can be visualized passing over the CMC joint. Scan from one side of the joint to the other to evaluate for any bony joint changes (Fig. 4.16).

Injection Techniques: Out-of-Plane Longitudinal Approach

Patient positioning: Sit the patient with the affected arm resting comfortably on a table. Place the hand in neutral position with the thumb facing up.

Probe positioning: Place the transducer in the longitudinal plane centered over CMC joint (Fig. 4.17a).

Markings: Identify and mark the APL and EPB tendon to avoid inadvertent needle puncture.

Needle position: The needle should be inserted at a steep angle at the center of the transducer aimed directly at the joint space. The needle tip should be visible within the joint. Proper placement can be confirmed by seeing capsular distention upon injection.

Injection Techniques: In-Plane Longitudinal Approach

Patient positioning: The patient should sit with the affected arm resting comfortably on a table with the wrist and hand in pronation.

Probe positioning: Start by placing the transducer longitudinal over the CMC joint (Fig. 4.18a).

Markings: Identify and mark the APL and EPB tendon to avoid inadvertent needle puncture.

Needle position: The needle should be inserted parallel to the transducer for optimal needle visualization.

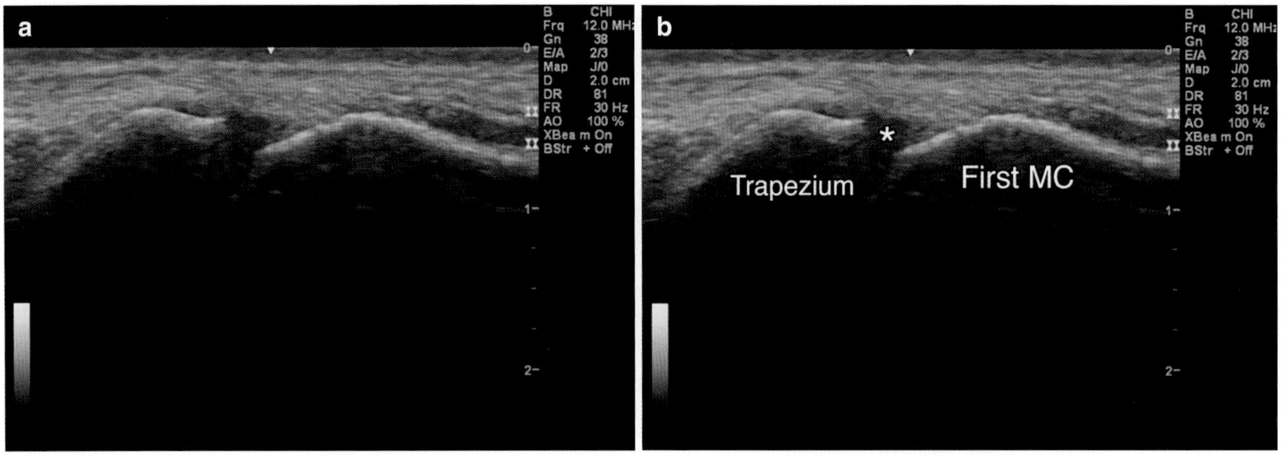

Fig. 4.16 (**a**) Sagittal view over CMC joint. (**b**) *Asterisk* indicates joint space. Trapezium and first metacarpal bone labeled

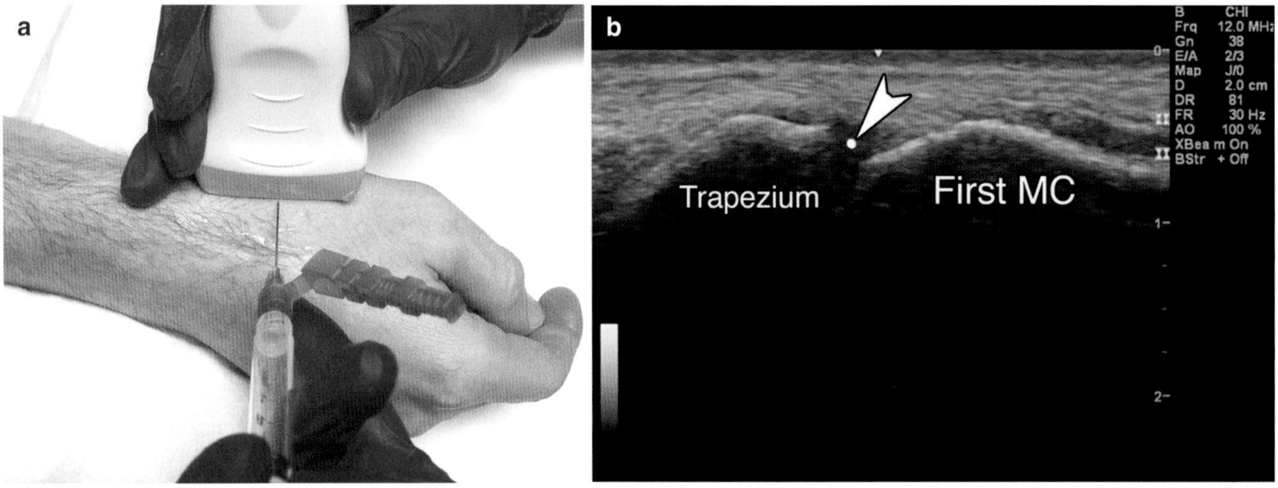

Fig. 4.17 (**a**) Example of longitudinal probe position over CMC joint. (**b**) Example of out-of-plane approach. *White arrowhead* points to needle tip. Trapezium and first metacarpal bone labeled

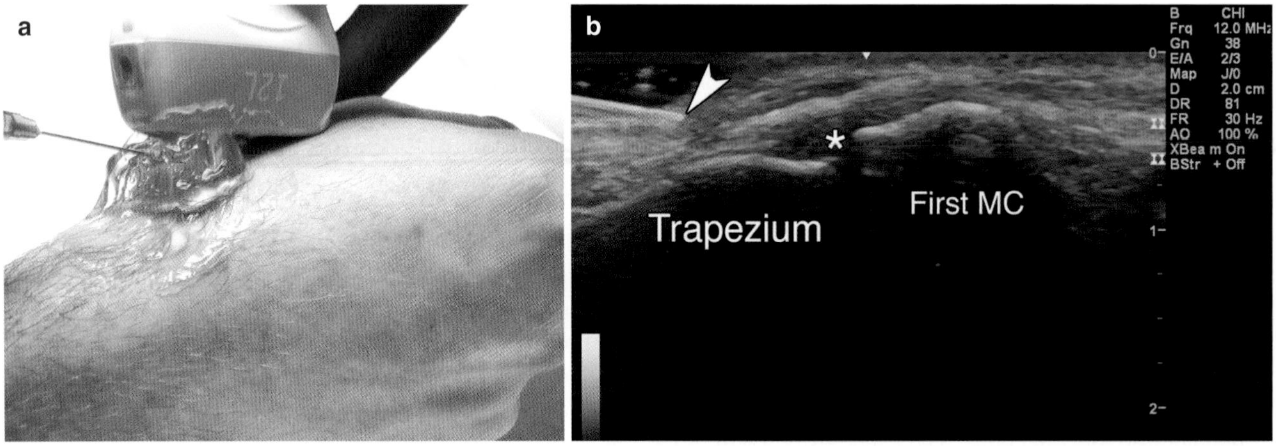

Fig. 4.18 (**a**) Example of probe position over CMC joint with gel standoff technique. (**b**) Example of in-plane approach. *White arrowhead* points to needle tip approaching joint. *Asterisk* indicates CMC joint space. Trapezium and first metacarpal bone labeled

Safety considerations: Do not inject the extensor tendons.

Pearls:

- An oblique standoff technique may be used.
- Flexing the thumb may help to open the CMC joint.

Equipment needed:

- High-frequency linear array transducer (10 MHz+)
- 25G 1.5″ needle
- 0.5 mL of steroid preparation
- 1–3 mL local anesthetic

References

1. Katz JN, Simmons BP. Clinical practice: carpal tunnel syndrome. N Engl J Med. 2002;346:1807–12.
2. Cartwright MS, Hobson-Webb LD, Boon AJ, et al. Evidence-based guideline: neuromuscular ultrasound for the diagnosis of carpal tunnel syndrome. AANEM practice guideline. Muscle Nerve. 2012;46:287–93.
3. Dammers JW, Veering MM, Vermuelen M. Injection with methylprednisolone proximal to the carpal tunnel: randomized double blind trial. Br Med J. 1999;319:884–6.
4. Gelberman RH, Aronson D, Weismen MH. Carpal-tunnel syndrome: results of a prospective trial of steroid injection and splinting. J Bone Joint Surg Am. 1980;62:1181–4.
5. Clinical practice guideline on the treatment of carpal tunnel syndrome. American Academy of Orthopaedic Surgeons. 2008. http://www.aaos.org/research/guidelines/ctstreatmentguideline.pdf.
6. McNally E. Musculoskeletal interventional ultrasound. In: McNally E, editor. Practical musculoskeletal ultrasound. New York: Elsevier; 2005. p. 293.
7. Jamadar DA, Jacobson JA, Hayes CW. Sonographic evaluation of the median nerve at the wrist. J Ultrasound Med. 2001;20:1011–4.
8. Smith J, Wisniewski SJ, Finnoff JT, Payne JM. Sonographically guided carpal tunnel injections the ulnar approach. J Ultrasound Med. 2008;27:1485–90.
9. Grassi W, Farina A, Filipucci E, Cervini C. Intralesional therapy in carpal tunnel syndrome: a sonographic-guided approach. Clin Exp Rheumatol. 2002;20:73–6.
10. Matloub HS, Yan JG, Mink Van Der Molen AB, Zhang LL, Sanger JR. The detailed anatomy of the palmar cutaneous nerves and its clinical implications. J Hand Surg [Br]. 1998;23:373–9.
11. Gassner EM, Schocke M, Peer S, Schwabegger A, Jaschke W, Bodner G. Persistent median artery in the carpal tunnel: color Doppler ultrasonographic findings. J Ultrasound Med. 2002;21:455–61.
12. Murray PM, Adams JE, Lam J, Osterman AL, Wolfe S. Disorders of the distal radioulnar joint. Instr Course Lect. 2010;59:295–311.
13. DeSmet L. The distal radioulnar joint in rheumatoid arthritis. Acta Orthop Belg. 2006;72:381–6.
14. Yoshida R, Beppu M, Ishii S, Hirata K. Anatomical study of the distal radioulnar joint: degenerative changes and morphological measurement. Hand Surg. 1999;4:109–15.
15. Jacobson JA. Fundamentals of musculoskeletal ultrasound. Philadelphia: Elsevier; 2007. p. 144.
16. Lourie GM, King J, Kleinman WB. The transverse radioulnar branch from the dorsal sensory ulnar nerve: its clinical and anatomical significance further defined. J Hand Surg [Am]. 1994;19:241–5.
17. Wolf JM, Sturdivant RX, Owens BD. Incidence of de Quervain's tenosynovitis in a young, active population. J Hand Surg [Am]. 2009;34:112–5.
18. Zingas C, Failla JM, Van Holsbeeck M. Injection accuracy and relief of De Quervain's tendinitis. J Hand Surg [Am]. 1998;23(1):89–96.
19. Avci S, Yilmaz C, Sayli U. Comparison of nonsurgical treatment measure for de Quervain's disease of pregnancy and lactation. J Hand Surg [Am]. 2002;27:322–4.
20. Trentanni C, Galli A, Melucci G, Stasi G. Ultrasonic diagnosis of De Quervain's stenosing tenosynovitis. Radiol Med. 1997;93(3):194–8.
21. De Maeseneer M, Marcelis S, Jager T, Girard C, Gest T, Jamadar D. Spectrum of normal and pathologic findings in the region of the first extensor compartment of the wrist: sonographic findings and correlations with dissections. J Ultrasound Med. 2009;28(6):779–86.
22. Kapoutsis DV, Dardas A, Day CS. Carpometacarpal and scaphotrapeziotrapezoid arthritis: arthroscopy, arthroplasty, and arthrodesis. J Hand Surg [Am]. 2011;36:354–66.
23. Carro LP, Golano P, Farinas O, Cerezal L, Hidalgo C. The radial portal for scaphotrapeziotrapezoid arthroscopy. Arthroscopy. 2003;19:547–53.
24. Crosby EB, Linscheid RL, Dobyns JH. Scaphotrapezial trapezoid arthritis. J Hand Surg [Am]. 1978;3:223–34.
25. White L, Clavijo J, Gilula LA, Wollstein R. Classification system for isolated arthritis of the scaphotrapeziotrapezoid joint. Scand J Plast Reconstr Surg Hand Surg. 2010;44:112–7.
26. Gude W, Morelli V. Ganglion cysts of the wrist: pathophysiology, clinical picture, and management. Curr Rev Musculoskelet Med. 2008;1:205–11.
27. Breidahl WH, Adler RS. Ultrasound-guided injection of ganglia with corticosteroids. Skeletal Radiol. 1996;25(7):635–8.
28. Angelides AC, Wallace PF. The dorsal ganglion of the wrist: its pathogenesis, gross and microscopic anatomy, and surgical treatment. J Hand Surg [Am]. 1976;1(3):228–35.
29. Teefey S, Dahiya N, Middleton W, Gelberman R, Boyer M. Ganglia of the hand and wrist: a sonographic analysis. AJR Am J Roentgenol. 2008;191:716–20.
30. Teh J, Vlychou M. Ultrasound-guided interventional procedures of the wrist and hand. Eur Radiol. 2009;19:1002–10.
31. Akhtar S, Bradley MJ, Quinton DN, Burke FD. Management and referral for trigger finger/thumb. BMJ. 2005;331:30–3.
32. Ebrahim FS, De Maeseneer M, Jager T, et al. US diagnosis of UCL tears of the thumb and Stener lesions: technique, pattern-based approach, and differential diagnosis. Radiographics. 2006;26:1007–20.
33. Shin EK, Osterman AL. Treatment of thumb metacarpophalangeal and interphalangeal joint arthritis. Hand Clin. 2008;24:239–50.
34. Carr MM, Freiberg A. Osteoarthritis of the thumb: clinical aspects and management. Am Fam Physician. 1994;50:995–1000.
35. Smith J, Rizzo M, Sayeed YA, Finnoff JT. Sonographically guided distal radioulnar joint injection. Technique and validation in a cadaveric model. J Ultrasound Med. 2011;30:1587–92.
36. Jeyapalan K, Choudhary S. Ultrasound-guided injection of triamcinolone and bupivacaine in the management of De Quervain's disease. Skeletal Radiol. 2009;38(11):1099–103.
37. Smith J, Brault JS, Rizzo M, Sayeed YA, Finnoff JT. Accuracy of sonographically guided and palpation guided scaphotrapeziotrapezoid joint injections. J Ultrasound Med. 2011;30:1509–15.
38. Lee DH, Han SB, Park JW, Lee SH, Kim KW, Jeong WK. Sonographically guided tendon sheath injections are more accurate than blind injections. J Ultrasound Med. 2011;30:197–203.
39. Fleisch SB, Spindler KP, Lee DH. Corticosteroid injections in the treatment of trigger finger: a level I and II systematic review. J Am Acad Orthop Surg. 2007;15:166–71.
40. Peters-Veluthamaningal C, Winters JC, Groenier KH, Meyboom-de JB. Corticosteroid injections effective for trigger finger in adults in general practice: a double-blinded randomized placebo controlled trial. Ann Rheum Dis. 2008;67:1262–6.
41. Bodor M, Flossman T. Ultrasound-guided first annular pulley injection for trigger finger. J Ultrasound Med. 2009;28:737–43.

5 Hip

Mahmud M. Ibrahim, Yolanda Scott, David A. Spinner, and Joseph E. Herrera

Ultrasound can be used in the hip to diagnose both intra-articular and extra-articular hip pathology, such as bursitis, joint effusions, and tendinopathy [1]. It also provides dynamic real-time images which can be compared to the contralateral side. Dynamic ultrasound can be useful in pathologies such as snapping hip syndrome [2]. In addition, Doppler can be used to identify any vasculature in the area when performing an interventional procedure. Ultrasound-guided nerve blocks in the hip region have been shown to be more efficacious than blocks performed blindly [3]. With proper technique, the ultrasound-guided injections have been shown to be safe and effective [4].

Hip Joint

Intra-articular hip joint injections are indicated for diagnostic or therapeutic purposes. Hip pain can occur from femoral acetabular impingement, avascular necrosis, labral tears, and synovitis but usually occurs from osteoarthritis. Groin pain is the principal symptom, usually exacerbated by activity and relieved by rest. Patients with osteoarthritis typically are older than 50 and have decreased and painful hip internal rotation and morning stiffness lasting less than 60 min [4]. Radiographic criteria include the presence of osteophytes (femoral or acetabular) and joint space narrowing (superior, axial, and/or medial) [1]. Intra-articular corticosteroid and hyaluronic acid injections have been shown to be useful in improving pain associated with hip osteoarthritis (Table 5.1) [10, 11].

M.M. Ibrahim, MD
Performance Spine and Sports Medicine, Lawrenceville, NJ, USA
e-mail: mibrahim926@gmail.com

Y. Scott, MD
Department of Rehabilitation Medicine,
Icahn School of Medicine at Mount Sinai, New York, NY, USA
e-mail: yscott80@gmail.com

D.A. Spinner, DO, RMSK (✉)
Department of Anesthesiology – Pain Medicine,
Arnold Pain Management Center, Beth Israel Deaconess
Medical Center, Harvard Medical School, Brookline, MA, USA
e-mail: dspinnerny@gmail.com

J.E. Herrera, DO, FAAPMR
Interventional Spine and Sports Medicine Division,
Department of Rehabilitation Medicine,
Icahn School of Medicine at Mount Sinai,
New York, NY, USA

Scanning Technique and Anatomy to Identify

The patient is placed supine with the leg in the neutral position. The anterior superior iliac spine (ASIS) is palpated and the transducer is placed in the transverse (axial) plane with the lateral end over the ASIS. The transducer is then slowly moved medially and inferiorly until the femoral head is visualized. The femoral neurovascular structures are just medial to the transducer in this position. In order to visualize these structures, the transducer is rotated in the transverse plane and moved medially to identify the femoral nerve, artery, and vein. The use of Doppler can make it easier to visualize the vessels. Once the location of these structures is confirmed, the transducer can be moved back to the femoral head. While maintaining the medial portion of the transducer on the femoral head, the lateral end of the transducer is rotated inferiorly approximately 40° to visualize the femoral neck. In this view, there should be a clear picture of the femoral head/neck junction, the overlying hyperechoic iliofemoral ligament, and hip capsule. While maintaining this orientation, the transducer is moved slightly superolaterally to place the transducer as far laterally while keeping the femoral head/neck junction in view (Fig. 5.1) [12].

Injection Technique: In-Plane Sagittal Oblique Approach

Patient positioning: Lay the patient supine with the leg in the neutral position. The hip can be slightly flexed for patient comfort by placing a knee roll under the ipsilateral knee.

Probe positioning: Place the lateral end of the probe in the axial plane over the ASIS and scan medially and inferiorly

D.A. Spinner et al. (eds.), *Atlas of Ultrasound Guided Musculoskeletal Injections*, Musculoskeletal Medicine,
DOI 10.1007/978-1-4614-8936-8_5, © Springer Science+Business Media, LLC 2014

until the femoral head/neck junction comes into view. Rotate the lateral end of the transducer approximately 40°. At this point, the transducer should be parallel to the femoral neck (Fig. 5.2a). Be sure to identify the femoral neurovascular structures medial to the head/neck junction in the transverse plane prior to injection.

Markings: Once the joint space is identified, the probe is moved as far lateral while still keeping the joint space in view. Mark this probe location. Rotate to the axial plane to scan medially, identify and mark the femoral neurovascular bundle, and then return to the previously marked probe position. Mark the skin a few centimeters distal to the inferior end of the transducer. By placing the needle in this location, it will help to increase needle visibility by keeping the needle more parallel to the transducer. The area is then prepped in the usual manner.

Needle position: A 25 g needle can be used to anesthetize the area using a layer-by-layer technique with 4–6 mL of 1 % lidocaine [12]. Alternatively ethyl chloride spray may be used. A 22 or 25 gauge spinal needle with the stylet in place is then advanced under direct ultrasound visualization to the femoral head/neck junction. A slight increase in resistance is felt as the needle traverses through the iliofemoral ligament into the hip joint. Once inside the joint, a test injection of 1–2 mL of local anesthetic can help confirm the intra-articular placement. Alternatively, a small amount of air can be injected to confirm needle placement into the joint space. If the air collects in a nondependent fashion along the hip joint, then the needle is believed to be intra-articular. However, if the air bubbles collect around the needle tip, then the needle is likely in an extra-articular position and needs to be adjusted. The remainder of the injectate can then be injected while visualizing the distension of the capsule under ultrasound.

Safety considerations: It is important to identify the femoral nerve, artery, and vein prior to inserting the needle in order to avoid piercing these structures. Care should be taken to avoid femoral nerve block from excessive local anesthesia.

Pearls:

- Gently pushing the probe into the skin (heel-toe maneuver) may help to better visualize deeper structures in larger patients.
- In thinner patients a linear transducer may be used at a lower frequency or "virtual convex" setting. Using heel-toe maneuver may be easier to maintain constant needle visualization.
- For larger patients a curvilinear transducer may be needed. Because of the curve, it is more difficult to visualize the needle in its entirety as some of the ultrasound beams will point away from the needle. It is important to use the heel-toe maneuver to maintain visualization of the needle tip.

Equipment needed:

- Wide-bandwidth linear array transducer (virtual convex mode may be helpful, if available) *or* low-frequency curvilinear transducer
- 22–25 gauge 3.5–5″ spinal needle
- 1–2 mL of steroid preparation
- 4–5 mL local anesthetic

Table 5.1 Accuracy of blind versus ultrasound guided hip injections

Study hip joint injection	Author	Accuracy
Ultrasound guided	Smith et al. [5]	97 % fluoro confirmed
Ultrasound guided	Pourbagher et al. [6].	100 % CT confirmed
Ultrasound guided	Levi [7]	100 % fluoro confirmed
Blind anterior approach	Leopold et al. [8]	60 % dissection
Blind anterior approach	Dobson [9]	61 % dissection

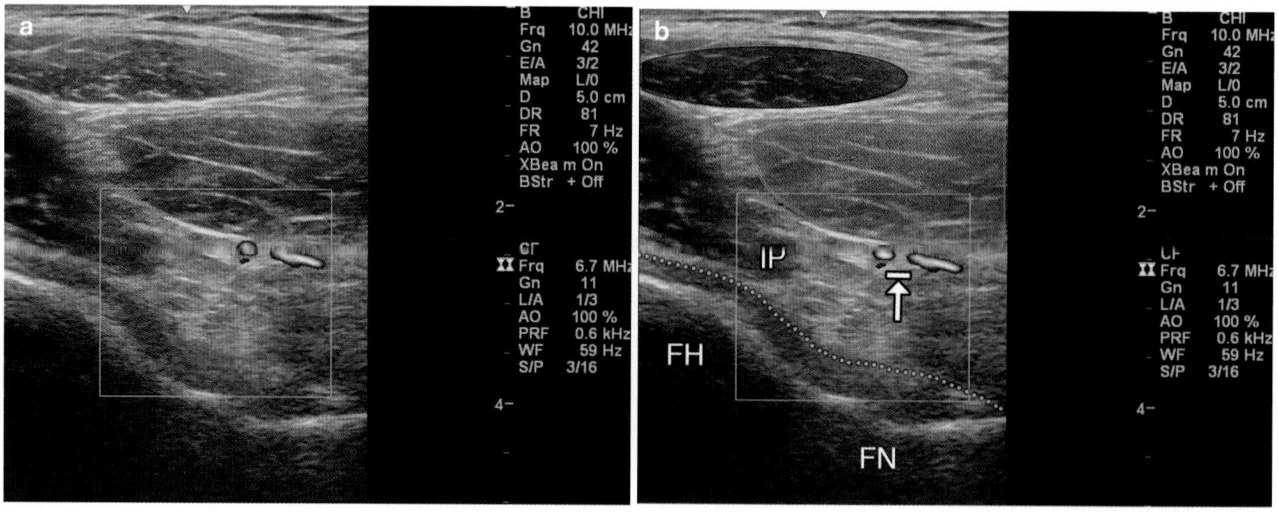

Fig. 5.1 (**a**) Sagittal oblique view of the femoral head/neck junction with Doppler visualizing artery. (**b**) *Purple* indicates sartorius muscle. *Orange* indicates rectus femoris. *IP* iliopsoas muscle, *FH* femoral head, *FN* femoral neck. *Arrow with stop* indicates vasculature. *Dotted green line* indicates hip joint capsule

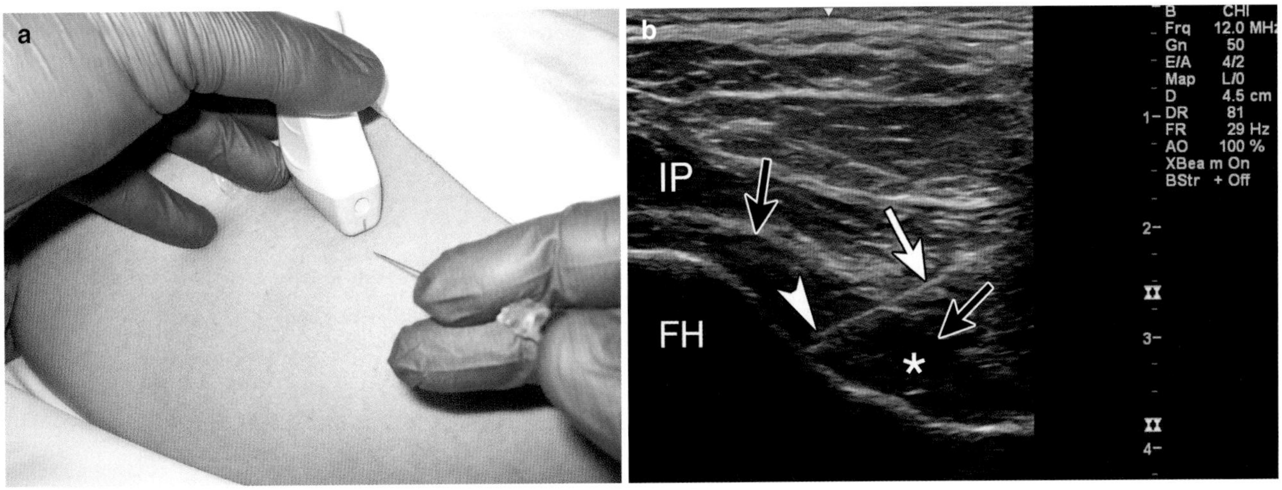

Fig. 5.2 (**a**) Example of sagittal oblique probe position over femoral head/neck junction with in-plane needle position. (**b**) Example of in-plane long-axis approach. *White arrow* indicates needle. *Arrowhead* indicates needle tip. *Black arrows* indicate joint capsule. *Asterisk* indicates effusion. *IP* iliopsoas muscle, *FH* femoral head

Greater Trochanteric Pain Syndrome

Greater trochanteric pain syndrome (GTPS) is a common cause of lateral hip pain [13]. Tenderness to palpation over the affected greater trochanter defines the diagnosis. The syndrome has been associated with low back pain, slight female predominance, and obesity [14]. It is usually due to a tendinopathy of the gluteus medius and minimus or inflammation of the greater trochanteric bursa (gluteus maximus) or gluteus medius bursae. The gluteus medius tendon inserts at two different locations on the greater trochanter: the superoposterior facet and the lateral facet. The gluteus minimus inserts on the anterior facet of the greater trochanter [15]. There are several bursae within this region. Between the gluteus minimus tendon and the anterior facet lies the subminimus bursa. The submedius bursa is located deep to the lateral insertion of the gluteus medius tendon. Typically, the greater trochanteric bursa is actually deep to the gluteus maximus tendon and superficial to the gluteus medius tendon. Clinically this is more tender posteriorly. Typical lateral pain is due to subgluteus minimus or medius bursitis [16]. Evidence supports that gluteus medius tendinopathy is the predominant finding in patients with GTPS and not bursitis [17]. Therefore, injections should be directed above and below the gluteus medius tendon, as well as into the greater trochanteric bursa, if seen (Table 5.2).

Table 5.2 GTPS relief following ultrasound guided versus blind injections

Study	Author	Accuracy
Ultrasound	Labrosse et al. [11]	72 % reported symptomatic relief at follow-up
Blind	Cohen et al. [12]	45 % reported symptomatic relief at follow-up

Scanning Technique and Anatomy to Identify

The patient is placed lying on the unaffected side in the lateral decubitus position with both hips slightly flexed. The trochanteric bursae are not typically visualized. Even when inflamed, fluid collection in the bursa may be difficult to appreciate. The transducer is placed longitudinally, parallel to the femoral diaphysis and scanned anterior to posterior to view the gluteus minimus and medius tendon insertion [18]. The gluteus minimus tendon can be visualized as it attaches on the anterior facet of the greater trochanter. The lateral and posterior parts of the gluteus medius tendon can also be evaluated as they insert on the lateral and superoposterior facets of the greater trochanter [19]. Signs of gluteus medius and minimus tendinopathy can also be assessed in this view. Look for tendon thickening, hypoechogenicity, loss of fibrillar pattern, cortical irregularity, calcifications, enthesophytes, or tears [20]. One can also view the greater trochanter in the transverse view with the probe subsequently moved anterior to posterior. The gluteus minimus and medius tendons will be viewed as a fibrillar hyperechoic structure (Fig. 5.3) [18].

Injection Technique: In-Plane Axial Approach

Patient positioning: Lay the patient on the unaffected side in the lateral decubitus position with both hips slightly flexed.

Probe positioning: The transducer is positioned in the transverse (axial) plane over the greater trochanter (Fig. 5.4a). A fluid-filled bursal sac may be seen just superficial to the greater trochanter or superficial to the gluteus medius or minimus tendons.

Markings: No special markings are needed.

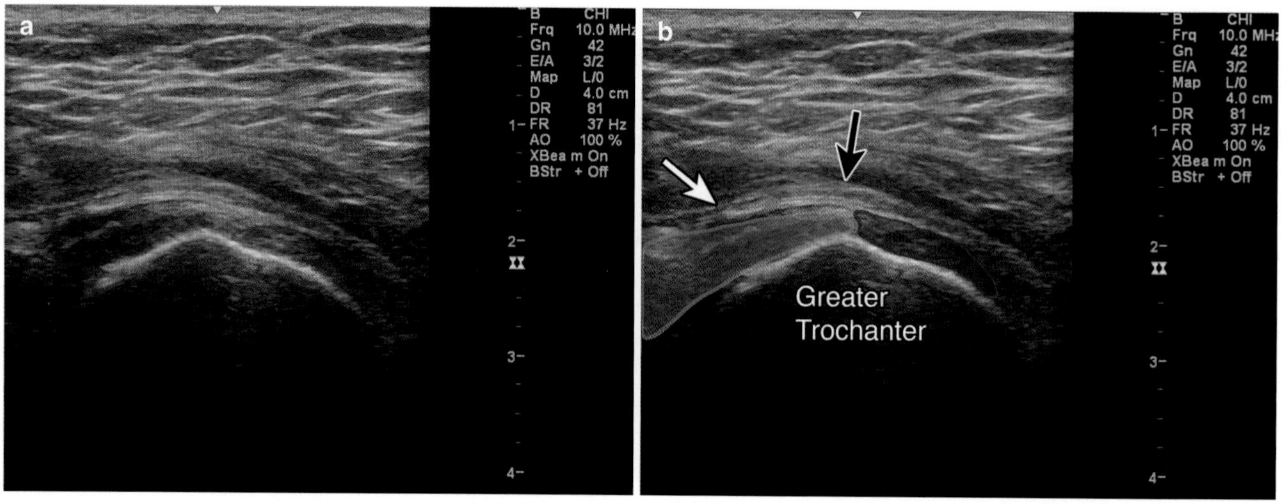

Fig. 5.3 (**a**) Transverse view of the greater trochanter. (**b**) *Purple* indicates gluteus minimus attaching to anterior facet. *Orange* indicates gluteus medius attaching to lateral facet. *Black arrow* indicates iliotibial tract. *White arrow* indicates subgluteus maximus bursa (trochanteric bursa). Greater trochanter labeled

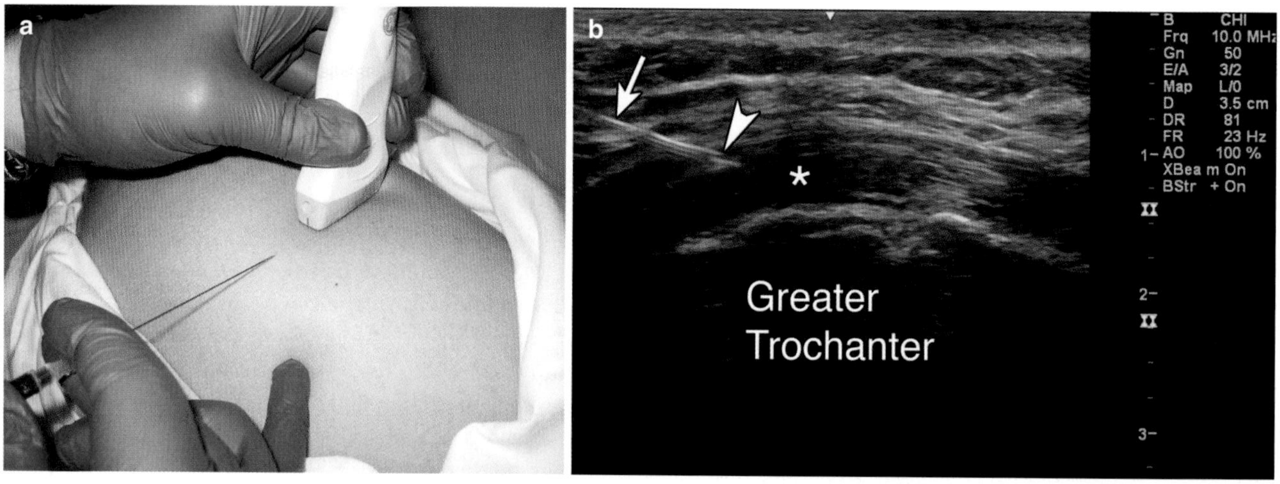

Fig. 5.4 (**a**) Example of probe position over greater trochanter with in-plane injection technique. (**b**) Example of in-plane axial approach. *White arrow* indicates needle. *Arrowhead* indicates needle tip. *Asterisk* indicates anisotropy within tendon. Greater trochanter labeled

Needle position: The needle is advanced under ultrasound guidance into the fluid-filled bursal sac if visualized; otherwise, it is placed both superficial and deep to the gluteus medius tendon, in the subtrochanteric or subgluteus medius bursa, respectively. Half of the medication may be injected into each site to cover both bursae.

Safety considerations: There are no major overlying blood vessels or nerves to avoid.

Pearls:

- Be careful not to apply too much force on the transducer as you may compress the inflamed bursa and cause pain during the procedure.

Equipment needed:

- High-frequency linear array transducer (8 MHz+)
- 22–25 gauge 1.5–3″ needle
- 1 mL of steroid preparation
- 4–5 mL local anesthetic

Hip Adductor Tendinosis/Obturator Nerve

Groin pain is a common complaint in many sports. Adductor tendinopathy accounts for 2/3 of all sports related groin injuries, most commonly in hockey, soccer, and running [3, 20]. Patients typically complain of groin or pelvic pain exacerbated by sport-specific activities. Provocative physical exam maneuvers may include a positive squeeze test and pain at the adductor origin with passive stretch or resisted adduction. Treatment is typically conservative with relative rest, pain medications, and physical therapy. If the pain is not relieved, different injections have been proposed to help with pain and/or healing [21].

The obturator nerve is derived from the ventral rami of L2, 3, and 4. As the nerve courses inferiorly through the pelvis, it divides into an anterior and posterior division. The anterior division provides motor innervation to the adductor longus, adductor brevis, and gracilis muscles while also supplying cutaneous innervation to the medial thigh [22]. The posterior division innervates the adductor magnus and provides a sensory branch to the medial side of the knee joint [3]. Obturator nerve blocks are important for providing pain relief or motor blockade in cases of preventing obturator jerk reflex during transurethral bladder tumor resections, obturator neuralgia, or adductor spasticity as seen in cerebral palsy, spinal cord injury, and other upper motor neuron syndromes. They may also be useful in assisting in the treatment or diagnosis of hip pain (Table 5.3) [18].

Scanning Technique and Anatomy to Identify

The patient is placed in the supine position, with the leg external rotated. Start by placing the probe in the transverse view over the pubic tubercle. Then move the transducer laterally until the three layers of adductor muscles appear. The superficial layer represents the adductor longus laterally and the gracilis medially. The middle layer represents the adductor brevis. In between the fascia of the adductor longus and adductor brevis muscles is the anterior division of the obturator nerve. The obturator nerve does not have the "honeycomb" appearance under ultrasound as do other nerves. Instead, it is localized by its distinct appearance passing through the fascial planes of the adductor brevis. It is important to visualize the medial femoral circumflex artery and vein which traverses between the pectineus muscle and iliopsoas muscle which then continues to travel intrafascially between the obturator externus and adductor brevis muscle [3]. Deep to the adductor brevis, the posterior division of the obturator nerve can be seen traversing the fascia. The anterior and posterior divisions of the obturator nerve can be localized approximately 2–3 cm lateral and 2–4 cm distal from the pubic tubercle. The anterior division is located about 1.2–2 cm deep, while the posterior division is located about 2.3–3.6 cm deep. The deep layer of muscle represents the adductor magnus. Scan proximally toward the pubis to view the insertion of these muscles. The insertion of the adductor longus tendon can be seen with its triangular hypoechoic shape. Although much more difficult to visualize, the common obturator nerve can be found approximately 1–3.5 cm lateral and 1–3 cm distal from the pubic tubercle (Fig. 5.5) [18].

Table 5.3 Accuracy of ultrasound guided obturator nerve injections

Study	Author	Accuracy
Ultrasound	Soong et al. [16]	85 % – anterior division 87.5 % – posterior division
Ultrasound	Sinha et al. [17]	93 % – using interfascial injection approach

Injection Technique: In-Plane Coronal Approach

Patient positioning: Lay the patient supine with the leg in slight external rotation; the affected hip can be slightly flexed for comfort.

Probe positioning: Place the probe in the transverse view over the ipsilateral pubic tubercle and scan laterally until the

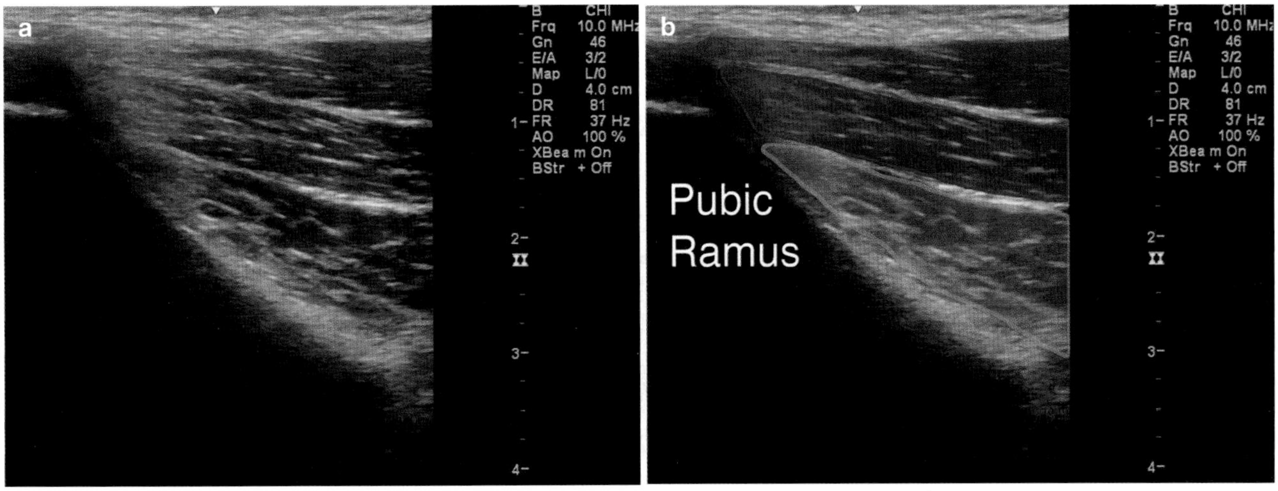

Fig. 5.5 (**a**) Coronal view off of the pubic ramus. (**b**) *Magenta* indicates adductor longus. *Purple* indicates adductor brevis. *Orange* indicates adductor magnus. Pubic ramus labeled

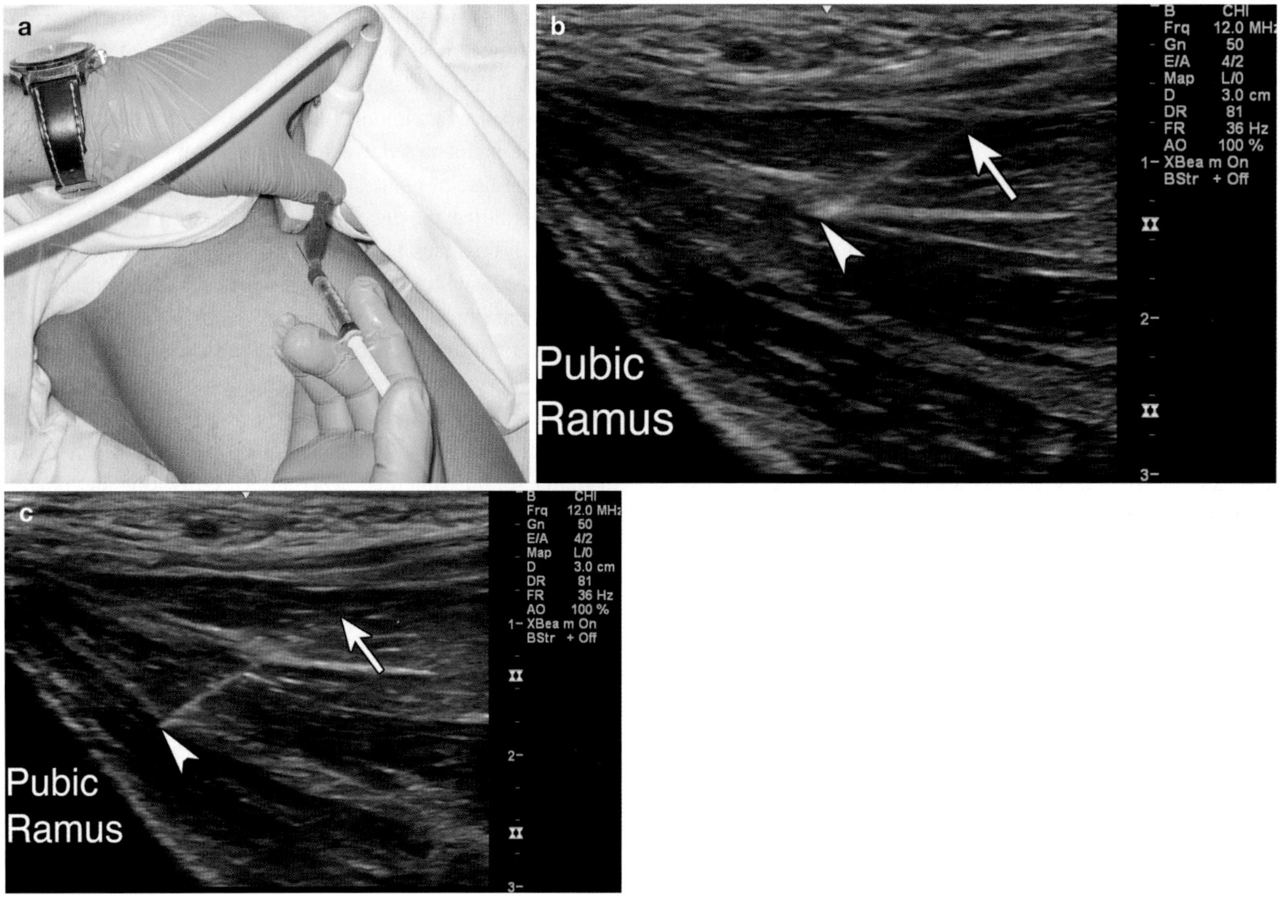

Fig. 5.6 (**a**) Example of probe position over adductor musculature and obturator nerve with in-plane injection technique. (**b**) Example of in-plane coronal approach. *Arrow* indicates needle. *Arrowhead* indicates needle tip in the fascial plane between the adductor longus and brevis for the anterior division. Pubic ramus labeled. (**c**) Example of in-plane long-axis approach. *Arrow* indicates needle. *Arrowhead* indicates needle tip in the fascial plane between the adductor brevis and magnus for the posterior division. Pubic ramus labeled

three layers of adductor muscles come into view. Turn the probe until a longitudinal view of the adductor musculature is attained (Fig. 5.6a). The anterior division of the obturator nerve will be seen traversing the fascial plane between the adductor longus and adductor brevis muscles, while the posterior division will be seen traversing the fascial plane between the adductor brevis and adductor magnus muscles. The medial femoral circumflex artery can be seen between the obturator externus and the adductor brevis [18]. The obturator artery usually divides into anterior and posterior branches which encircle the obturator foramen.

Markings: Obturator and medial femoral circumflex arteries and veins if noted.

Needle position: Advance the needle under direct ultrasound visualization so that the needle tip is directed just outside the desired adductor tendon or to the fascial plane of the obturator nerve division of interest. Even if nerve visualization is difficult, spread of local anesthetic in the appropriate fascial plane under direct ultrasound guidance confirms an accurate block.

Safety considerations: It is important to identify the obturator and medial femoral circumflex arteries and veins prior to inserting the needle in order to avoid piercing these structures [18].

Pearls:

- Externally rotating the leg with the knee flexed can result in poor nerve imaging.
- Given the probe compression needed to visualize the obturator nerve, the walls of the obturator vein may be collapsed and therefore not visible. Doppler mode can help visualize the obturator artery which lies in close proximity, or the probe pressure can be released to visualize rebound flow.

Equipment needed:

- High-frequency linear array transducer (8 MHz+)
- 22–25 gauge 1.5–3″ needle
- 1 mL of steroid preparation if desired
- 3–5 mL of local anesthetic or alcohol or phenol solution

Lateral Femoral Cutaneous Nerve

The lateral femoral cutaneous nerve is a pure sensory nerve that arises from the L2 and L3 spinal nerve roots. The nerve travels downward lateral to the psoas muscle and then crosses the iliacus muscle. Near the anterior superior iliac spine (ASIS), the nerve courses in contact with the lateral border of the inguinal ligament [23]. It is susceptible to compression as it courses from the lumbosacral plexus, through the abdominal cavity, under the inguinal ligament, and into the subcutaneous tissue of the thigh [24].

Meralgia paresthetica is used to describe the clinical syndrome of pain, burning, numbness, and paresthesia in the anterolateral thigh associated with compression of the nerve [25]. This more commonly occurs in obese or pregnant patients because of the abdomen bulging over the inguinal ligament. However, in some cases, it can also be idiopathic or caused by trauma [26]. Symptoms may be worse with walking, prolonged sitting, or prolonged standing and typically improve with weight loss or the loosening of belts or clothing. In some cases, surgery may be needed to release the nerve [25]. However, local anesthetics or steroid can also be used to anesthetize the nerve and provide pain relief and avoid the need for surgery (Table 5.4).

Scanning Technique and Anatomy to Identify

The patient is placed supine with the leg in the neutral position. The anterior superior iliac spine is palpated and the lateral end of the transducer is placed over it in the transverse position. The medial end can then be turned slightly caudally so that the probe lies directly over the inguinal ligament. The probe is then moved medially and caudally to search for the "honeycomb" appearance of the lateral femoral cutaneous nerve deep to the fascia lata [25]. However, the nerve may be difficult to identify. In a thin patient, the nerve may be seen proximal to the inguinal ligament lying over the iliacus muscles. At the level of the inguinal ligament, the nerve can be seen medial to the ASIS between the iliacus muscle and the inguinal ligament. Distal to the inguinal ligament, the course of the nerve may vary. If the nerve continues superficial to the iliacus muscle, then it may be appear as a hyperechoic structure between the fascia iliaca and fascia lata approximately 2–3 cm from the ASIS. Alternatively, it may travel laterally and be found superficial to the sartorius muscle or pass through the sartorius and posterior to the ASIS (Fig. 5.7) [24].

Table 5.4 Accuracy of blind versus ultrasound guided LFCN injections

Study	Author	Accuracy
Ultrasound	Peng et al. [27]	70 %
Blind	Shannon et al. [28]	40 %
Ultrasound vs blind	Ng et al. [29]	84.2 % vs. 5.3 %

Injection Technique: In-Plane Axial Approach

Patient positioning: Lay the patient supine with the leg in the neutral position.

Probe positioning: Axial plane with the nerve centered (Fig. 5.8a).

Markings: Once the nerve is located, the transducer is moved medially to allow easier needle access. The location of the probe can be marked on the skin along with the location of the initial needle puncture.

Needle position: The needle is advance in-plane from lateral to medial under direct ultrasound guidance. If the ASIS does not allow for this approach, a medial to lateral approach can be utilized. In cases where the nerve is difficult to visualize, one may use hydro-dissection deep to the level of the

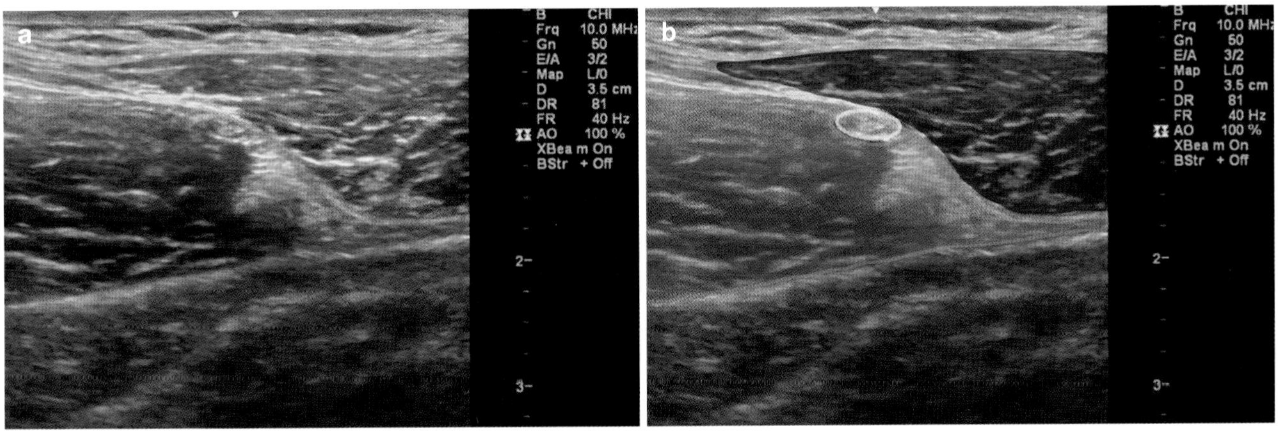

Fig. 5.7 (**a**) Axial view of the lateral femoral cutaneous nerve. (**b**) *Purple* indicates rectus femoris muscle. *Orange* indicates vastus lateralis muscle. *Yellow circle* surrounds lateral femoral cutaneous nerve

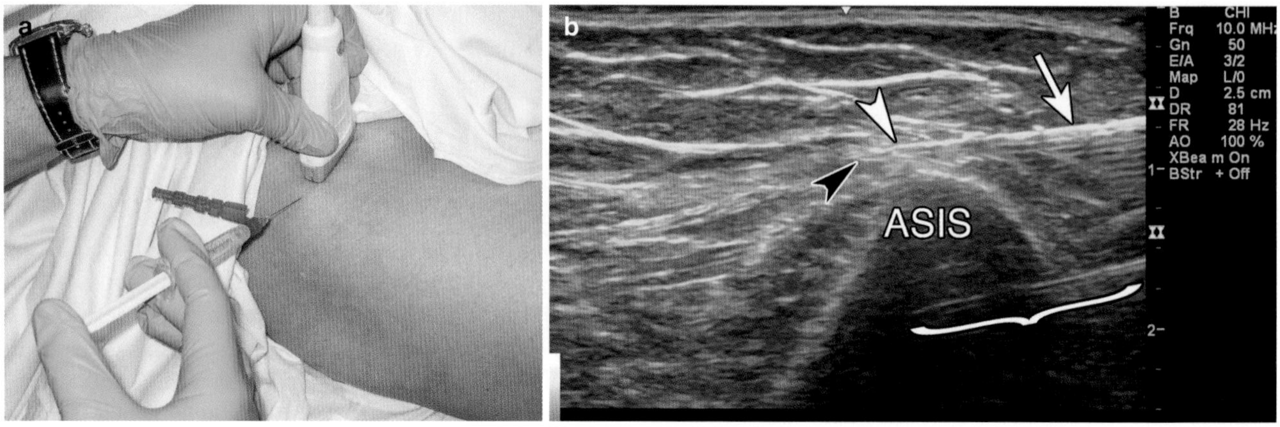

Fig. 5.8 (**a**) Example of axial probe position adjacent to ASIS over the lateral femoral cutaneous nerve with in-plane needle position. (**b**) Example of in-plane axial approach. *White arrow* indicates needle. *White arrowhead* indicates needle tip. *Black arrowhead* indicates lateral femoral cutaneous nerve. *Bracket* indicates needle reverberation. *ASIS* anterior superior iliac spine

fascia lata just medial to the ASIS to improve visualization of the nerve. If the lateral femoral cutaneous nerve is still not found, then the probe should be placed over the ASIS, scanning along the sartorius muscle medially and distally to locate the nerve as it crosses the muscle superficially. Once the nerve is located, the medication is injected and the perineural spread can be visualized under ultrasound.

Safety considerations: It is important to identify the femoral nerve, artery, and vein prior to inserting the needle in order to avoid piercing these structures. If injection of the nerve is superficial to the inguinal ligament, avoid bowel or bladder puncture.

Pearls:

- If the nerve is difficult to see, identify the fascial plane where the nerve is known to lie and ensure that the injectate spreads appropriately.

Equipment needed:

- High-frequency linear array transducer (10 MHz+)
- 22–25 gauge 1.5 or 3″ spinal needle
- 1 mL of steroid preparation
- 3–5 mL local anesthetic

Iliopsoas Bursitis/Tendinopathy

Iliopsoas tendinopathy is another source of anterior hip pain [30]. Directly anterior to the hip joint is the iliopsoas muscle complex, which is composed of the iliacus, the psoas major, and the psoas minor. The iliopsoas tendon inserts onto the lesser trochanter [31]. Iliopsoas tendinopathy can lead to snapping hip syndrome, which is characterized by pain and snapping of the hip with movement. The snapping is caused by an abnormal interposition of the medial fibers of the iliacus muscle between the psoas major tendon and the superior pubic ramus, which corrects abruptly during hip movement, thus creating the snapping sensation [32]. In many cases, it will be associated with an iliopsoas bursitis [33]. The iliopsoas bursa is located at the posteromedial aspect of the distal iliopsoas. The bursa may communicate with the hip joint in up to 15 % of the population [34]. Treatment options include rest, analgesics, physical therapy, and corticosteroid injections into the iliopsoas bursa. In addition, surgical lengthening or release of the iliopsoas tendon can also be performed [1].

Scanning Technique and Anatomy to Identify

The patient is placed supine with the leg in the neutral position. The ASIS is palpated and the transducer is placed in the transverse (axial) plane with the lateral end just medial to the ASIS. The transducer is then moved medially until the femoral head is visualized. The femoral neurovascular structures are just medial to the transducer in this position. The use of Doppler can make it easier to visualize the vessels. Just lateral to these structures is the iliopsoas tendon [35]. The tendon can be followed up to the acetabular brim. At this level, the iliopsoas bursa can be seen lying deep to the tendon [33].

To visualize the snapping of the iliopsoas tendon, the transducer is placed parallel to the inguinal ligament over the iliopsoas at the level of the pelvis. The patient is asked to flex and externally rotate the hip and then slowly straighten the leg. Normally, the muscles will rotate slowly without any abrupt snapping. However, with snapping hip syndrome, the medial fibers of the iliacus are interposed between the psoas major and the ilium. Therefore, as the leg is straightened, the iliopsoas tendon abruptly snaps toward the ilium as the iliacus fibers move and are no longer interposed (Fig. 5.9) [32].

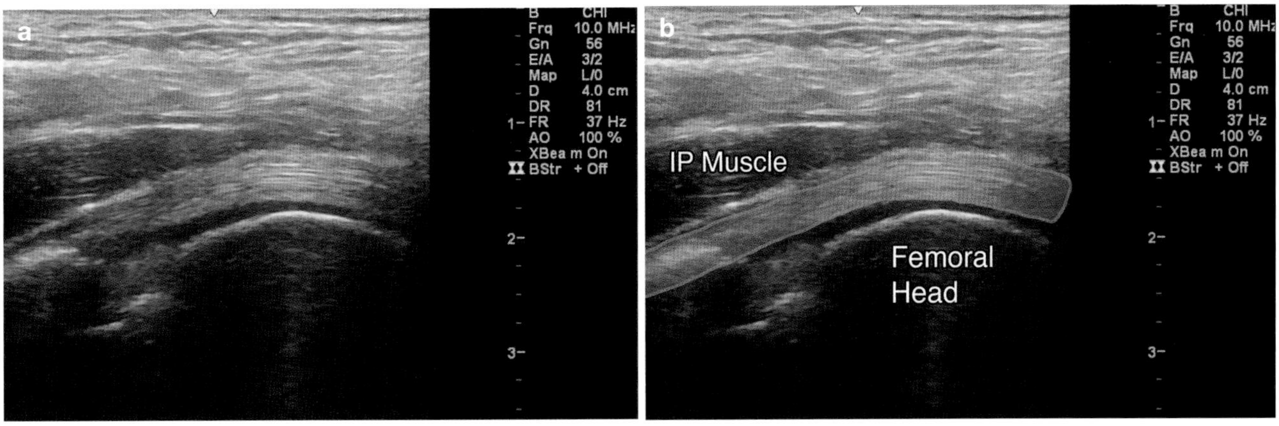

Fig. 5.9 (**a**) Sagittal view of the iliopsoas muscle over femoral head. (**b**) IP, iliopsoas muscle and tendon (*orange*) anterior to the femoral head

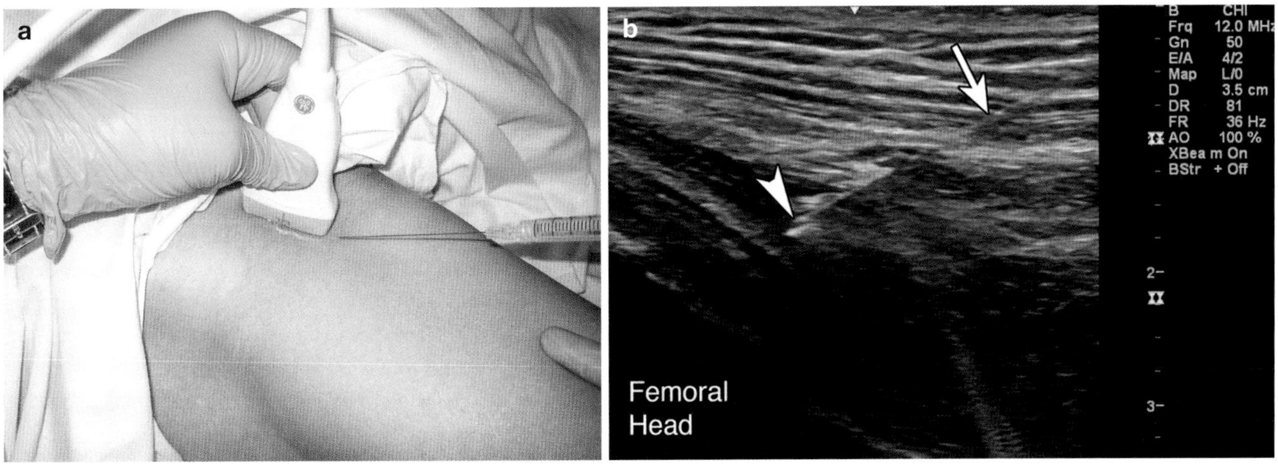

Fig. 5.10 (**a**) Example of probe position over femoral head with in-plane injection technique. (**b**) Example of in-plane sagittal approach. *Arrow* indicates needle. *Arrowhead* indicates needle tip. Femoral head labeled

Injection Technique: In-Plane Sagittal Approach

Patient positioning: Lay the patient supine with the leg in the neutral position.

Probe positioning: Place the lateral end of the probe in the transverse (axial) position just medial to the ASIS and scan medially until the femoral head comes into view. Be sure to identify the femoral neurovascular structures medial to the femoral head in the transverse plane prior to inserting the needle. Lying just lateral to the neurovascular bundle is the iliopsoas tendon. The tendon can be followed proximally to the acetabular brim, where deep to the tendon, the bursa is located. Rotate the probe 90° to obtain a longitudinal or sagittal view of the iliopsoas muscle crossing the femoral head (Fig. 5.10a).

Markings: Identify the femoral neurovascular bundle.

Needle position: The needle is advanced under direct ultrasound visualization into the iliopsoas tendon using a distal to proximal approach. A lateral to medial approach can also be utilized to gain access to the iliopsoas bursa deep to the tendon. The needle tip is positioned between the iliopsoas muscle-tendon complex and the ilium at the level of the iliopectineal eminence [32].

Safety considerations: It is important to identify the femoral nerve, artery, and vein prior to inserting the needle in order to avoid piercing these structures.

Pearls:

- If the goal of the injection is to diagnose extra-articular pathology, then it is important to keep the needle tip superior to the femoral head. This will ensure that the injection remains outside of the hip joint capsule.
- Similarly, avoid injecting into the iliopsoas bursa as the medication may gain access to the hip joint if a communication exists between these two spaces.

Equipment needed:

- Linear array transducer (8–4 MHz)
- 22–25 gauge 3.5–5″ spinal needle
- 1 mL of steroid preparation
- 4–5 mL local anesthetic

Iliohypogastric and Ilioinguinal Nerves

The nerves that supply the skin between the abdomen and the thigh are called the border nerves; they consist of the iliohypogastric, ilioinguinal, and genitofemoral nerves. These nerves are oftentimes damaged after surgeries such as appendectomies, inguinal hernia repairs, or cesarian sections. The nerves may be of interest to help diagnose and treat chronic inguinal and lower abdominal pain.

The iliohypogastric and the ilioinguinal nerves stem from the anterior rami of L1 and runs subperitoneally. The iliohypogastric nerve pierces the internal oblique muscles and provides motor fibers to the internal oblique muscles. It travels between the internal and external obliques distributing sensory fibers to the skin over the rectus abdominus. The ilioinguinal nerve travels under the psoas, pierces the abdominal muscle, and gives sensory fibers to the inguinal region and anterosuperior thigh (Table 5.5).

Scanning Techniques and Anatomy to Identify

For the ilioinguinal/iliohypogastric block, locate the ASIS and draw a line connecting the ASIS with the umbilicus. Slowly move the transducer along that line, perpendicular to the inguinal ligament. Rotate the transducer until three layers of muscle are visualized. These three muscles are the internal oblique, external oblique, and transverse abdominis (IO, EO, TA). One should be able to observe splitting of the fascia between the TA and IO which is where the ilioinguinal and iliohypogastric nerve traverses through. It can typically be found 1–3 cm medially from the ASIS. The iliohypogastric nerve is typically located more medially (Fig. 5.11) [33].

Table 5.5 Accuracy of blind versus ultrasound guided II and IH injections

Study of the II and IH injection	Author	Accuracy
Blind injection for II and IH	Thibaut et al. [36]	68 % dissection
Ultrasound-guided injection	Eichenberger et al. [37]	95 % dissection

Injection Techniques: In-Plane Axial Oblique Approach

Patient positioning: Place the patient in the supine position. Drape appropriately.

Probe positioning: Place the lateral end of the probe in a transverse (axial) plane over the ASIS, and rotate (oblique) until the nerve is identified (Fig. 5.12a). Visualize the TA and IO medially.

Markings: Once the nerve is identified, mark the probe location. Identify and mark the femoral neurovascular bundle, then return to the previously marked probe position. Mark the skin a few centimeters distal to the inferior end of the transducer.

Needle position: A 25 g needle can be used to anesthetize the area using a layer-by-layer technique with 4–6 mL of 1 % lidocaine.7 Alternatively ethyl chloride spray may be used. A 22 or 25 gauge needle is then advanced under direct ultrasound visualization. Direct the needle toward the separation between the internal oblique and transverse abdominus muscles. Inject up to 5 mL of local anesthetic between both muscles. The patient should soon feel numbness in the groin region [34].

Safety considerations: It is important to identify any vasculature prior to inserting the needle in order to avoid piercing these structures.

Pearls:

- The II and IH can be found between the transverse abdominal muscle and internal oblique muscle with 90 % probability [32].

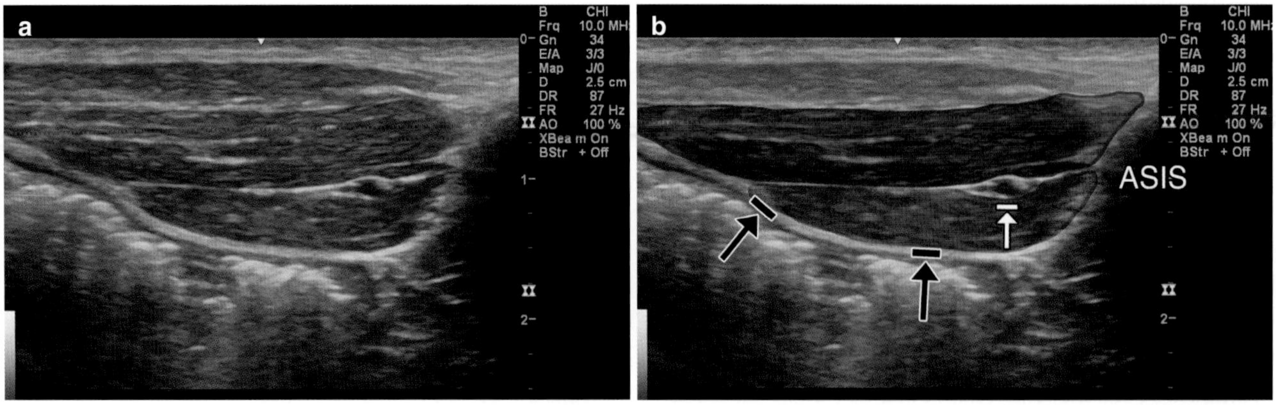

Fig. 5.11 (**a**) Axial oblique of the ilioinguinal nerve. (**b**) *Orange* indicates internal oblique muscle. *Purple* indicates external oblique muscle. *Magenta* indicates transverse abdominis muscle. *White arrow with stop* indicates neurovascular bundle. *Black arrows with stops* indicate peritoneum

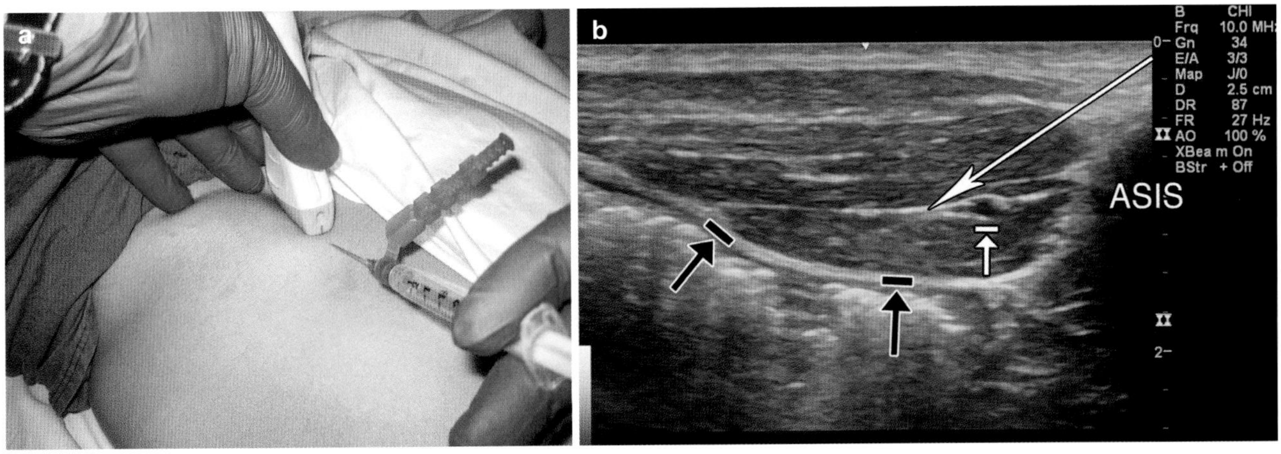

Fig. 5.12 (**a**) Example of axial oblique probe position medial to the ASIS over the ilioinguinal and iliohypogastric nerves with in-plane needle position. (**b**) Example of in-plane approach. *Long white arrow* indicates needle trajectory. *White arrow with stop* indicates neurovascular bundle. *Black arrows with stops* indicate peritoneum. *ASIS* anterior superior iliac spine

- The size of the ilioinguinal nerve is inversely proportional to the iliohypogastric nerve [38].
- A nerve stimulator may be helpful in addition to ultrasound guidance

Equipment needed:

- Linear array transducer (7 MHz+)
- 22–25 gauge 1.5–3″ spinal needle
- 1 mL of steroid preparation
- 4–5 mL local anesthetic

Piriformis

The piriformis muscle lies deep to the gluteus maximus, originating from the anterior sacrum at S1–3 and inserting onto the superolateral facet of the greater trochanter. The function of the piriformis is to abduct the flexed thigh and to externally rotate the extended thigh. The sciatic nerve normally exits the greater sciatic foramen beneath the piriformis muscle, but there are anatomical variants in which the nerve can exit above or through the piriformis. A patient may complain of pain in the gluteal region with palpation, sciatica, or pain noticed more with sitting as compared to standing. Piriformis syndrome may arise due to overuse (such as excessive exercise) or prolonged sitting. Between 1 and 2 % of lower back pain can be attributed to piriformis syndrome [35]. Provocative tests include the FAIR test where the patient is placed in the contralateral decubitus position and the ipsilateral hip is flexed, adducted, and internally rotated. This should reproduce concordant buttock pain and possibly sciatica if present. Freiberg, Beatty, and Pace maneuvers can also be helpful, but physical exam alone is difficult (Table 5.6) [35].

Table 5.6 Accuracy of ultrasound guided versus fluoroscopic piriformis injections

Study of piriformis injection	Author	Accuracy
Ultrasound guided	Finnoff et al. [39]	95 % confirmed
Fluoroscopic	Thibaut et al. [36]	30 % confirmed

Scanning Techniques and Anatomy to Identify

Palpate the posterior superior iliac spine (PSIS) and place the transducer horizontally over the bone. Move caudally until the posterior inferior iliac spine is visualized. Move slightly inferior to the PIIS remaining lateral to the sacrum; the image will show the greater sciatic notch. The piriformis muscle will appear deep to the lateral sacral border. The muscle superficial to the sacrum is the gluteus maximus. To confirm the location of the piriformis muscle, laterally follow the muscle to its insertion into the superior greater trochanter (Fig. 5.13) [38].

Injection Techniques: In-Plane Axial Approach

Patient positioning: Lay the patient in the prone position. Drape appropriately.

Probe positioning: Place the medial side of the transducer axially over the S2–4 portion of the sacrum and then move laterally over the piriformis (Fig. 5.14a).

Markings: The intersection between the inferior border of the SI joint and the greater trochanter is the presumed location of the piriformis [27]. Mark the sciatic nerve is visible to avoid inadvertent puncture.

Needle position: Insert the needle from medial to lateral under direct ultrasound visualization [8]. As the needle goes through the gluteus maximus and approaches the piriformis,

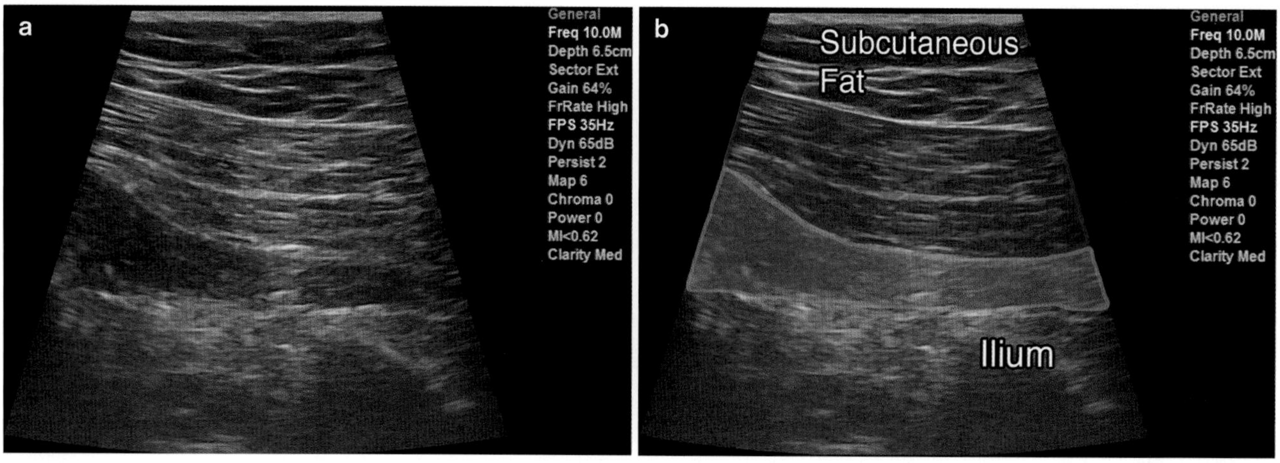

Fig. 5.13 (**a**) Axial view of the piriformis muscle. (**b**) *Purple* indicates gluteus maximus. *Orange* indicates piriformis muscle. Subcutaneous fat and ilium labeled

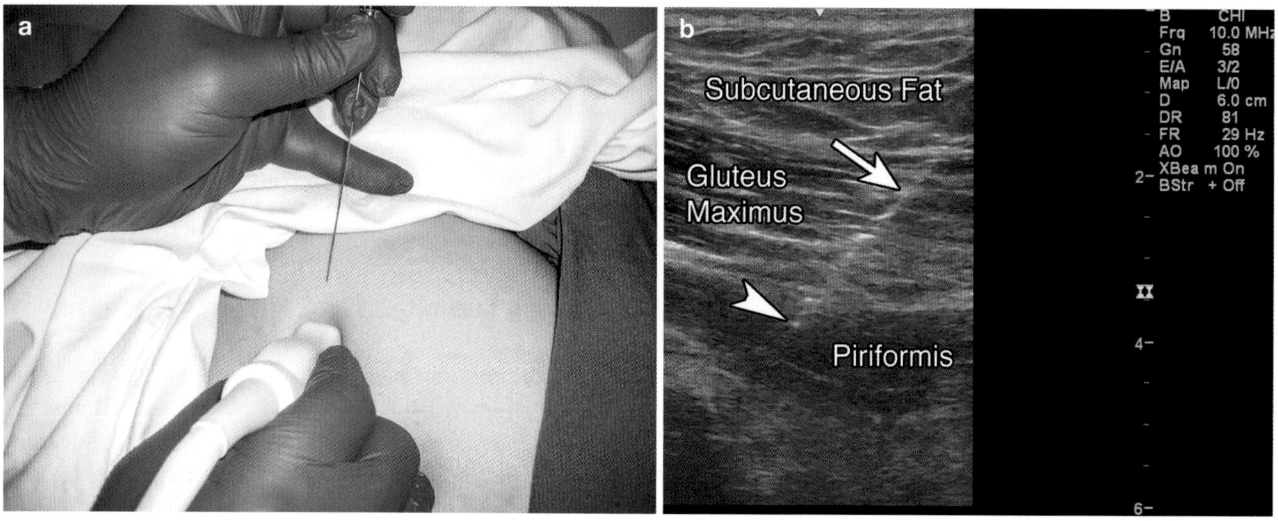

Fig. 5.14 (**a**) Example of axial probe position over piriformis muscle with in-plane needle injection technique. (**b**) Example of in-plane axial approach. *Arrow* indicates needle. *Arrowhead* indicates needle tip. Piriformis, gluteus maximus, and subcutaneous fat labeled

internally and externally rotating the leg will help identify the muscle.

Safety considerations: Due to anatomical variations with regard to the course of the sciatic nerve, it is important to ensure that the anatomical landmarks are confirmed.

Pearls:

- The most common anatomical variant associated with the piriformis is called Beaton Type B, which occurs when the common peroneal nerve pierces the piriformis muscle.
- Three muscles forming the tricipital tendons (superior and inferior gemellus muscles and the obturator internus) are also attached to the greater trochanter and can resemble the piriformis muscles. These are inferior to the piriformis, so it is important to locate the muscle by starting at the PSIS and scanning inferiorly. Flexing the knee and internally and externally rotating the leg can also help to delineate the piriformis muscle.
- Injecting <0.5 mL of normal saline, which will appear hypoechoic in the muscle, can help to confirm that the correct structure is located [29].
- A nerve or muscle stimulator may be helpful, to stimulate the piriformis or sciatic nerve, respectively. When the needle is in close proximity to the nerve, ankle and knee flexion will be seen; when the needle is retracted into the muscle belly, only local contraction or hip abduction or external rotation may be noted.

Equipment needed:

- Low to medium-frequency linear or curvilinear transducer
- 22–25 gauge needle
- 1 mL of steroid preparation
- 2–4 mL local anesthetic

References

1. Rowbotham EL, Grainer AJ. Ultrasound-guided intervention around the hip joint. AJR Am J Roentgenol. 2011;197(1):122–7.
2. O'Neill J, Girish G. The adult hip. In: O'Neill J, editor. Musculoskeletal ultrasound: anatomy and technique. New York: Springer; 2008.
3. Sinha SK, Abrams JH, Houle TT, et al. Ultrasound-guided obturator nerve block: an interfascial injection approach without nerve stimulation. Reg Anesth Pain Med. 2009;34(3):261–4.
4. Altman R, Alarcón G, Appelrouth D, et al. The American College of Rheumatology criteria for the classification and reporting of osteoarthritis of the hip. Arthritis Rheum. 1991;34(5):505.
5. Smith J, Hurdle MF, Weingarten TN. Accuracy of sonographically guided intra-articular injections in the native adult hip. J Ultrasound Med. 2009;28(3):329–35.
6. Pourbagher MA, Ozalay M, Pourbagher A. Accuracy and outcome of sonographically guided intra-articular sodium hyaluronate injections in patients with osteoarthritis of the hip. J Ultrasound Med. 2005;24(10):1391–5.
7. Levi DS. Intra-articular hip injections using ultrasound guidance: accuracy using a linear array transducer. PM R. 2013;5(2):129–34.
8. Leopold SA, Battista V, Oliverio JA. Safety and efficacy of intraarticular hip injections using anatomic landmarks. Clin Orthop Relat Res. 2001;391:192–7.
9. Dobson MM. A further anatomical check on the accuracy of intra-articular hip injections in relation to the therapy of coxarthritis. Ann Rheum Dis. 1950;9:237–40.
10. Lambert RG, Hutchings EJ, Grace MG, et al. Steroid injection for osteoarthritis of the hip: a randomized, double-blind, placebo-controlled trial. Arthritis Rheum. 2007;56(7):2278–87.
11. Migliore A, Massafra U, Bizzi E, et al. Intra-articular injection of hyaluronic acid in symptomatic osteoarthritis of the hip: a prospective cohort study. Arch Orthop Trauma Surg. 2011;131(12):1677–85.
12. Smith J, Hurdle MF. Office-based ultrasound-guided intra-articular hip injection: technique for physiatric practice. Arch Phys Med Rehabil. 2006;87(2):296–8.
13. Lustenberger DP, Ng VY, Best TM, et al. Efficacy of treatment of trochanteric bursitis: a systematic review. Clin J Sport Med. 2011;21(5):447–53.
14. Segal NA, Felson DT, Torner JC, et al. Greater trochanteric pain syndrome: epidemiology and associated factors. Arch Phys Med Rehabil. 2007;88(8):988–92.
15. Lequesne M, Mathieu P, Vuillemin-Bodaghi V, et al. Gluteal tendinopathy in refractory greater trochanter pain syndrome: diagnostic value of two clinical tests. Arthritis Rheum. 2008;59(2):241–6.
16. Kong A, Van der Vliet A, Zadow S. MRI and US of gluteal tendinopathy in greater trochanteric pain syndrome. Eur Radiol. 2007;17(7):1772–83.
17. Labrosse JM, Cardinal E, Leduc BE, et al. Effectiveness of ultrasound-guided corticosteroid injection for the treatment of gluteus medius tendinopathy. AJR Am J Roentgenol. 2010;194(1):202–6.
18. Paraskeuopoulos T, Saranteas T. Ultrasound-guided obturator nerve block: the importance of the medial circumflex femoral vessels. Reg Anesth Pain Med. 2012;37(5):565.
19. Nestorova R, Vlad Violeta V, Petranova T, et al. Ultrasonography of the hip. Med Ultrason. 2012;14(3):217–24.
20. Holmich P. Long-standing groin pain in sports people falls into three primary patterns, a "clinical entity" approach: a prospective study of 207 patients. Br J Sports Med. 2007;41(4):247–52.
21. Robertson IJ, Curran C, McCaffrey N, et al. Adductor tenotomy in the management of groin pain in athletes. Int J Sports Med. 2011;32(1):45–8.
22. Soong J, Schafhalter-Zoppoth I, Gray AT. Sonographic imaging of the obturator nerve for regional block. Reg Anesth Pain Med. 2007;32(2):146–51.
23. Tagliafico A, Serafini F, Lacelli F, et al. Ultrasound-guided treatment of meralgia paresthetica (lateral femoral cutaneous neuropathy). J Ultrasound Med. 2011;30(10):1341–6.
24. Aszmann OC, Dellon ES, Dellon AL. Anatomical course of the lateral femoral cutaneous nerve and its susceptibility to compression and injury. Plast Reconstr Surg. 1997;100(3):600–4.
25. Hurdle MF, Weingarten TN, Crisostomo RA, et al. Ultrasound-guided blockade of the lateral femoral cutaneous nerve: technical description and review of 10 cases. Arch Phys Med Rehabil. 2007;88(10):1362–4.
26. Kim JE, Lee SG, Kim EJ, et al. Ultrasound-guided lateral femoral cutaneous nerve block in meralgia paresthetica. Korean J Pain. 2011;24(2):115–8.
27. Peng PW, Narouze S. Ultrasound-guided interventional procedures in pain medicine: a review of anatomy, sonoanatomy, and procedures: Part I: nonaxial structures. Reg Anesth Pain Med. 2009;34(5):458–74.
28. Shannon J, Lang SA, Yip RW, et al. Lateral femoral cutaneous nerve block revisited. A nerve stimulator technique. Reg Anesth. 1995;20(2):100–4.
29. Ng I, Vaghadia H, Choi PT, et al. Ultrasound imaging accurately identifies the lateral femoral cutaneous nerve. Anesth Analg. 2007;107(3):1070–4.
30. Adler RS, Buly R, Ambrose R, et al. Diagnostic and therapeutic use of sonography-guided iliopsoas peritendinous injections. AJR Am J Roentgenol. 2005;185(4):940–3.
31. Jacobson JA, Bedi A, Sekiya JK, et al. Evaluation of the painful athletic hip: imaging options and imaging-guided injections. AJR Am J Roentgenol. 2012;199(3):516–24.
32. Eichenberger U, Greher M, Kirchmair L, et al. Ultrasound-guided blocks of the ilioinguinal and iliohypogastric nerve: accuracy of a selective new technique confirmed by anatomical dissection. Br J Anaesth. 2006;97(2):238–43.
33. Peng P, Tumber P. Ultrasound-guided interventional procedures for patients with chronic pelvic pain – a description of techniques and review of literature. Pain Physician. 2008;11(2):215–24.
34. Gofeld M, Christakis M. Sonographically guided Ilioinguinal nerve block. J Ultrasound Med. 2006;25(12):1571–5.
35. Kirschner JS, Foye PM, Cole JL. Piriformis syndrome, diagnosis and treatment. Muscle Nerve. 2009;40(1):10–8.
36. Thibaut D, de la Cuadra-Fontaine JC, Bravo MP, et al. Ilioinguinal/iliohypogastric blocks: where is the anesthetic injected? Anesth Analg. 2008;107(2):728–9.
37. Eichenberger U, Greher M, Kirchmair L, et al. Ultrasound-guided blocks of the ilioinguinal and iliohypogastric nerve: accuracy of a selective new technique confirmed by anatomical dissection. Br J Anaesth. 2006;97(2):238–43.
38. Huerto A, Yeo SN, Ho K. Piriformis muscle injection using ultrasonography and motor stimulation – report of technique. Pain Physician. 2007;10:687–90.
39. Finnoff JT, Hurdle MF, Smith J. Accuracy of ultrasound-guided versus fluoroscopically guided contrast-controlled piriformis injection. A cadaveric study. J Ultrasound Med. 2008;27(8):1157–63.

Knee

6

David A. Spinner, Houman Danesh, and Waheed S. Baksh

Various pathologies afflict the knee including overuse injuries, tendinopathies, ligament sprains, nerve injuries, bursitis, meniscal tears, and various arthritides. Ultrasound guidance is particularly useful in this region for aspiration and injection of the tibiofemoral and tibiofibular joint spaces, pes anserine bursa, and Baker's cysts. It is also a valuable tool for popliteus, iliotibial band, patellar and quadriceps tendon tenotomies, prolotherapy, and PRP injection.

Knee Osteoarthritis (OA) and Joint Effusion

Knee osteoarthritis is one of the most commonly seen conditions in a musculoskeletal practice. Musculoskeletal ultrasound is becoming the gold standard for diagnosing synovitis and/or effusion in chronic painful OA [1]. Recent studies have demonstrated improved accuracy of injections, increased responder rate to treatment, decreased pain scores, and a reduction in overall cost per year with ultrasound guidance [1–4]. Inaccurate steroid injections can result in steroid articular cartilage atrophy, crystal synovitis, and postinjection pain (Tables 6.1, 6.2, 6.3) [2].

D.A. Spinner, DO, RMSK (✉)
Department of Anesthesiology – Pain Medicine, Arnold Pain Management Center, Beth Israel Deaconess Medical Center, Harvard Medical School, Brookline, MA, USA
e-mail: dspinnerny@gmail.com

H. Danesh, MD
Department of Anesthesiology – Pain Medicine, Icahn School of Medicine at Mount Sinai, New York, NY, USA
e-mail: houmanmd@gmail.com

W.S. Baksh, MD, DPT
Advanced Pain Relief Center, Winchester Medical Center, Winchester, VA, USA
e-mail: waheed.baksh@gmail.com

Scanning Technique and Anatomy to Identify

Lay the patient supine with the knee flexed 20–30°. Place the probe longitudinally on the midline superior pole of the patella. From deep to superficial, visualize the femur, prefemoral fat pad, hypoechoic suprapatellar joint space, suprapatellar fat pad, and quadriceps tendon inserting onto the patella. Rotate the probe 90° to the axial (transverse) plane. From deep to superficial, view the femur, prefemoral fat pad, hypoechoic suprapatellar and parapatellar joint spaces, suprapatellar fat pad, and quadriceps tendon. Glide medial and lateral here to assess for fluid in the medial and lateral parapatellar recesses. Milking or compressing those areas may help delineate the joint space (Fig. 6.1).

Injection Techniques: In-Plane Superolateral Approach

Patient positioning: Lay the patient supine, knee flexed 20–30°. Place a towel or pillow underneath the knee.

Probe positioning: Place the probe axial (transverse) over the distal thigh, superior to the patella (Fig. 6.2a). Suprapatellar joint fluid may be visualized directly under the quadriceps tendon or deep to the suprapatellar fat pad.

Markings: Identify the quadriceps tendon and muscles, periosteum, and fat pads to avoid these structures when injecting.

Needle position: Insert the needle in-plane from lateral to medial in the superolateral region of the knee.

Safety considerations: Identify and avoid any obvious vessels.

Pearls:

- Fluid in the parapatellar recesses is dependent: Keeping the knee flexed allows joint fluid to collect in the suprapatellar space. Alternatively, one may milk the fluid from the parapatellar recesses into the suprapatellar pouch.

D.A. Spinner et al. (eds.), *Atlas of Ultrasound Guided Musculoskeletal Injections*, Musculoskeletal Medicine,
DOI 10.1007/978-1-4614-8936-8_6, © Springer Science+Business Media, LLC 2014

Table 6.1 Utility of ultrasound guided knee injections

Study	Author	Outcomes
Clinical utility of ultrasound guidance for intra-articular knee injections	Berkoff et al. [2]	Image-guided Accuracy 96.7 % vs. anatomic (blind) 81.0 %, 75 % reduction in significant pain and 26 % increase in responder rate
A randomized controlled trial evaluating the cost-effectiveness of sonographic guidance for intra-articular injection of the osteoarthritic knee	Sibbitt et al. [5]	48 % less procedural pain, 42 % reduction in pain scores, 36 % increase in therapeutic duration, 58 % reduction in cost per responder per year

Table 6.2 Accuracy of knee joint injections

Author	Image-guided (%)	Anatomical (blind) (%)
Cunnington et al. [6]	91.4	81.8
Park et al. [7]	96	83.7
Balint et al. [8]	94.7	40.0

Table 6.3 Comparing location of ultrasound guided knee injections

Study	Approach	Accuracy (%)
Comparison of sonographically guided intra-articular injections at three different sites of the knee [9]	Superolateral	100
	Midlateral	95
	Medial	75

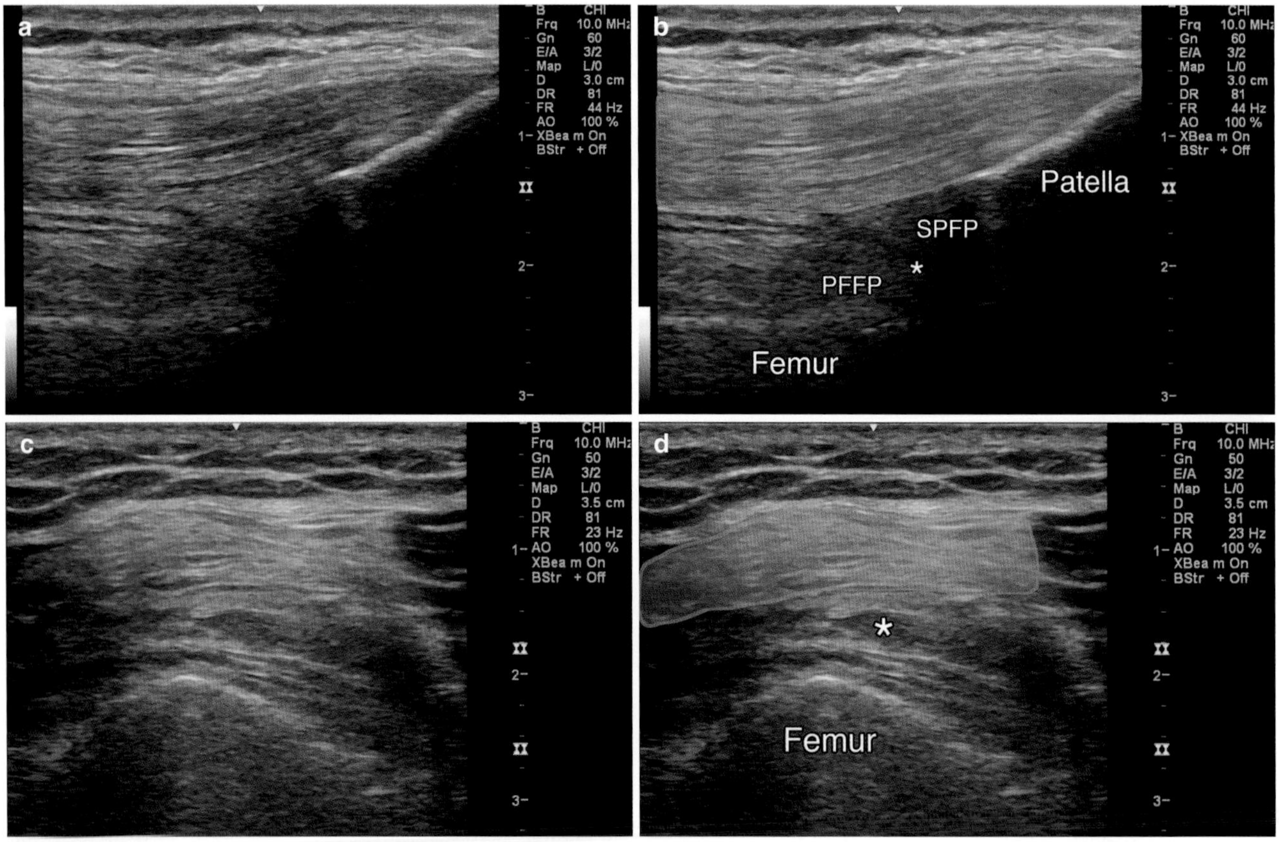

Fig. 6.1 (**a**) Sagittal view over suprapatellar joint recess. (**b**) *Orange* indicates quadriceps tendon, *SPFP* suprapatellar fat pad, *PFFP* prefemoral fat pad, *asterisk* indicates joint recess, patella and femur labeled. (**c**) Axial view over suprapatellar recess. (**d**) *Orange* indicates quadriceps tendon, *asterisk* indicates joint space, femur labeled

- Insert the needle deep to the quadriceps tendon through the vastus lateralis, and keep the needle at a flat angle to avoid needling the tendon and allow for optimal visualization.
- Vary the pressure on the transducer and use local anesthetic to hydrodissect the suprapatellar space if no effusion is present.

Equipment needed:

- High-frequency linear array transducer (8 MHz+)
- 22G–25G 1.5″ needle (3″ for morbidly obese)
- 1 mL of steroid preparation
- 3–5 mL local anesthetic

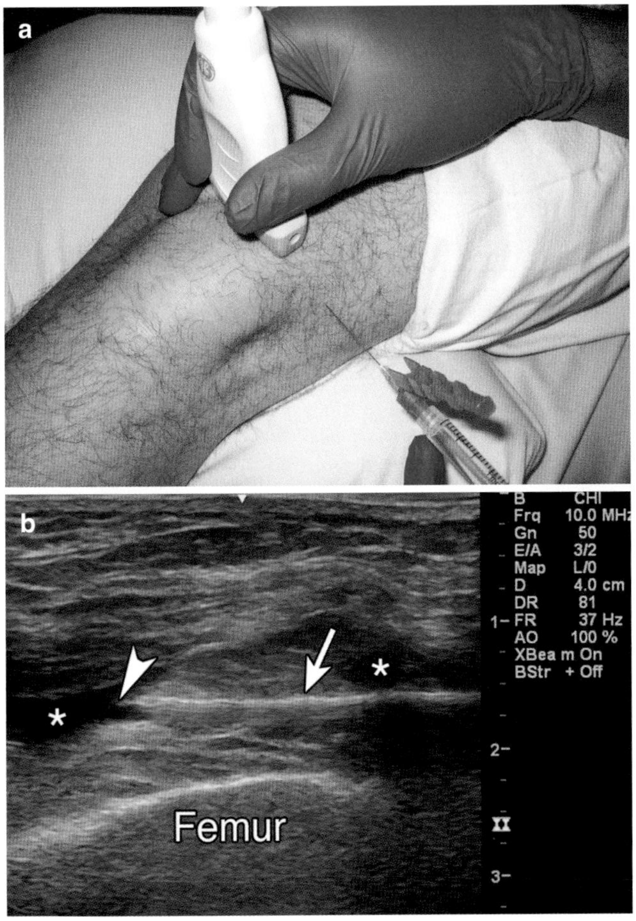

Fig. 6.2 (**a**) Example of probe position over suprapatellar joint recess with in-plane injection technique. (**b**) *Arrowhead* indicates needle tip within joint recess, *arrow* points to needle, *asterisk* indicates effusion, femur labeled

Patellar Tendinosis

Patellar tendinosis or "jumper's knee" is a common source of focal anterior knee pain for active, high-impact activity individuals [3]. Treating chronic patellar tendinosis is challenging given the low capacity for tendons to heal [4]. It is not clear why tendinosis develops. Histologically, there is evidence of tissue degeneration with failed reparative response and absence of inflammatory cells. Research on patellar tendinopathy does not support any one treatment as the most effective. Patellar tendon needling has been described using no injectate (needle alone), with sclerosing agents, autologous blood or platelet-rich plasma (PRP), and corticosteroids [10–13].

Scanning Technique and Anatomy to Identify

Lay the patient supine, knee flexed approximately 30°, with a pillow or rolled towel underneath the knees. Place the transducer longitudinally over the patellar tendon. Proximally, visualize the hyperechoic patella with the fibrillar patellar tendon coming off it and Hoffa's fat pad immediately deep to the tendon. In patellar tendinosis, there will be tendon irregularity, thickening, areas of hypoechoic swelling, and potentially neovascularization [14]. Scan the entire width and entire length of the tendon from the inferior pole of the patella to its insertion onto the tibial tuberosity, in both short and long axis (Fig. 6.3).

Injection Techniques: In-Plane Axial Approach

Patient positioning: Lay the patient supine, knee flexed about 30° with a pillow or rolled towel placed underneath.

Probe positioning: Place the transducer over the middle of the patella to obtain an axial view (Fig. 6.4a).

Markings: No significant vascular or neural structures need to be marked.

Needle position: Insert the needle in-plane from a lateral to medial or medial to lateral direction, aiming at the areas of greatest tendinosis.

Safety considerations: Care should be taken when injecting a tendon, as this may increase susceptibility to tendon rupture [15, 16].

Pearls:

- Use a larger gauge needle to break up calcium deposits.
- Increasing the gain on Doppler may help identify neovascularization.
- Switch between long and short axis to visualize the entire area of tendinosis while redirecting the needle in all directions, both in and out of plane.
- Use the "K-turn" – insert the needle, then retract, then adjust clockwise or counterclockwise, insert, then retract, and continue in this manner in order to increase the amount of tendon covered without having to reinsert the needle through the skin.

Equipment needed:

- High-frequency linear array transducer (10 MHz+).
- 25 gauge, 1.5″ needle.
- 0.5 mL of steroid preparation or 2–4 mL of PRP or autologous whole blood.
- 1–3 mL of local anesthetic.
- For PNT, use a larger (18–20 gauge) needle.

Pes Anserine Bursitis

Pes anserine bursitis is a common source of medial-sided knee pain, frequently associated with worsening knee OA, overuse, or repetitive trauma [17]. It typically presents with pain with walking and climbing or descending stairs [18]. Patients typically have tenderness to palpation over the

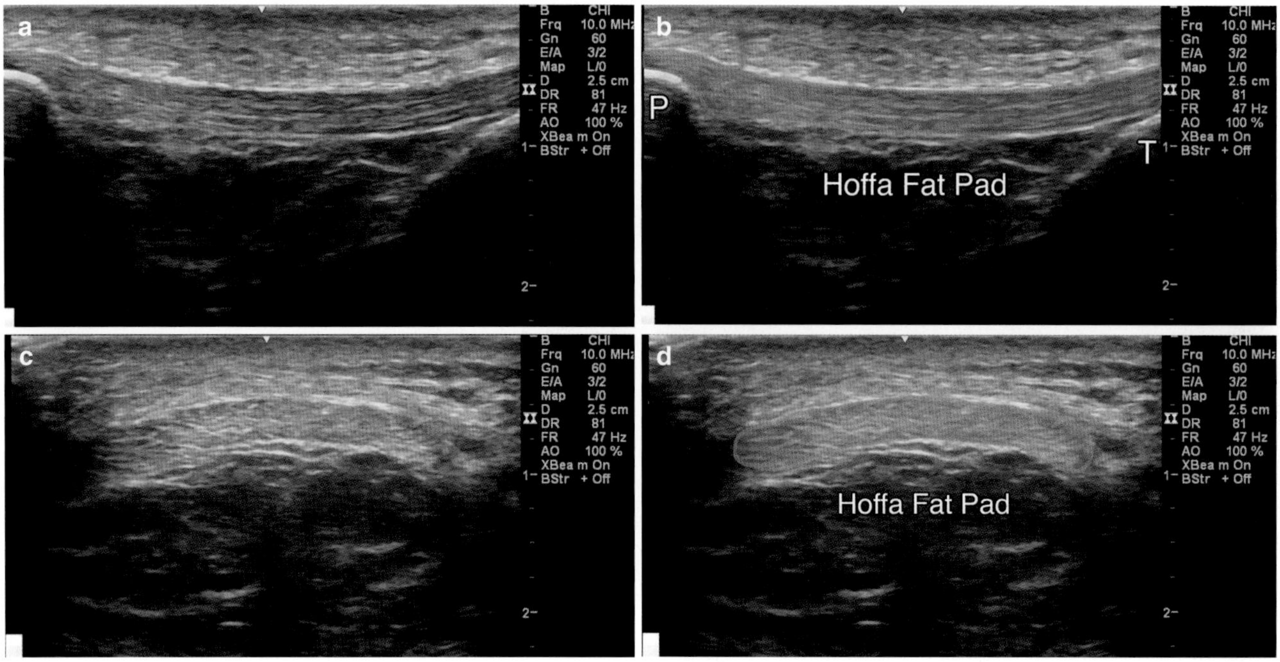

Fig. 6.3 (**a**) Sagittal view of patellar tendon. (**b**) *Orange* indicates patellar tendon, P patella, T tibial tuberosity, Hoffa fat pad labeled. (**c**) Axial view of patellar tendon. (**d**) *Orange* indicates patellar tendon, Hoffa fat pad labeled

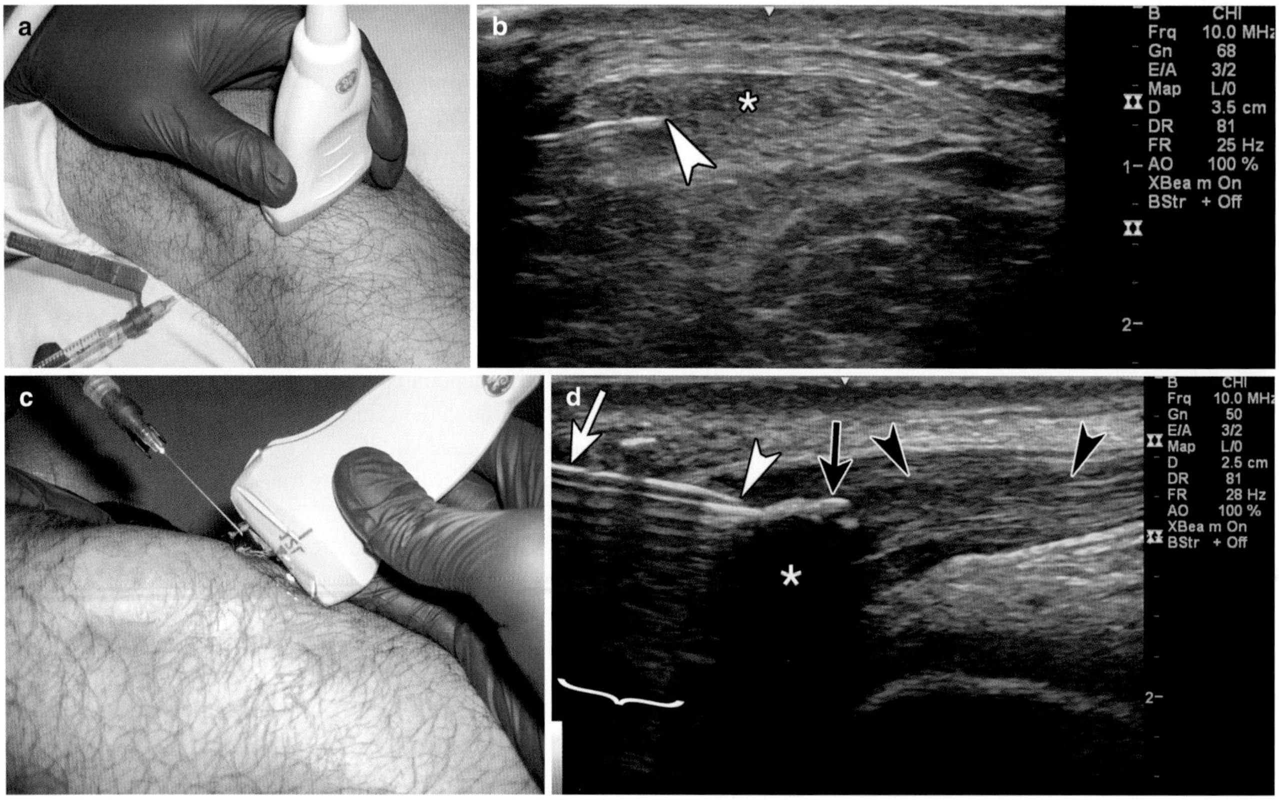

Fig. 6.4 (**a**) Example of axial probe position over patellar tendon with in-plane injection technique. (**b**) *Arrowhead* indicates needle tip, *asterisk* indicates patellar tendon. (**c**) Example of sagittal probe position with gel standoff over patellar tendon with in-plane injection approach .(**d**) Example of sagittal in-plane needling of a calcium deposition within patella tendon, *white arrowhead* indicates needle tip, *white arrow* indicates needle, *bracket* indicates reverberation, *black arrow* indicates calcium deposition, *black arrowheads* indicates patellar tendon, *asterisk* indicates acoustic shadowing

Table 6.4 Accuracy of ultrasound guided versus blind pes anserine bursa injections

Study: pes anserine bursitis	Author	Accuracy
Ultrasound-guided vs. blind	Finnoff et al. [19]	100 % vs. 50 %

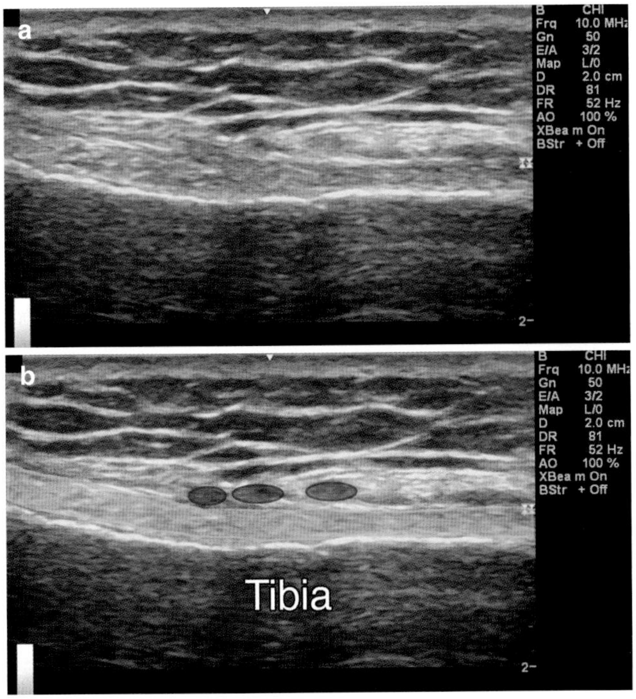

Fig. 6.5 (**a**) Sagittal view of the pes anserine bursa. (**b**) *Green* indicates medial collateral ligament, *purple circles* indicate pes anserine tendons, tibia labeled

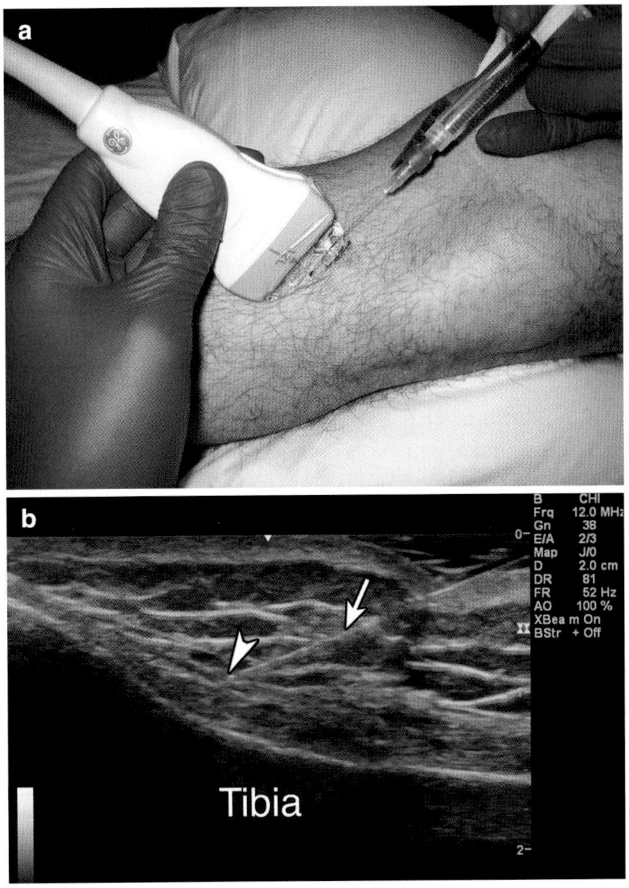

Fig. 6.6 (**a**) Example of sagittal transducer position with gel standoff over pes anserine bursa with in-plane needle approach. (**b**) *Arrowhead* indicates needle tip, *arrow* indicates needle, tibia labeled

conjoined tendon insertion of the sartorius, gracilis, and semitendinosus. Treatment typically consists of rest, nonsteroidal anti-inflammatory medications, physical therapy, and corticosteroid injections. The literature describes varying benefit from injections; however, prior injections were performed with an anatomical (blind) method. Finnoff et al. injected the pes anserine bursae under ultrasound guidance with an accuracy of 100 % compared to 50 % unguided [19]. It is not clear how well this translates to clinical improvement, however (Table 6.4).

Scanning Technique and Anatomy to Identify

Place the probe in a transverse oblique orientation over the posterior medial knee. The semitendinosus, gracilis, and sartorius muscles can be seen in cross section and traced distally towards their insertion. From deep to superficial, identify the hyperechoic proximal tibia, fibers of the medial collateral ligament (MCL) oriented obliquely, pes anserine bursa, and three ovoid tendons superficially. This bursa is rarely seen, even when the patient is symptomatic, suggesting that "pes anserine bursitis" may more likely be a distal tendinopathy, medial geniculate neuritis, or tibial stress reaction (Fig. 6.5).

Injection Technique: In-Plane Sagittal Approach

Patient positioning: Place the patient supine, knee extended and leg externally rotated with a towel underneath the knee to allow slight flexion.

Probe positioning: Place the transducer short axis (transverse) on the posteromedial aspect of the distal thigh. Move the transducer distally along the semitendinosus tendon, which helps with visualizing the gracilis and sartorius tendons. Identify the tendons as the transducer is moved distally and anteromedially. Rotate the transducer longitudinally relative to the fibers of the MCL, sagittal over the anteromedial tibia (Fig. 6.6a).

Markings: To identify the central area of the pes anserine bursa, mark the skin over the middle of pes anserinus, where it crosses the anterior margin of the MCL.

Needle position: Insert the needle in-plane on the proximal or distal side of the transducer, targeting the bursa between the MCL and the pes anserinus.

Safety considerations: This is a superficial injection which increases the risk of steroid depigmentation and fat atrophy at the site of injection. Avoid injecting steroids directly into the MCL [15].

Pearls:

- The pes anserine bursa is typically located 2.5–3 cm distal to the medial joint line [4].
- The bursae lay between the pes anserine tendons and the MCL.

Equipment needed:

- High-frequency linear array transducer (10 MHz+)
- 25G 1.5″ needle
- 1 mL of steroid preparation
- 2 mL local anesthetic

Tibiofibular Joint

The proximal tibiofibular joint (PTFJ) is an arthrodial sliding joint with great morphological variability. The PTFJ has been categorized into two main types by anatomic orientation: horizontal, with increased joint surface area and rotary mobility, and oblique, with less joint surface area and mobility. The joint supports 1/6 of the axial load of the leg. It is often overlooked as a potential cause of lateral knee pain, frequently mistaken for a lateral collateral ligament injury [20, 21]. Symptoms are nonspecific; patients may complain of joint instability or anterolateral knee and lateral calf pain that can be referred proximally or distally. Exacerbating factors may include stair climbing, hamstring pain or tightness, and knee and ankle movements [22]. Physical examination including manual pressure or grading laxity of the PTFJ did not correlate with the degree of arthritis seen in one study [23, 24].Therefore, an injection may provide both diagnostic and therapeutic benefits (Table 6.5).

Table 6.5 Accuracy of sonographically and palpation-guided PTFJ injections

Technique	Accurate (%)	Accurate with overflow (%)	Inaccurate (%)
Sonographically guided	67	33	0
Palpation guided	17	42	42

Scanning Technique and Anatomy to Identify

Place the patient in an oblique side-lying position with the lateral aspect of the affected knee towards the ceiling [25]. Slight flexion of the knee to 20–30° will widen the joint space. Palpate the PTFJ and place the transducer in a transverse–oblique view. Rotate the transducer for the best view of the PTFJ [26]. From deep to superficial, identify the joint space between the hyperechoic bony tibia and fibula, the anterior superior proximal tibiofibular ligament connecting the two bones, and superficial subcutaneous tissue (Fig. 6.7).

Injection Technique: Out-of-Plane Transverse Oblique Approach

Patient positioning: Place the patient in an oblique side-lying position, knee slightly flexed with a rolled towel underneath for comfort.

Probe positioning: Place the transducer in a transverse–oblique orientation with the lateral end of the transducer over the fibular head. The medial end of the transducer should be oriented towards the inferior patellar pole, over the tibia. With the lateral end of the transducer anchored on the fibular head, rotate the medial end to optimize visualization of the joint space (Fig. 6.8a).

Markings: Identify the anterior superior proximal tibiofibular ligament connecting the fibula and tibia. This ligament sits superficial to the joint space.

Needle position: Insert the needle out-of-plane perpendicular to the long axis of the transducer, targeting the joint space between the fibula and tibia.

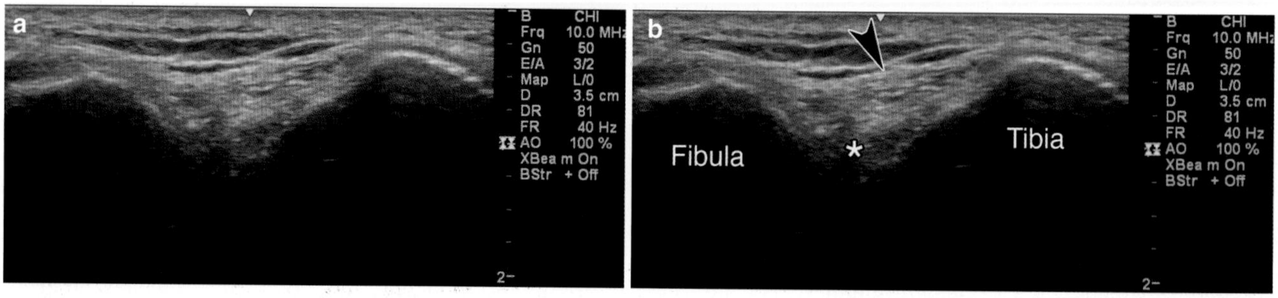

Fig. 6.7 (**a**) Transverse–oblique view over the PTFJ. (**b**) *Asterisk* indicates joint space, *arrowhead* indicates tibiofibular ligament, fibula and tibia labeled

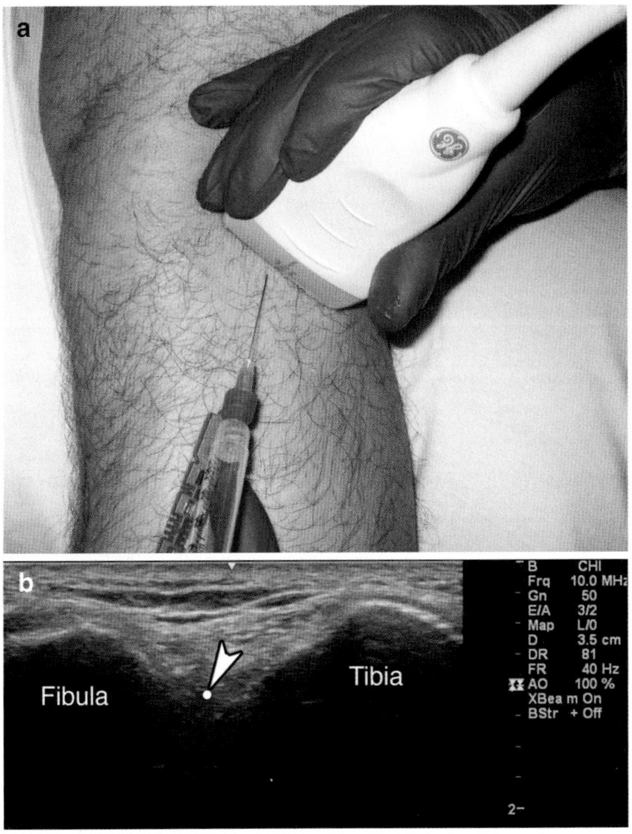

Fig. 6.8 (**a**) Example of transverse–oblique probe position over PTFJ with out-of-plane needle position. (**b**) *Arrowhead* indicates needle tip within joint space, tibia and fibula labeled

Safety considerations: Be careful when touching or walking off the painful bony surfaces.

Pearls:

- Rotate the transducer over the joint space to find the widest area.
- Once the needle is inserted, rotating the bevel may help to visualize the bright hyperechoic white dot representing the needle tip.

Equipment needed:

- High-frequency linear array transducer (8 MHz+)
- 25 gauge, 1.5″ needle
- 0.5 mL of steroid preparation
- 1–3 mL of local anesthetic

Popliteus

The evaluation and treatment of lateral knee pain can be challenging, particularly in the absence of major trauma. The popliteus muscle–tendon unit (PMTU) arises primarily from the lateral femoral condyle and proximal fibula and inserts in a triangular fashion onto the posteromedial surface of the proximal tibia. The PMTU serves to maintain dorsolateral knee stability and aids in controlling tibial rotation [27].

Table 6.6 Accuracy of sonographically guided popliteus tendon sheath injections [29]

Technique	Accurate (%)	Accurate with overflow (%)	Inaccurate (%)
Longitudinal approach	33	67	0
Transverse approach	25	58	17

PMTU injuries are uncommon and may arise from an osteophyte causing impingement and a snapping sensation, rotational injuries to the distal femur/proximal tibia, tendinosis, or chronic overuse especially in runners [28]. Ultrasound-guided popliteal tendon sheath injections can play a substantial role in providing both diagnostic and therapeutic information for pain arising from the PMTU, as there are no clinical exam maneuvers with a high degree of sensitivity or specificity to isolate PMTU pain (Table 6.6).

Scanning Technique and Anatomy to Identify

Place the patient in an oblique side-lying position, with the affected PMTU facing the ceiling. The knee should be positioned with slight flexion, with a rolled towel underneath for comfort. Place the probe in an oblique plane over the lateral knee from the lateral femoral condyle to the fibular head. Identify the lateral collateral ligament connecting the lateral femoral condyle to the fibular head. It lays superficial to the popliteus tendon, which is visualized short axis in the popliteal groove. The popliteofibular ligament can be seen attaching to the fibular head [30]. Rotate the probe 90° and view the popliteus tendon longitudinally (Fig. 6.9).

Injection Technique: In-Plane Short-Axis (Coronal) Approach

Patient positioning: Place the patient in a lateral decubitus position, knee flexed 20–30°, with the leg slightly internally rotated.

Probe positioning: Palpate the lateral femoral epicondyle, and place the probe with the cephalad end there and the caudal end over the fibula. The PMTU is seen transversely within the groove; it is highly subject to anisotropy (Fig. 6.10a).

Markings: Identify and avoid injection into the lateral collateral ligament, ITB, or joint space.

Needle position: Insert the needle in-plane from superior to inferior aiming at the superior margin of the PMTU (tendon sheath).

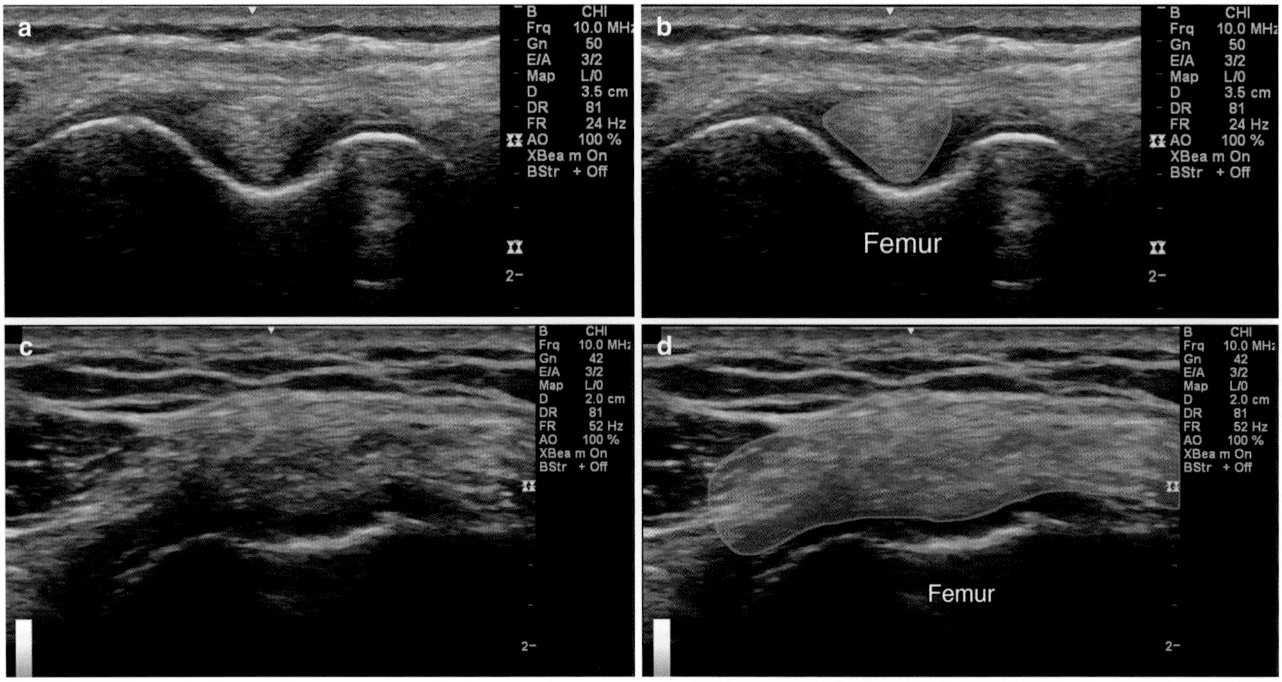

Fig. 6.9 (**a**) Oblique cross-section view of the PMTU. (**b**) *Orange* indicates popliteus tendon within popliteal groove, femur labeled. (**c**) Longitudinal view of popliteus tendon. (**d**) *Orange* indicates longitudinal view of popliteus tendon, femur labeled

Safety considerations: Avoid directly injecting the tendon, as this may increase susceptibility to tendon rupture [15, 16]. If corticosteroids are used, there is a risk of local fat atrophy and depigmentation at the site of injection.

Pearls:

- Identify the lateral collateral ligament when planning the needle trajectory to help avoid injection into that ligament.
- Stay as anterior as possible to help avoid the more posterior common fibular nerve.

Equipment needed:

- High-frequency linear array transducer (10 MHz+)
- 25 gauge, 1.5″ needle
- 0.5 mL of steroid preparation
- 1–3 mL of local anesthetic

Iliotibial Band Syndrome (ITBS)

Iliotibial band (ITB) friction syndrome is a common cause of lateral knee pain. It occurs most commonly in runners and cyclists and was first reported to occur in military recruits [31]. The ITB is formed proximally by the

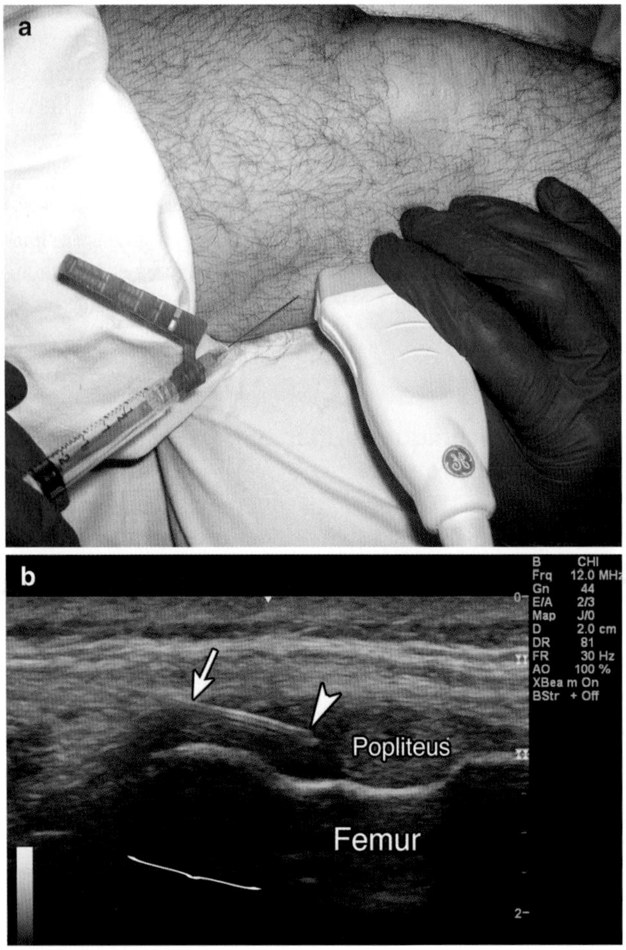

Fig. 6.10 (**a**) Example of coronal probe position relative to the PMTU with in-plane injection technique. (**b**) *Arrowhead* indicates needle tip, *arrow* points to needle. *Bracket* indicates needle reverberations, popliteus and femur labeled

Table 6.7 Normative values for ITB thickness

Study	Imaging modality	Patients	ITB thickness (mm)	Anatomical level
Goh et al. [32]	Ultrasound	Healthy controls	1.9±0.3	Lateral femoral epicondyle
Wang et al. [33]	Ultrasound	Healthy controls	1.9±0.2	Lateral femoral epicondyle
Gyaran et al. [34]	Ultrasound	Healthy controls	1.1±0.2	Level of knee joint
Ekman et al. [35]	MRI	Patients with ITBS	5.4±2.1	Lateral femoral epicondyle

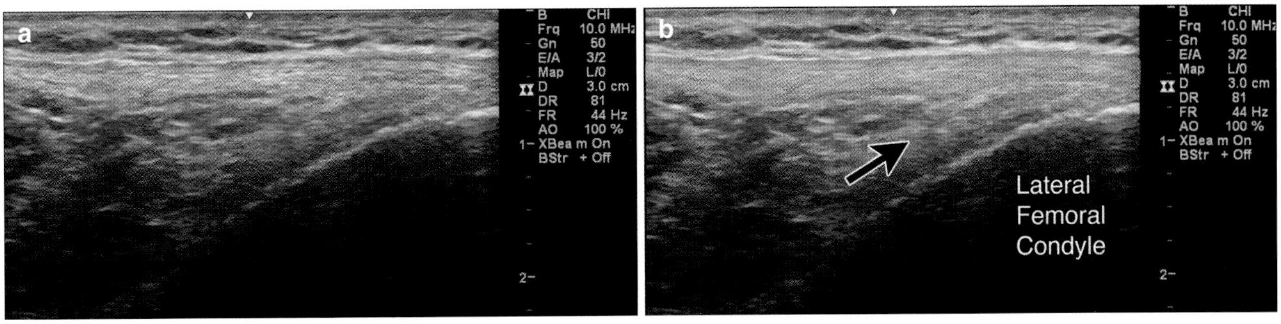

Fig. 6.11 (**a**) Coronal view of the iliotibial band. (**b**) *Orange* indicates iliotibial band, *arrow* indicates fat pad, lateral femoral condyle labeled

convergence of the tensor fascia latae, gluteus maximus, and gluteus medius at the level of the trochanteric bursa. The ITB then travels distally along the lateral femur and inserts distally by forming an inverted U with two main insertions, the lateral epicondyle and Gerdy's tubercle. ITBS is thought to be caused by repetitive friction and abrasion of the iliotibial tract across the lateral femoral epicondyle or from chronic inflammation of the iliotibial band bursa. Training factors, including sudden increases in mileage, frequency, or intensity, have also been suggested to play a role in the development of this condition. Patients commonly present with pain and tenderness over the lateral femoral epicondyle approximately 3 cm above the lateral joint line [26]. Evaluation for ITBS is typically performed with Ober's test or direct palpation to evaluate for tightness and pain. Ultrasound and MRI have provided some normative values for ITB thickness in healthy and affected patients. Corticosteroid injections have shown to provide pain relief versus a lidocaine alone (Table 6.7) [27].

Scanning Technique and Anatomy to Identify

Lay the patient on their side or supine with affected leg internally rotated. Visualize the ITB by scanning in the coronal plane from above the lateral femoral epicondyle and then inferiorly across the lateral knee joint to its insertion onto Gerdy's tubercle, a bony prominence at the anterior lateral condyle of the tibia, lateral to the distal margin of patellar tendon. Try to identify an ITB bursa between the ITB and lateral femoral condyle. Gyaran et al. found the sonographic mean ITB thickness at the level of the lateral femoral condyle to be 1.1±0.2 mm in healthy subjects, regardless of age, weight, height, or gender (Fig. 6.11) [34].

Injection Technique: In-Plane Coronal Approach

Patient positioning: Lay the patient on their side, knee flexed 30°.

Probe positioning: Place the transducer on the lateral aspect of the knee in a coronal plane. Look for hypoechoic bursal fluid between the hyperechoic femur and overlying dense fibrillar ITB (Fig. 6.12a).

Markings: Identify the lateral femoral epicondyle and Gerdy's tubercle. Measure the thickness of the ITB at the level of the lateral knee.

Needle position: Insert the needle in-plane from either proximal to distal or distal to proximal, targeting the inflamed bursa or thickened ITB.

Safety considerations: Due to the superficial nature of the ITB, there is a risk of local fat atrophy and depigmentation with corticosteroid injection or superficial hematoma with tenotomy or platelet-rich plasma. Care should be taken to avoid directly injecting the tendon, as this may increase susceptibility to tendon rupture [11].

Pearls:

- Ultrasound measurements of the ITB may help to monitor asymmetric thickening.

Equipment needed:

- High-frequency linear array transducer (10 MHz+).
- 25 gauge, 1.5″ needle.
- 0.5 mL of steroid preparation or 2–4 mL of PRP or autologous whole blood.
- 1–3 mL of local anesthetic.
- For PNT, use a larger (20–22 gauge) needle.

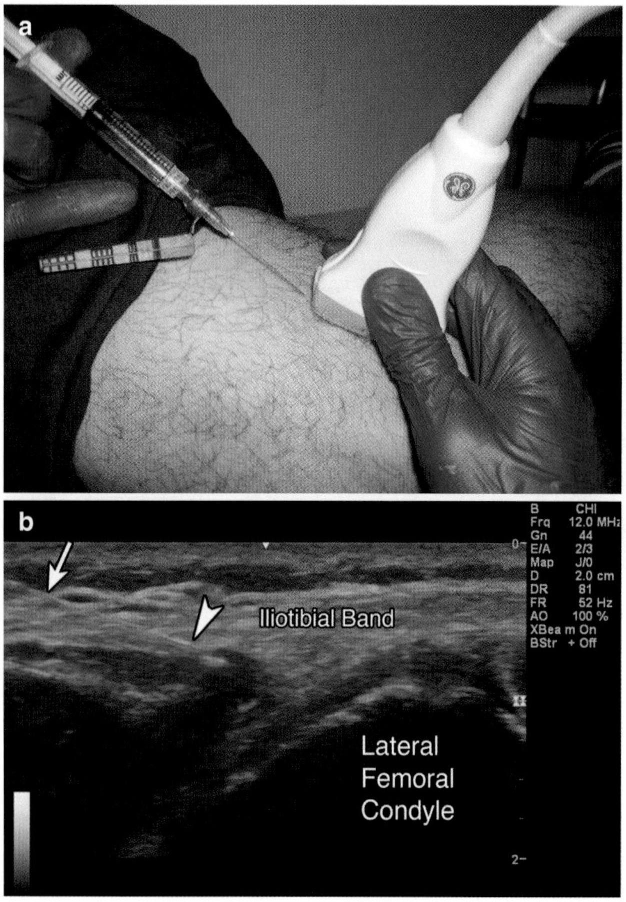

Fig. 6.12 (**a**) Example of coronal probe position over ITB with in-plane needle position. (**b**) *Arrowhead* indicates needle tip just deep to iliotibial band, *arrow* indicates needle, iliotibial band and lateral femoral condyle labeled

Baker's Cyst

Baker's cysts are popliteal cysts bordered by the semimembranosus and medial gastrocnemius. They are formed by the posterior extension of the semimembranosus–gastrocnemius bursa and communicate with the subgastrocnemius bursa [36]. Primary Baker's cysts do not communicate with the knee joint and are more common in children. The vast majority of Baker's cysts are secondary cysts (due to osteoarthritis, meniscal tears, trauma) that communicate with the knee joint proper [37]. Patients typically complain of posterior knee pain, stiffness, and swelling. Ruptured cysts can cause significant pain and calf swelling, easily mistakable for deep vein thrombosis (DVT). Ultrasound provides a fast, accurate, and cost-effective imaging tool to differentiate Baker's cysts [38]. Ultrasound guidance is important because of the neurovascular structures in the area, and the often complex nature of the cysts, to ensure maximal volume is aspirated.

Scanning Technique and Anatomy to Identify

Lay the patient prone with knee extended. Place the probe axially (transverse) over the upper third of the calf. Move medially and laterally to visualize the medial and lateral gastrocnemius. Scan to the medial border of the medial gastrocnemius, visualizing the semimembranosus tendon medial to the gastrocnemius tendon, and then scan superiorly to the knee joint. The cyst should appear crescent-shaped and hypoechoic or anechoic with well-defined borders. Chronic cysts may have a heterogeneous appearance. The base or stalk of the cyst may be visualized between and deep to the medial gastrocnemius and semimembranosus. Turn the probe 90° to evaluate the cyst longitudinally for size and shape and to assess for rupture. A sharp, pointed end can signify a ruptured Baker's cyst, which typically occurs inferiorly. Scanning the posterior knee laterally in the axial plane will reveal the popliteal artery, vein, and tibial nerve (Fig. 6.13).

Injection Technique: In-Plane Sagittal Approach

Patient positioning: Lay the patient prone with legs extended.

Probe positioning: Place the transducer transversely (short axis) at the upper third of the calf. Move the probe to the medial border of the medial gastrocnemius, then superiorly to the knee joint. Identify the semimembranosus and medial gastrocnemius tendon. A Baker's cyst appears typically as a circumferential, thin-walled, anechoic structure in this location. Rotate the transducer into the longitudinal (long axis) position to assess its extent superiorly and inferiorly. Place the probe longitudinally over the center of the cyst (Fig. 6.14a).

Markings: Scan laterally and mark the popliteal artery, vein, and tibial nerve.

Needle position: Insert the needle in-plane from distal to proximal.

Safety considerations: Avoid placing the needle in the middle and lateral popliteal fossa. Doppler should be used to avoid the popliteal artery and vein.

Pearls:

- Toggle the probe to avoid anisotropy. The medial gastrocnemius and semimembranosus tendons are not truly parallel to one another; therefore, the normally hyperechoic tendons may appear hypoechoic.
- Sharp tapering of one end of the cyst usually represents a rupture [14].
- Doppler can confirm the absence of vascular flow to exclude a popliteal artery aneurysm or venous ectasia [39].

Equipment needed:

- High-frequency linear array transducer (8 MHz+)
- 16–20G spinal needle
- 1 mL of corticosteroid preparation
- 3–5 mL local anesthetic

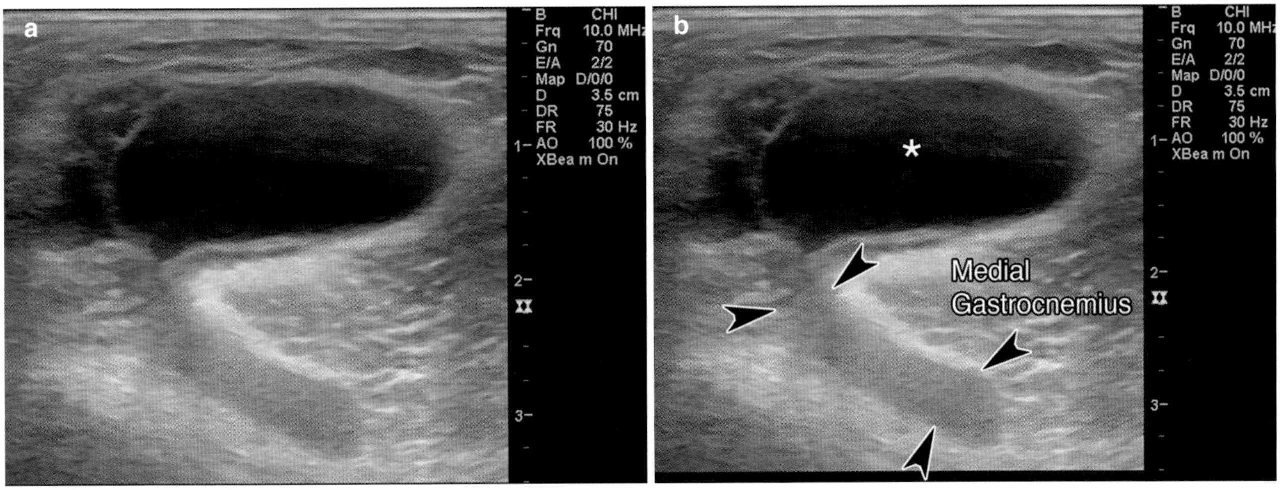

Fig. 6.13 (**a**) Axial view of Baker's cyst. (**b**) *Black arrowheads* outline stalk or communication with joint, *asterisk* indicates Baker's cyst, Medial Gastrocnemius labeled

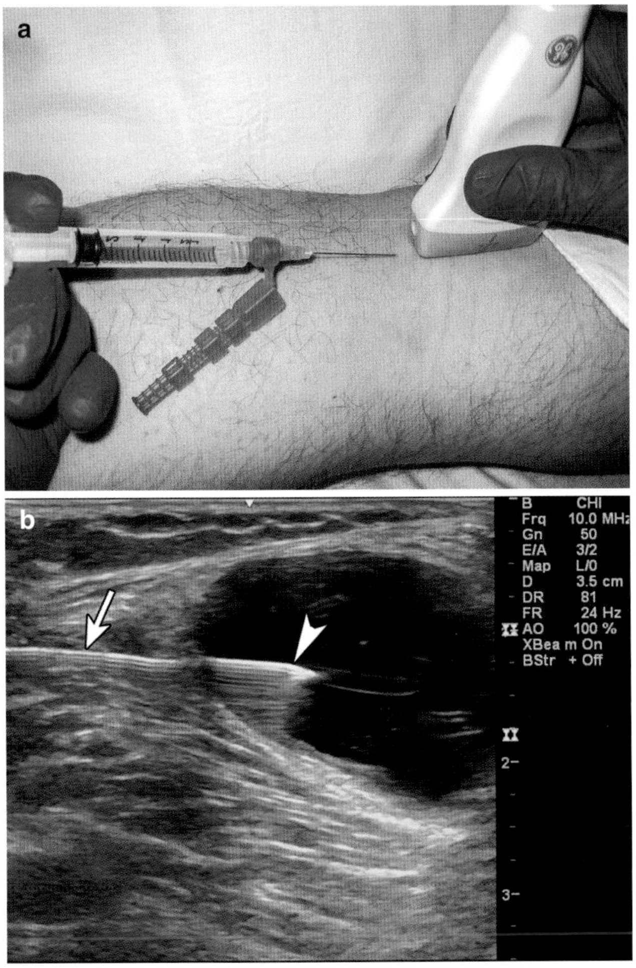

Fig. 6.14 (**a**) Example of sagittal probe position over posterior knee with in-plane injection technique. (**b**) *Arrow* indicates needle, *arrowhead* indicates needle tip within Baker's cyst

References

1. Esen S, Akarirmak U, Aydm FY, et al. Clinical evaluation during the acute exacerbation of knee osteoarthritis: the impact of diagnostic ultrasonography. Rheumatol Int. 2013;33:711–7.
2. Berkoff DJ, Miller LE, Block JE. Clinical utility of ultrasound guidance for intra-articular knee injections: a review. Clin Interv Aging. 2012;7:89–95.
3. Kettunen JA, Kvist M, Alanen E, et al. Long-term prognosis for jumper's knee in male athletes. A prospective follow-up study. Am J Sports Med. 2002;30:689–92.
4. Ark M, Zwerver J, Akker-Scheek I. Injection treatments for patellar tenidonpathy. Br J Sports Med. 2011;45:1068–76.
5. Sibbitt Jr WL, Band PA, Kettwich LG, et al. A randomized controlled trial evaluating the cost-effectiveness of sonographic guidance for intra-articular injection of the osteoarthritis knee. J Clin Rheumatol. 2011;17(8):409–15.
6. Cunnington J, Marshall N, Hide G, et al. A randomized, double-blind, controlled study of ultrasound-guided corticosteroid injection into the joint of patients with inflammatory arthritis. Arthritis Rheum. 2010;62(7):1862–9.
7. Bum Park Y, Ah Choi W, Kim YK, et al. Accuracy of blind versus ultrasound-guided suprapatellar bursal injection. J Clin Ultrasound. 2012;40(1):20–5.
8. Balint PV, Kane D, Hunter J, et al. Ultrasound guided versus conventional joint and soft tissue fluid aspiration in rheumatology practice: a pilot study. J Rheumatol. 2002;29(10):2209–13.
9. Park Y, Lee SC, Nam HS, et al. Comparison of sonographically guided intra-articular injections at 3 different sites of the knee. J Ultrasound Med. 2011;30:1669–76.
10. Filardo G, Kon E, Villa SD, et al. Use of platelet rich plasma for the treatment of refractory jumper's knee. Int Orthop. 2010;34(6): 909–15.
11. De Vos RJ, Van Veldhoven PLJ, Moen MH, et al. Autologous growth factor injections in chronic tendinopathy; a systematic review. Br Med Bull. 2010;95(1):63–77.
12. Hoksrud A, Torgalsen T, Harstad H, et al. Ultrasound-guided sclerosis of neovessels in patellar tendinopathy. Am J Sports Med. 2012;40(3):542–6.

13. James SL, Ali K, Pocock C, et al. Ultrasound guided dry needling and autologous blood injection for patellar tendinosis. Br J Sports Med. 2007;41:518–22.
14. Hoksrud A, Ohberg L, Alfredson H, et al. Color Doppler ultrasound findings in patellar tendinopathy (Jumper's knee). Am J Sports Med. 2008;36(9):1813–20.
15. Haraldsson BT, Langberg H, Aagaard P, Zuurmond AM, van El B, Degroot J, Kjaer M, Magnusson SP. Corticosteroids reduce the tensile strength of isolated collagen fascicles. Am J Sports Med. 2006;34:1992–7.
16. Carpenito G, Gutierrez M, Ravagnani V, Raffeiner B, Grassi W. Complete rupture of biceps tendons after corticosteroid injection in psoriatic arthritis "Popeye sign": role of ultrasound 2. J Clin Rheumatol. 2011;17:108.
17. Biundo JJ. Regional rheumatic pain syndromes. In: Shumacher HR, editor. Primer on the rheumatic diseases. 11th ed. Atlanta: Arthritis Foundation; 1997. p. 144.
18. Yoon HS, Kim SE, Suh YR, et al. Correlation between ultrasonographic findings and the response to corticosteroid injection in pes anserinus tendinobursitis syndrome in knee osteoarthritis patients. J Korean Med Sci. 2005;20:109–12.
19. Finnoff JT, Nutz DJ, Henning PT. Accuracy of ultrasound-guided versus unguided pes anserinus bursa injections. PM R. 2010;2:732–9.
20. Proximal tibiofibular joint injuries. In: Wheeless' textbook of orthopaedics. Online at http://www.wheelessonline.com/ortho/proximal_tibiofibular_joint_injuries
21. Andersen K. Dislocation of the superior tibiofibular joint. Injury. 1985;16:494–8.
22. Oztuna V, Yildiz A, Ozer C, Milcan A. Involvement of the proximal tibiofibular joint in osteoarthritis of the knee. Knee. 2003;10: 347–9.
23. Ozcan O, Boya H, Oztekin H. Clinical evaluation of the proximal tibiofibular joint in knees with severe tibiofemoral primary osteoarthritis. Knee. 2009;16:248–50.
24. Nadaud MC, Ewing JW. Proximal tibiofibular joint arthritis; an unusual cause of lateral knee pain. Orthopedics. 2001;24:397–8.
25. Smith J, Finnoff JT, Lvey BA, et al. Sonographically guided proximal tibiofibular joint injection. J Ultrasound Med. 2010;29:783–9.
26. McNally E. Musculoskeletal interventional ultrasound. In: McNally E, editor. Practical musculoskeletal ultrasound. 1st ed. New York: Elsevier; 2005. p. 300–1.
27. Gunter P, Schwellnus MP. Local corticosteroid injection in iliotibial band friction syndrome in runners: a randomized controlled trial. Br J Sports Med. 2004;38(3):269–72.
28. Gain WJ, Mohammed A. Osteophyte impingement of the popliteus tendon as a cause of lateral knee joint pain. Knee. 2002;9:249–52.
29. Smith J, Finnoff JT, Santaella-Sante B, et al. Sonographically guided popliteus tendon sheath injection techniques and accuracy. J Ultrasound Med. 2010;29:775–82.
30. Sekiya JK, Jacobson JA, Wojtys EM. Sonographic imaging of the posterolateral structures of the knee: findings in human cadavers. Arthroscopy. 2002;18(8):872–81.
31. Renne JW. The iliotibial band friction syndrome. J Bone Joint Surg Am. 1975;57(8):1110–1.
32. Goh LA, Chhem RK, Wang SC. Iliotibial band thickness: sonographic measurements in asymptomatic volunteers. J Clin Ultrasound. 2003;31:239–44.
33. Wang TG, Jan MH, Lin KH, et al. Assessment of stretching of the iliotibial tract with Ober and modified Ober tests: an ultrasonographic study. Arch Phys Med Rehabil. 2006;87:1407–11.
34. Gyaran IA, Spiezia F, Hudson Z. Sonographic measurement of iliotibial band thickness: an observational study in healthy adult volunteers. Knee Surg Sports Traumatol Arthrosc. 2011;19:458–61.
35. Ekman EF, Pope T, Martin DF. Magnetic resonance imaging in iliotibial band syndrome. Am J Sports Med. 1994;22:851–4.
36. Rauschning W. Popliteal cysts and their relation to the gastrocnemio-semimembranous bursa: studies on the surgical and functional anatomy. Acta Orthop Scand. 1979;179:9–43.
37. Janzen DL, Peterfy CG, Forbes JR, et al. Cystic lesions around the knee joint: MR imaging findings. Am J Roentgenol. 1994;163: 155–61.
38. Chen CK, Lew HL, Liao RIH. Ultrasound-guided diagnosis and aspiration of Baker's cysts. Am J Phys Med Rehabil. 2012;91(11): 1002–4.
39. Koroglu M, Callioglu M, Eris HN, et al. Ultrasound guided percutaneous treatment and follow-up of Baker's cyst in knee osteoarthritis. Eur J Radiol. 2012;81:3466–71.

Foot and Ankle

7

Kiran Vadada, Richard G. Chang, Christopher Sahler, and Jonathan S. Kirschner

The foot and ankle function together in an extremely complex network of structures, each of which can be affected by injury. Multiplanar movement is achieved by interactions between the ankle, hindfoot, midfoot, and forefoot. Stability is provided primarily by the medial (deltoid) and lateral ligaments. The mobility and repetitive stress on the foot and ankle make them susceptible to injury. The bones and their cartilaginous articulations are subject to degeneration, fracture, and inflammation. The muscles, tendons, and ligaments can suffer from acute or chronic tearing or overuse. Peripheral neuropathy and vascular disease can lead to injury and impair healing.

The clinical utility and superiority of ultrasound guidance for technical accuracy when performing injections in the foot and ankle has been well reported and will be cited throughout the chapter. Given the high density of structures in this region, accuracy is key in ensuring diagnostic and therapeutic efficacy. More importantly, the ability to visualize the neurovascular structures and bony landmarks allows for increased patient safety and comfort.

Tibiotalar ("Ankle") Joint

The tibiotalar joint is a diarthrodial joint comprised of the talus inferiorly, the distal tibia superiorly and medially, and the distal fibula laterally. The medial and lateral malleoli articulate with the chondral surface of the talus on their respective sides. A capsular joint ligament surrounds the ankle and is strengthened by the medial and lateral ligament complexes. Although sprains and other soft tissue injuries to the surrounding structures of the joint are common, arthritis is the primary source of intra-articular pain. An anterior approach with the ankle in plantar flexion is preferred due to optimal visualization of effusions and needle access for aspiration and injection [1–3]. Ultrasound can detect as little as 2 mL of fluid in the tibiotalar joint; up to 3 mL can be considered normal (Table 7.1) [6, 7].

Scanning Techniques and Anatomy to Identify

Scan the anterior aspect of the joint in the sagittal plane to visualize the anterior recess. Identify the distal tibia, the talar head, and the talar dome in between them with its thin anechoic cartilage. The joint capsule extends as a hyperechoic line between the distal tibia and the talar head. Immediately deep to the capsule is the intra-articular fat pad, which is triangular shaped, like a wide arrowhead pointing posteroinferiorly into the joint space. Sweep medially and laterally to visualize the surface of the talar dome, exploring for effusion or osteochondral defects. Rotate the transducer 90° to the axial plane. Position it slightly inferior to the distal tibia, and identify the tendons of the tibialis anterior, extensor hallucis longus, and extensor digitorum longus muscles. Identify and avoid the anterior tibial artery and deep fibular nerve (Fig. 7.1).

Table 7.1 Accuracy of tibiotalar joint injections

Study – tibiotalar joint injection	Author	Accuracy (%)
Palpation	Wisniewski et al. [4]	88
Ultrasound guided	Kirk et al. [5]	100

K. Vadada, MD (✉) • R.G. Chang, MD, MPH • C. Sahler, MD
J.S. Kirschner, MD, FAAPMR, RMSK
Interventional Spine and Sports Medicine Division,
Department of Rehabilitation Medicine,
Icahn School of Medicine at Mount Sinai, New York, NY, USA
e-mail: kvadadamd@gmail.com; richard.chang@mountsinai.org; christophersahler@gmail.com; jonathan.kirschner@mountsinai.org

D.A. Spinner et al. (eds.), *Atlas of Ultrasound Guided Musculoskeletal Injections*, Musculoskeletal Medicine,
DOI 10.1007/978-1-4614-8936-8_7, © Springer Science+Business Media, LLC 2014

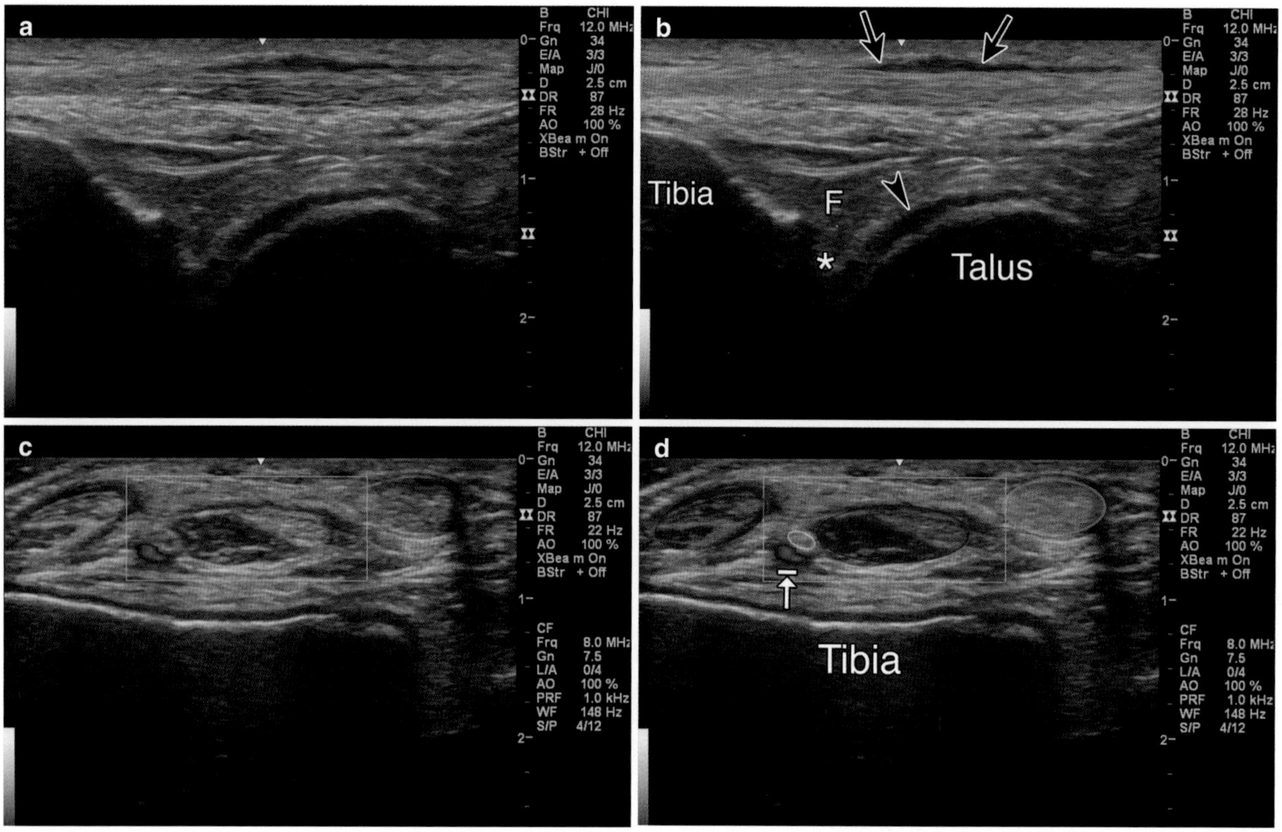

Fig. 7.1 (**a**) Sagittal view of tibiotalar joint. (**b**) *Orange* indicates tibialis anterior tendon. *Arrowhead* indicates hyaline cartilage. Arrows indicate fluid within tibialis anterior tendon sheath. *Asterisk* indicates joint space. *F* fat pad. Tibia and talus labeled. (**c**) Axial view of tibiotalar joint. (**d**) *Orange* indicates tibialis anterior muscle. *Purple* indicates extensor hallucis longus muscle. *Yellow* indicates deep peroneal nerve. *Arrow with stop* indicates the anterior tibial artery. *Magenta* indicates extensor digitorum longus muscle

Injection Technique: In-Plane Sagittal Anterior Approach [2, 8]

Patient positioning: Lay the patient supine, knee flexed with foot flat. Alternatively, the ankle can rest off the end of the table with the foot passively plantar flexed.

Probe positioning: Position the transducer so that the center of the screen is in between the extensor hallucis longus and tibialis anterior, and then rotate back to the sagittal plane for the injection (Fig. 7.2a).

Markings: Identify the dorsalis pedis artery, deep fibular nerve, tibialis anterior tendon, and extensor hallucis longus tendon.

Needle position: Enter in-plane and maintain a relatively steep angle to avoid scraping the talar dome, which can sometimes appear contiguous with an overlying effusion.

Safety considerations: Avoid the dorsalis pedis artery, deep fibular nerve, tibialis anterior tendon, and extensor hallucis longus tendon.

Pearls:

- There should be minimal resistance during injection.
- Superior migration of the overlying fat pad further confirms intra-articular spread of injectate.
- If visualization is poor, gel standoff can be used.

Equipment needed:

- Medium-frequency linear array transducer (8–12 MHz)
- 22–25G 1.5″ needle
- 0.5–1.0 mL of steroid preparation
- 1–3 mL local anesthetic

Subtalar Joint (Talocalcaneal Articulation)

The subtalar joint is comprised of three articulations between the talus and the calcaneus. The anterior facet is located above the anteromedial corner of the calcaneus, the middle facet is located medially, and the posterior facet is located posteriorly. The anterior and middle facets are contiguous and together comprise the anterior subtalar articulation [9, 10]. The current literature only focuses on the posterior articulation, perhaps because it is the largest of the three and presumably bears the majority of the weight across the joint. In one study blind injection using an anterolateral approach resulted in a 27 % rate of extravasation into the surrounding structures in an unpredictable distribution [9]. The posterolateral approach was found to be superior (91.2 % vs. 67.6 %) [10]. A study comparing ultrasound-guided anterolateral, posterolateral, and posteromedial approaches resulted in 100 % accuracy for all three methods, with rates of extravasation 25, 25, and 8.3 %, respectively [11]. Furthermore, using dynamic ultrasound may allow a smoother needle trajectory, minimizing contact with surrounding structures [12].

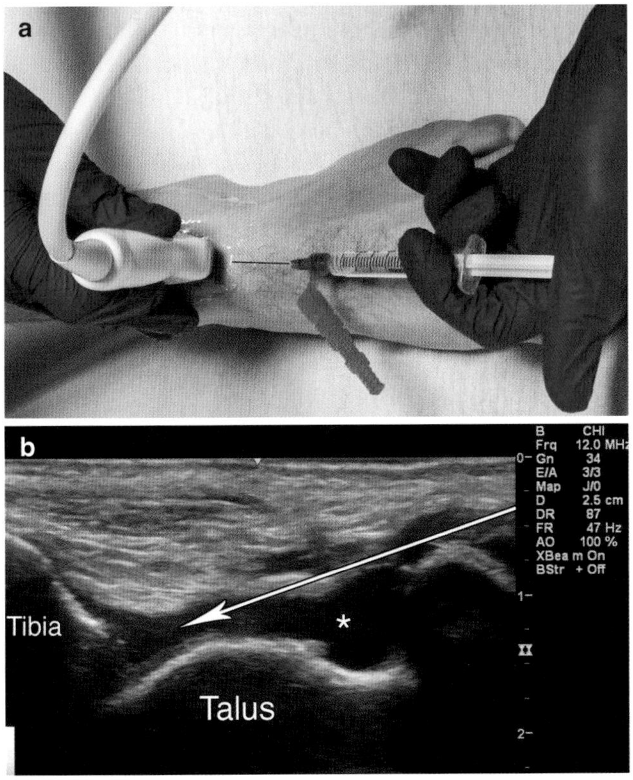

Fig. 7.2 (**a**) Example of sagittal probe position over anterior tibiotalar joint with in-plane needle position. (**b**) Sagittal view tibiotalar joint. *Arrow* indicates needle trajectory. *Asterisk* indicates effusion. Tibia and talus labeled

Scanning Techniques and Anatomy to Identify

The posteromedial approach has been shown to have the best accuracy (reference above). Position the patient side lying with the medial aspect of the affected joint upwards and a rolled towel beneath the lateral malleolus to place the ankle in subtalar eversion. Place the transducer in the coronal plane with the proximal end on the medial malleolus and the distal end over the sustentaculum tali of the calcaneus. Identify the middle subtalar facet, which appears as an anechoic space between the sustentaculum tali and the talus. Sweep the transducer posteriorly to locate the anechoic medial aspect of the posterior subtalar joint line (Fig. 7.3).

Injection Technique: Out-of-Plane Coronal Posteromedial Approach

Patient positioning: Lay the patient on their side with the medial aspect of the affected ankle facing upwards. A rolled-up towel can be placed below the lateral malleolus to promote subtalar eversion.

Probe positioning: Place the probe in the coronal plane just posterior to the sustentaculum tali and medial malleolus (Fig. 7.4a).

Markings: Identify and avoid the tarsal tunnel.

Needle position: Insert the needle out-of-plane, anterior to the transducer, and angle it posteriorly and laterally.

Safety considerations: Avoid the tibialis posterior, flexor digitorum, and flexor hallucis longus tendons and the plantar nerves and arteries.

Pearls:

- Subtalar alignment can vary based on the type of pathology
- Gel standoff can be used to optimize trajectory

Equipment needed:

- High-frequency linear array transducer

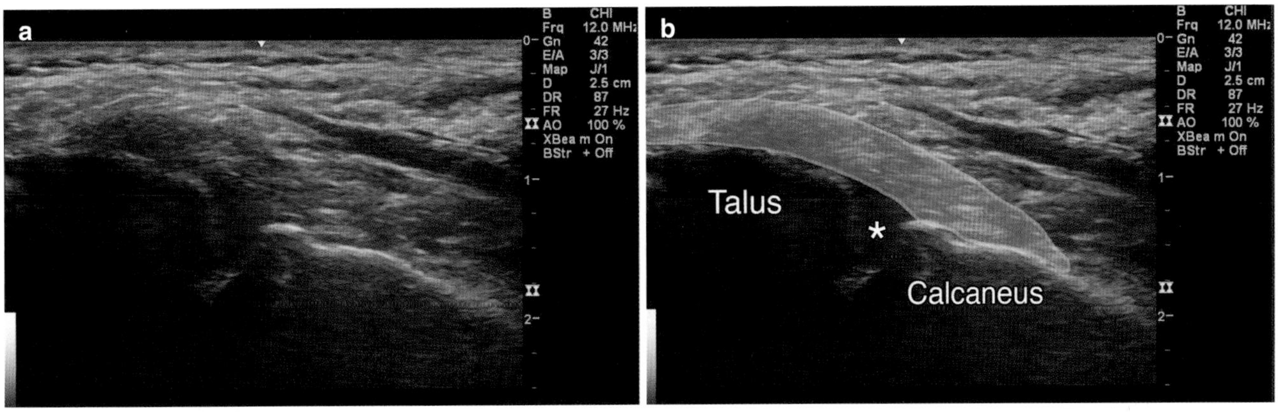

Fig. 7.3 (**a**) Coronal view of posterior subtalar joint. (**b**) *Green* deltoid ligament. *Asterisk* indicates subtalar joint. Talus and calcaneus labeled

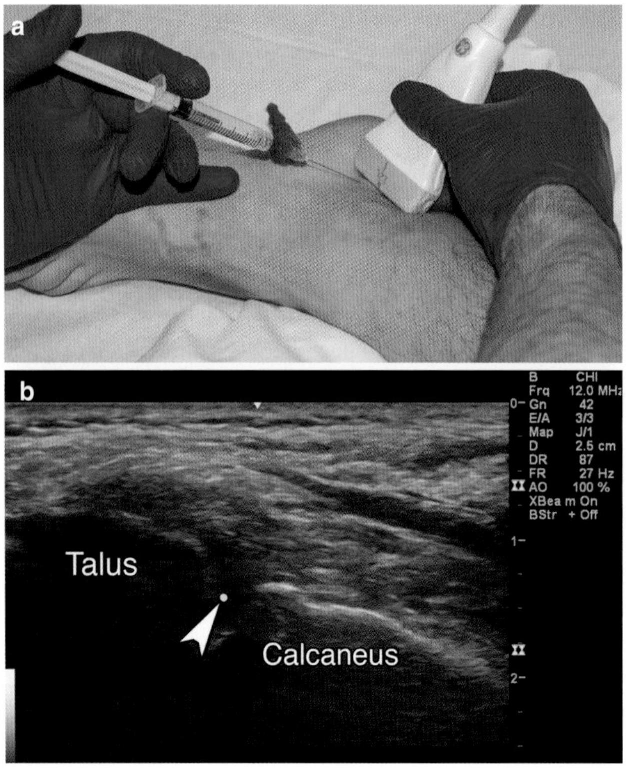

Fig. 7.4 (**a**) Example of coronal probe position over posteromedial subtalar joint with out-of-plane needle position. (**b**) Coronal view over subtalar joint. *Arrowhead* indicates needle tip. Talus and calcaneus labeled

- 22–25G 1.5″ needle
- 0.5 mL of steroid preparation
- 1–3 mL local anesthetic

Medial (Deltoid) Ligament

Ankle sprains have been found to account for 15–40 % of all athletic injuries [13–15]. The medial ligament is composed of the posterior tibiotalar, tibiocalcaneal, tibionavicular, and anterior talotibial ligaments. The complex is stronger, more stable, and less commonly injured than the lateral ligaments. It is a major contributor to ankle stability during weight bearing and is the primary limiter of lateral talar shift and talar external rotation. External rotation fractures at the lateral malleolus are associated with medial ligament injuries. Local swelling, tenderness, and ecchymosis have been shown to be unreliable in establishing a diagnosis. MRI is useful for visualization of ligament irregularity but is unable to demonstrate instability. A 2004 study found the most commonly used radiographic finding for deltoid ligament rupture and medial ankle instability (the medial clear space) to be unreliable [16]. In a prospective study of 12 patients with supination external rotation injuries, ultrasound accurately diagnosed acute deltoid ligament rupture with a sensitivity and specificity of 100 % [8]. No current evidence supports the use of local injections for medial ligament injuries. However, emerging studies seem promising for the eventual development of an appropriate injectate.

Scanning Techniques and Anatomy to Identify

Position the patient in side-lying position with the medial aspect of the affected joint facing upwards. Use a rolled-up towel below the lateral malleolus to place the ankle in subtalar eversion. Maintain the proximal end of the transducer over the medial malleolus and rotate the distal end to the neck of the talus for the anterior tibiotalar ligament, the navicular bone for the tibionavicular ligament, the sustentaculum tali for the tibiocalcaneal ligament, and the posterior process of the talus for the posterior tibiotalar ligament, which sits deep to the tibialis posterior tendon (Fig. 7.5).

Injection Technique: In-Plane Coronal Approach

Patient positioning: Lay the patient on their side with the medial aspect of the affected ankle facing upwards. A rolled-up towel can be placed below the lateral malleolus to promote subtalar eversion.

Probe positioning: Maintain the proximal end of the probe over the medial malleolus while rotating the distal end to the talar neck for the anterior tibiotalar ligament, the navicular bone for the tibionavicular ligament, the sustentaculum tali for the tibiocalcaneal ligament, and the posterior process of the talus for the posterior tibiotalar ligament, which sits deep to the tibialis posterior tendon (Fig. 7.6a).

Markings: Identify the tarsal tunnel and avoid inadvertent puncture.

Needle position: Enter with a superficial trajectory, in-plane with the probe.

Safety considerations: Avoid the posterior tibialis, flexor digitorum, and flexor hallucis longus tendons, and the plantar nerves and arteries.

Pearls:

- Manipulate the ankle to provide slack vs. tension to the structures of interest while scanning.
- Placing tension on the ligament may help the "feel" of the needle tip piercing its surface.
- Placing slack on the ligament may cause it to appear thicker, resulting in better visualization.

Equipment needed:

- High-frequency linear array transducer
- 25G 1.5″ needle
- 0.5 mL of injectate
- 1–3 mL local anesthetic

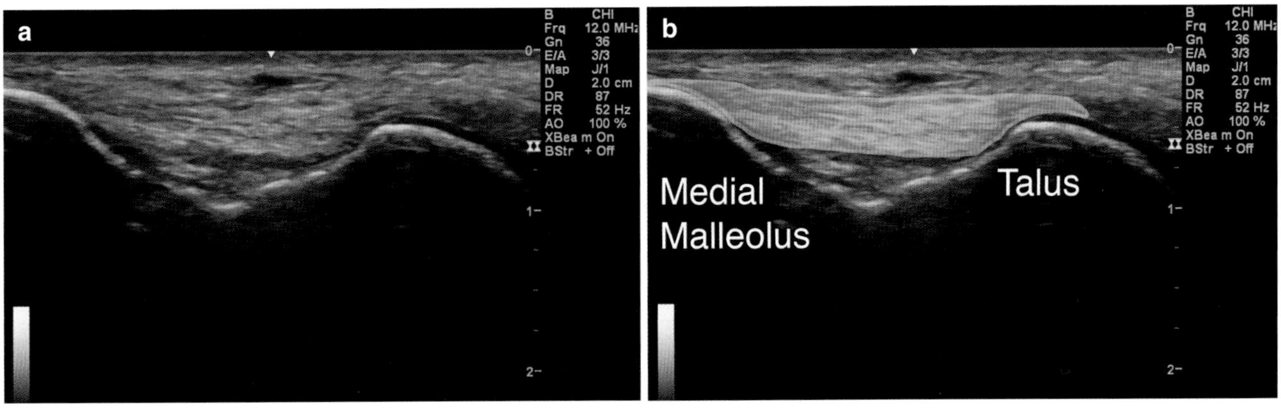

Fig. 7.5 (**a**) Coronal view of anterior tibiotalar ligament. (**b**) *Green* indicates tibiotalar component of deltoid ligament. Medial malleolus and talus labeled

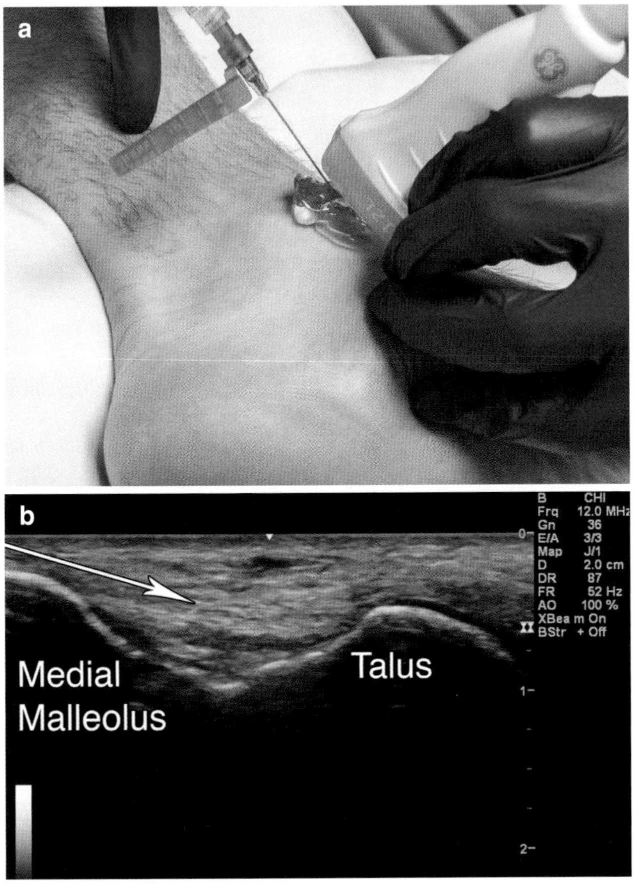

Fig. 7.6 (**a**) Example of coronal probe position with gel standoff over anterior tibiotalar ligament with in-plane needle position. (**b**) Coronal view of anterior tibiotalar ligament. *Arrow* indicates needle trajectory. Medial malleolus and talus labeled

Lateral Ligament Complex

The lateral ligament complex consists of the anterior talofibular ligament (ATFL), the calcaneofibular ligament (CFL), and the posterior talofibular ligament (PTFL) [17, 18]. In one study, point tenderness over the ATFL and CFL correlated with ligament rupture 52 and 72 % of the time, respectively. 71 % of patients with a positive anterior drawer sign, 68 % of patients with a positive talar tilt, 70 % of patients with ≥4 cm of swelling under the lateral malleolus, and 91 % of patients with such swelling in combination with point tenderness were shown to have lateral ligamentous injury [19]. Ultrasound has been shown to have the diagnostic accuracy of 95 % for ATFL tears and 90 % for CFL tears (Table 7.2) [17, 18].

Scanning Techniques and Anatomy to Identify

Position the patient on their side with the lateral aspect of the affected ankle facing upwards. Use a rolled-up towel under the medial malleolus to place the ankle in subtalar inversion. For the ATFL, passively plantar flex the ankle and place the proximal edge of the transducer over the anterior aspect of the lateral malleolus, with the distal edge over the talus, reaching horizontally towards the midfoot. Visualize the lateral malleolus, the talus, and the ligament between them. For the CFL place the ankle in neutral and position the proximal edge of the transducer over the lateral malleolus. Aim the distal edge inferiorly and slightly posteriorly. Dorsiflexing the ankle may help visualize the ligament by placing it in tension. Immediately superficial to the CFL at the level of the superior edge of the calcaneus, the fibular tendons appear in cross section. The sural nerve runs inferior to these tendons, at a similar depth (Fig. 7.7) [21].

Injection Techniques: In-Plane Axial Approach

Patient positioning: Lay the patient on their side with the lateral aspect of the affected ankle facing upwards. A rolled-up towel can be placed under the medial malleolus to promote subtalar inversion. Place the ankle in plantar flexion for ATFL and dorsiflexion for CFL.

Table 7.2 Anatomy of lateral ligament complex

Ligament [12, 20]	ATFL	CFL	PTFL
Origin	1 cm proximal to the distal tip of the fibula	Distal tip of the fibula	10 mm proximal to the distal tip of the fibula
Insertion	lateral talar neck	Calcaneus	Posterior talus
Size	6–10 mm wide × 10 mm long × 2 mm thick	Cylindrical in shape, 20–25 mm length × 6–8 mm diameter	
Notes	Weakest, most commonly injured	Attachment point of the peroneal tendon sheath	Strongest, least commonly injured

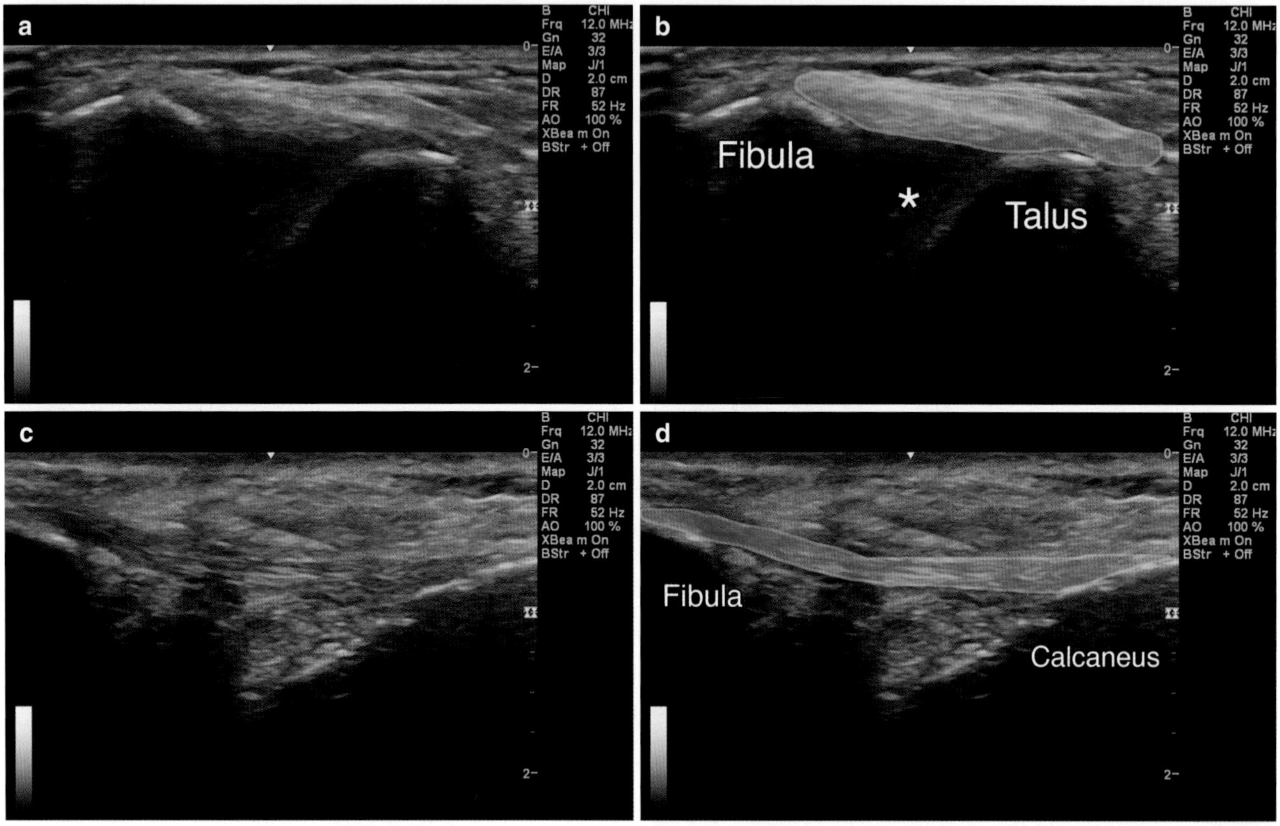

Fig. 7.7 (**a**) Axial view of the ATFL. (**b**) *Green* indicates the ATFL. *Asterisk* indicates joint space. Fibula and talus labeled. (**c**) Coronal oblique view of the CFL. (**d**) *Green* indicates the calcaneofibular ligament. Fibula and calcaneus labeled

Probe positioning: Maintain the proximal edge over lateral malleolus. Place the distal edge over the talus in the axial plane for the ATFL (Fig. 7.8a). Place the distal edge over the calcaneus in the coronal plane for the CFL.

Markings: Identify and avoid the sural nerve.

Needle position: Enter the skin with a superficial trajectory, in-plane with the probe.

Safety considerations: Avoid the sural nerve, peroneal tendons, and lesser saphenous vein.

Pearls:

- Manipulate the ankle to provide slack vs. tension to the structures of interest while scanning.
- Placing tension on the ligament may help the "feel" of the needle tip piercing its surface.
- Placing slack on the ligament may cause it to appear thicker, resulting in better visualization.
- The ATFL is contiguous with the ankle joint capsule and can appear as a discrete capsular thickening.
- The CFL is the only extra-articular ligament within the lateral complex.

Equipment needed:

- High-frequency linear array transducer
- 25G 1.5″ needle
- 0.5 mL of steroid preparation
- 1–3 mL local anesthetic

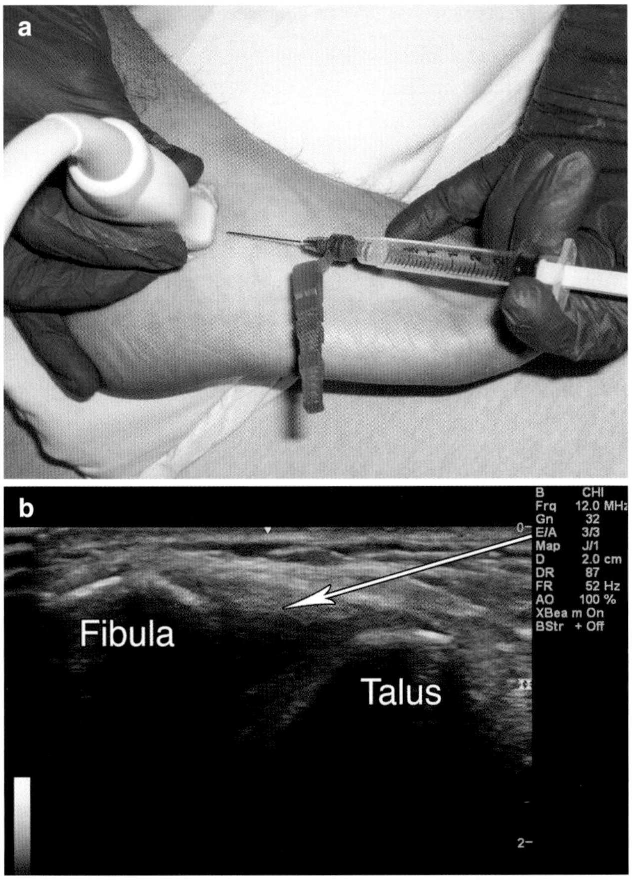

Fig. 7.8 (**a**) Example of axial probe position over ATFL with in-plane needle approach. (**b**) Axial view of ATFL with *arrow* indicating needle trajectory. Fibula and talus labeled

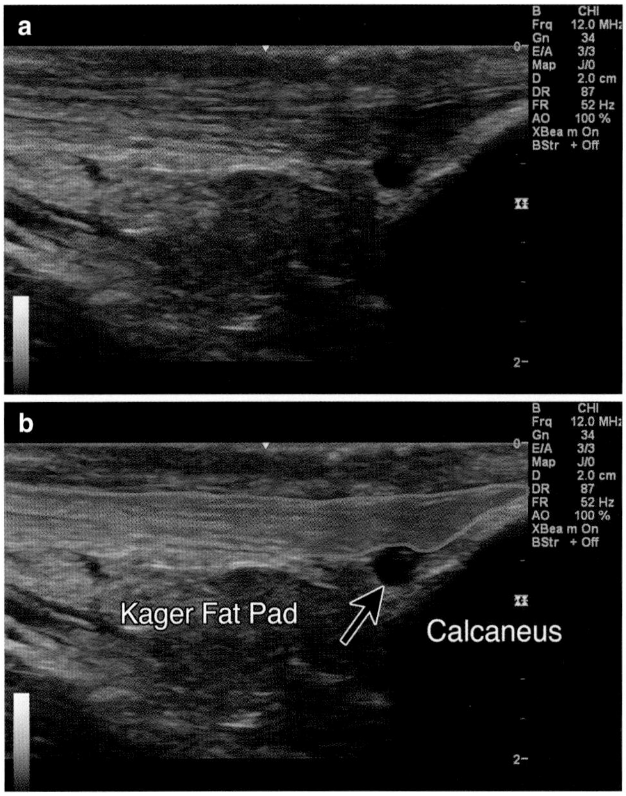

Fig. 7.9 (**a**) Sagittal view of Achilles tendon and retrocalcaneal bursa. (**b**) *Orange* indicates Achilles tendon. *Arrow* indicates retrocalcaneal bursitis. Kager's fat pad and calcaneus labeled

Retrocalcaneal Bursa

The retrocalcaneal bursa is located immediately superior and deep to the distal insertion of the Achilles tendon on the posterior calcaneus. Ultrasound has been shown to accurately visualize the bursa and guide targeted intervention [20]. One study suggests that merely visualizing the bursa on ultrasound suggests pathology [22]. An anterior to posterior diameter greater than 2.5 mm is generally considered abnormal [15]. The Achilles (retro-Achilles/subcutaneous calcaneal) bursa is larger and located superficial to the Achilles tendon at the same level. Any evidence of fluid here on ultrasound is pathologic.

Scanning Techniques and Anatomy to Identify

Position the patient prone with the ankle and foot hanging off the table edge. Place the transducer in the longitudinal plane directly over the Achilles tendon. Visualize the Achilles tendon, its calcaneal insertion, and Kager's fat pad, which is deep to the tendon immediately proximal to its insertion. The retrocalcaneal bursa sits in between these three structures and is not always visible. Rotate the transducer 90° into the axial plane and identify the aforementioned structures [23]. The fat pad should not be visible since it is directly superior to this viewing level, above the bursa. Moving the transducer superiorly and inferiorly will bring the fat pad and calcaneus into view, respectively (Fig. 7.9).

Injection Technique: In-Plane Axial Approach

Patient positioning: Lay the patient prone with the foot hanging off the table edge.

Probe positioning: Place the probe in the sagittal plane directly midline over the Achilles tendon at its calcaneal attachment. Center the bursa on the screen in the sagittal plane, then rotate into the axial plane. Use Doppler to identify any surrounding blood vessels and use a medial or lateral approach accordingly (Fig. 7.10a).

Markings:

Needle position: Enter the skin in-plane with the transducer from the medial or lateral side.

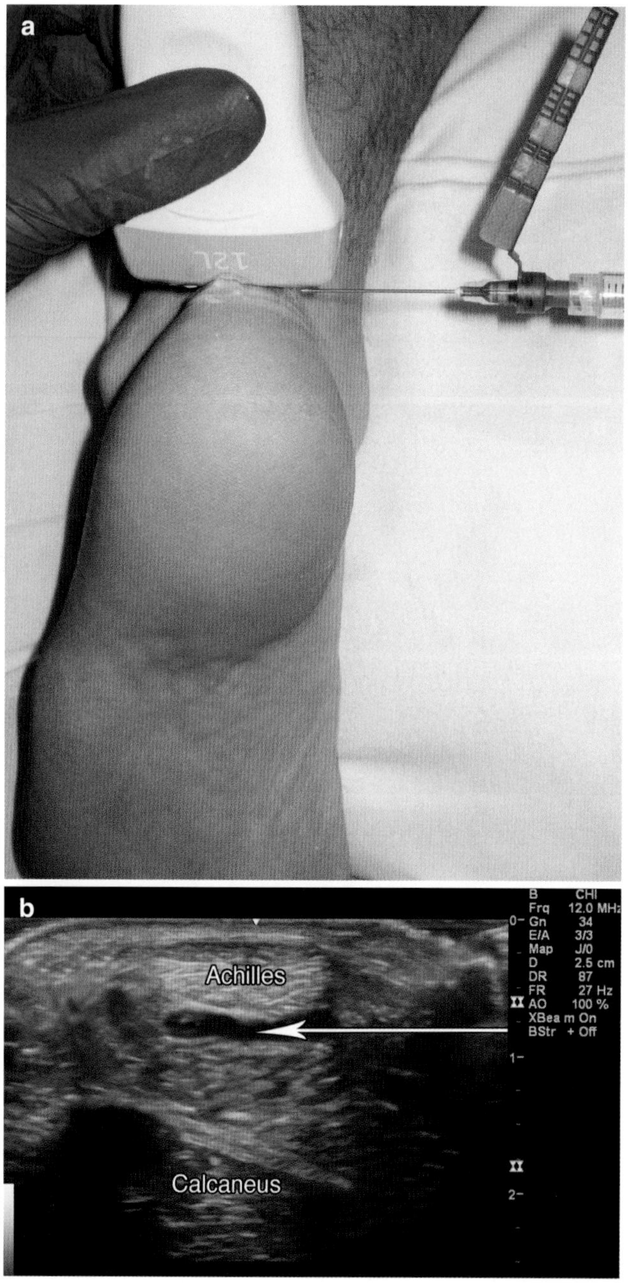

Fig. 7.10 (**a**) Example of axial probe position over retrocalcaneal bursa with in-plane needle position. (**b**) *Arrow* indicates needle trajectory into retrocalcaneal bursitis. Cross section of Achilles labeled. Calcaneus labeled

Safety considerations: Avoid the sural nerve and any obvious vessels with the lateral approach.

Pearls:

- Doppler can also be used to confirm hyperemia within the bursa.

Equipment needed:

- High-frequency linear array transducer
- 25G 1.5″ needle
- 0.5 mL of steroid preparation
- 1–3 mL local anesthetic

Table 7.3 Accuracy of achilles tendon injections

Study – Achilles tendon injection	Author	Accuracy (%)
Ultrasound guided (unblinded)	Reach et al. [2]	100

Achilles Tendon/Paratenon

Ultrasound is useful in identifying small tears, partial ruptures, retrocalcaneal bursitis, and chronic tendinosis [24–26]. Corticosteroid injection is generally not recommended due to the risk of rupture; however, in the setting of acute and/or chronic inflammation, corticosteroid injection to the surrounding paratenon sheath can alleviate symptoms. If symptoms become chronic, dry needling and injection of reparative substances are potential interventions (Table 7.3) [27].

Scanning Techniques and Anatomy to Identify

Position the patient prone with the foot hanging off the end of the examination table. A pillow under the distal tibia can be used for comfort. Scan both views of the tendon from the myotendinous junction to the calcaneus. In the transverse plane, scan on both sides of the tendon to visualize the paratenon envelope or peritendinous sheath [1, 8]. Passive plantar/dorsiflexion may improve visualization of the tendon [28]. Look for the retro-Achilles and retrocalcaneal bursae. Power Doppler settings may be utilized to visualize neovascularization and inflammation [1]. Tendinosis appears as areas of hypoechogenicity with intact fibrillar structure. Thickening of the tendon or a relatively diffuse convex shape at the attachment of the tendon is abnormal [29, 30]. Generally, the injection approach is medial to avoid injuring the sural nerve [31–33]. Alternatively, inject the paratenon at the midportion level (2–6 cm proximal to the Achilles tendon insertion into the calcaneus) (Fig. 7.11) [34].

Injection Technique: In-Plane Sagittal Approach

Patient positioning: Lay the patient prone with foot resting off the end of the table.

Probe positioning: Place the probe in the sagittal plane for initial visualization and scan proximally and distally, looking for focal thickening and/or fluid (Fig. 7.12a). The probe can also be rotated 90° to the axial plane for an in-plane axial approach.

Markings:

Needle position: Enter in-plane, from proximal to distal or distal to proximal, and maintain a shallow trajectory.

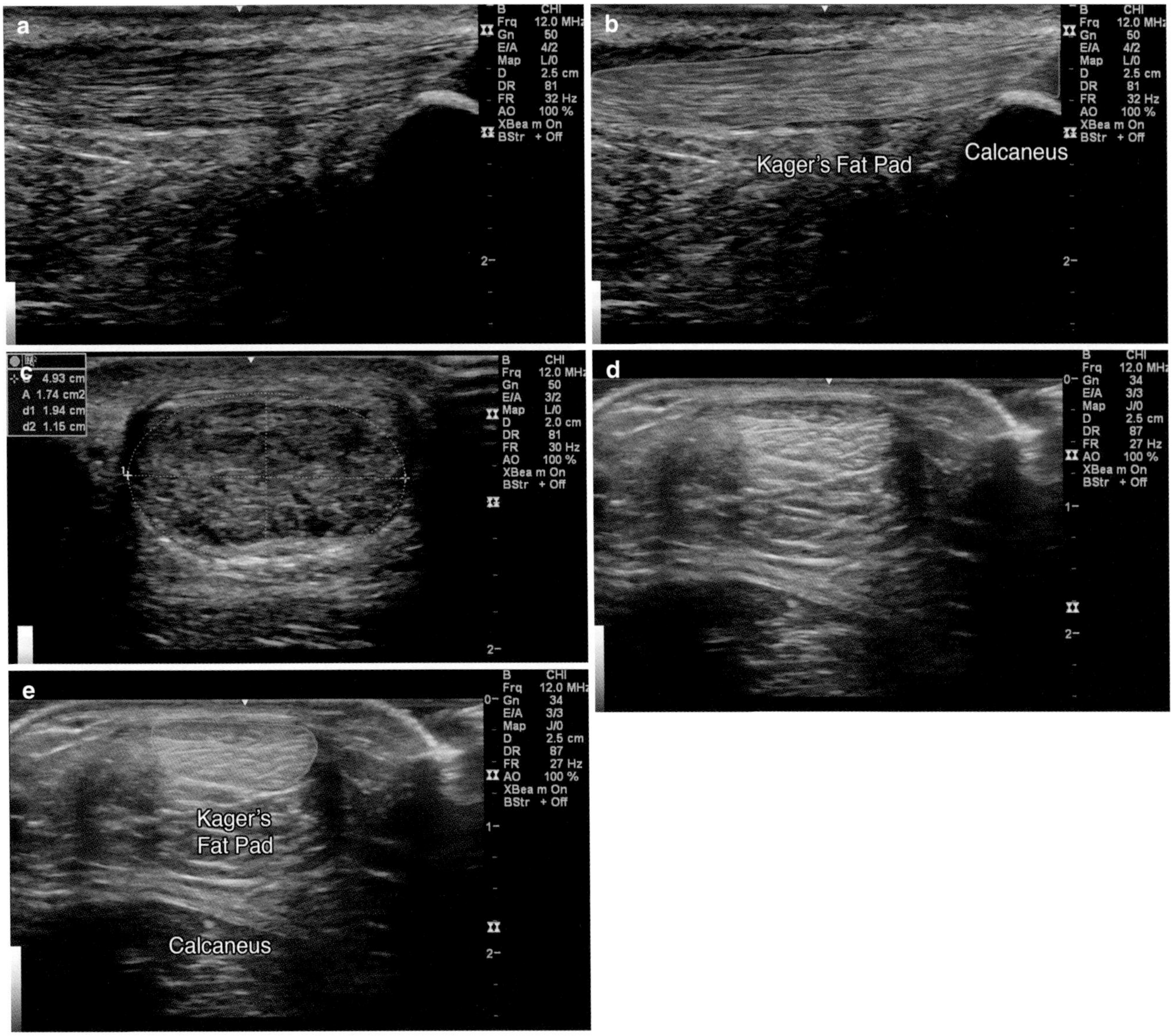

Fig. 7.11 (**a**) Sagittal view of Achilles tendon. (**b**) *Orange* indicates Achilles tendon, Kager's fat pad and calcaneus labeled. (**c**) Axial view of Achilles tendinosis. (**d**) Axial view of Achilles tendon (**e**) *Orange* indicates Achilles tendon. Kager's fat pad and calcaneus labeled

Safety considerations: Approach from medial to lateral to avoid damage to the sural nerve.

Pearls:

- Accurately measuring the depth of the target on the screen is important to maintain the trajectory parallel to the transducer.
- Ankle dorsiflexion stretches the Achilles tendon and may reduce anisotropy [30].
- Power Doppler may also be used to see areas of increased vascularity, representing inflammation [2, 35].

Equipment needed:

- High-frequency linear array transducer
- 25G 1.5″ needle
- 0.5 mL of steroid preparation
- 1–3 mL local anesthetic

Midtarsal Joint (Transverse Tarsal Joint)

The midtarsal or transverse tarsal joint, also known as the Chopart joint, is comprised of articulations between the talonavicular and calcaneocuboid joints. Ligaments that help to stabilize this joint are the dorsal talonavicular, dorsal and plantar calcaneocuboids, spring, and bifurcate ligaments. The spring ligament attaches from the sustentaculum tali of the calcaneus and attaches to the medial and plantar border of the navicular bone, providing strong plantar support for the talar head along with the short and long plantar ligaments (plantar calcaneocuboids and calcaneocuboid metatarsal ligaments, respectively), as well as maintaining the longitudinal arch of the foot [5].

Although injuries to the midtarsal joints are rare with the incidence estimated to be at 3.6 per 1,000,000 year, up to

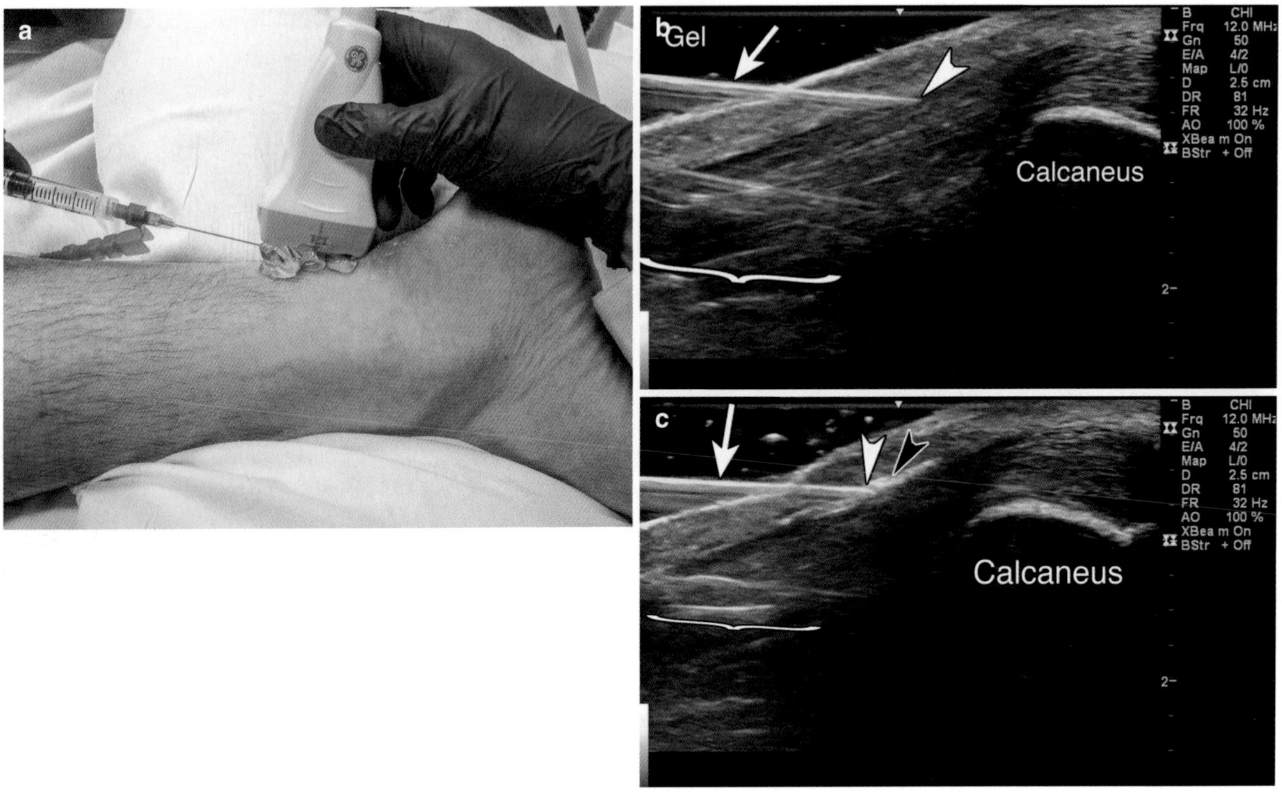

Fig. 7.12 (**a**) Example of sagittal probe position with gel standoff over Achilles tendon with in-plane needle position. (**b**) Example of in-plane injection with *arrowhead* in tendon sheath. *Arrow* indicates needle. Gel shows standoff positioning. *Bracket* indicates needle reverberation. Calcaneus labeled. (**c**) *Black arrowhead* indicates steroid flash within in sheath superficial to the Achilles tendon. *White arrowhead* indicates needle tip. *Arrow* indicates needle. *Bracket* indicates needle reverberation. Calcaneus labeled

41 % of these cases are misdiagnosed, possibly secondary to poor imaging choices [36]. In the detection of midfoot fractures, standard dorsoplantar and oblique radiographic views are reported to have low sensitivities ranging anywhere from 25 to 33 % [37]. In regard to tendinous injuries, insufficiency of the spring ligament is associated with increased risk for development of pes planus and dysfunction of the posterior tibial tendon [38]. Osteoarthritis of the midfoot may occur as a result of aging, trauma, and/or misalignment.

Scanning Techniques and Anatomy to Identify

Place the patient supine with the ipsilateral knee bent so that the foot is resting comfortably on the table. Use the medial and lateral malleoli as starting points for the proximal end of the transducer, and place the distal end sagittal, towards the midfoot. For the talonavicular joint, start at the medial malleolus and slide the transducer anteriorly while identifying the talus, then the navicular bone. For the calcaneocuboid joint, start at the lateral malleolus and slide the transducer anteriorly while identifying the talus, then calcaneus, then cuboid bone (Fig. 7.13).

Injection Technique: In-Plane Axial Approach

Patient positioning: Lay the patient supine with the knee bent and the foot resting comfortably on the table.

Probe positioning: For the talonavicular joint, start with proximal tip over the medial malleolus and the distal tip extending towards the midfoot. Slide distally while identifying the talus, and then the navicular bone. For the calcaneocuboid joint, start with proximal tip over the lateral malleolus and the distal tip extending towards the midfoot. Slide distally while identifying the talus, then calcaneus, then cuboid bone (Fig. 7.14a). Center the joints on the screen and build up adequate gel standoff.

Markings: None.

Needle position: Enter the skin in-plane with the probe, using gel standoff to optimize the trajectory (proximal to distal for the talonavicular joint and distal to proximal for the calcaneocuboid joint).

Safety considerations: Avoid the dorsalis pedis artery by using power Doppler to plan the needle entry point.

Pearls:

- The angle of needle entry must be fairly steep to steer clear of the medial and lateral malleoli. Improve the angle by performing the injection distal to proximal.

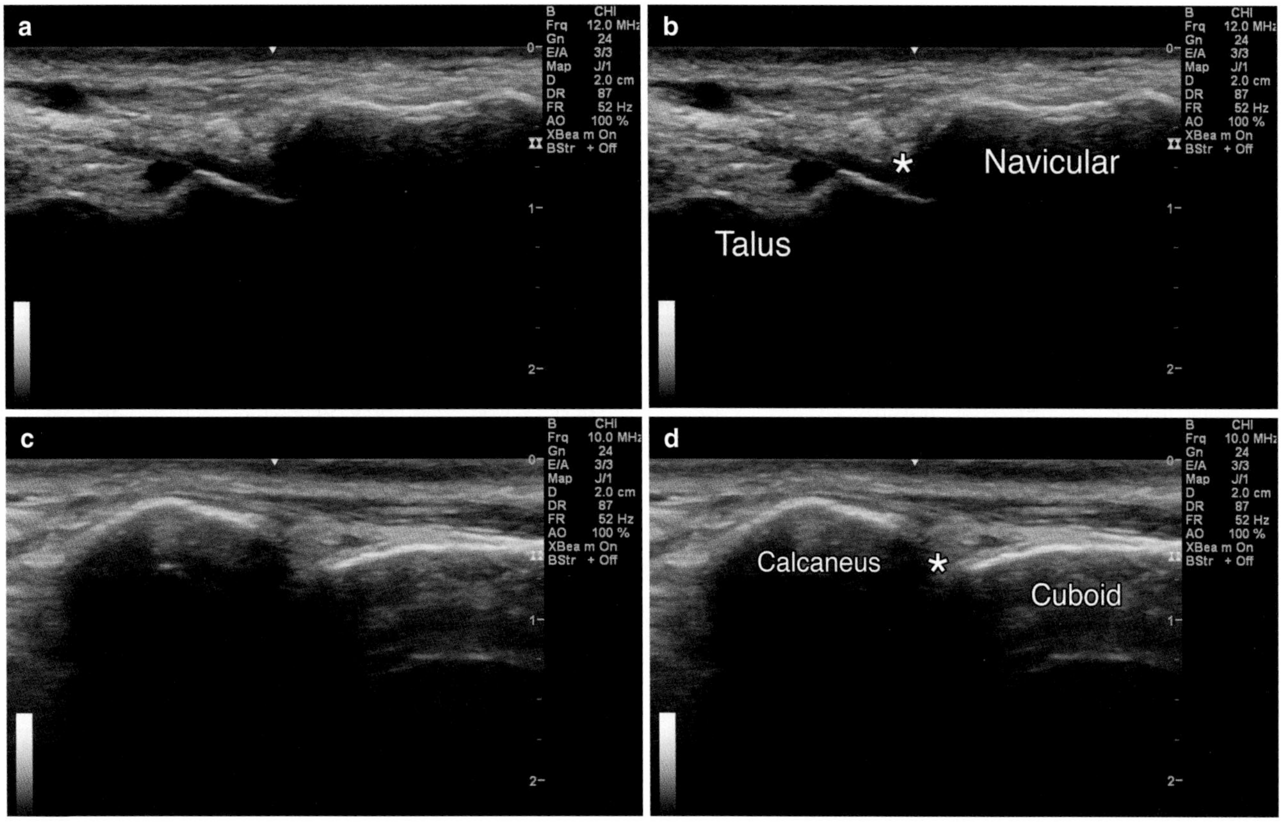

Fig. 7.13 (**a**) Axial view of talonavicular joint. (**b**) *Asterisk* indicates joint space. Talus and navicular labeled. (**c**) Axial view of calcaneocuboid joint. (**d**) *Asterisk* indicates joint space. Calcaneus and cuboid labeled

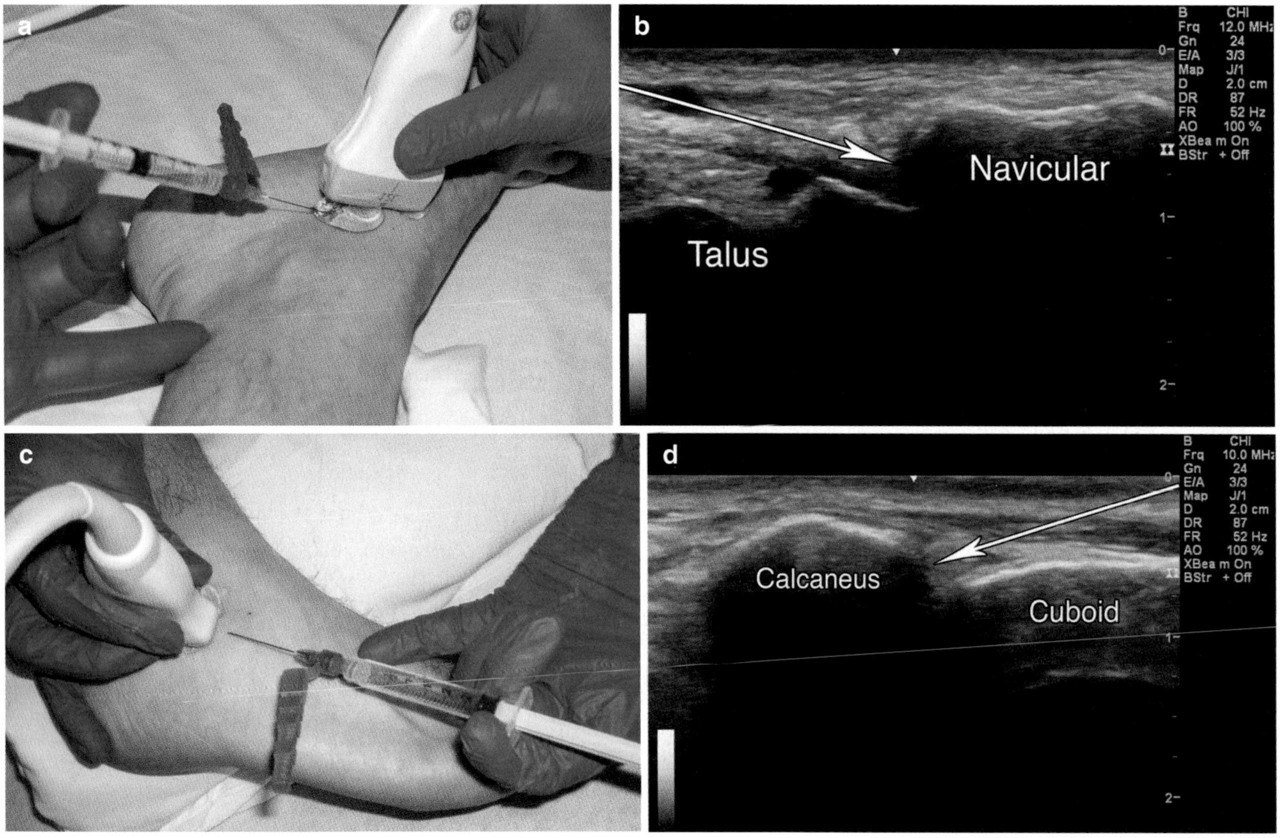

Fig. 7.14 (**a**) Example of axial probe position with gel standoff over talonavicular joint with in-plane needle position. (**b**) *Arrow* indicates needle trajectory into the talonavicular joint. Talus and navicular labeled. (**c**) Example of axial probe position over calcaneocuboid joint with in-plane needle position. (**d**) *Arrow* indicates needle trajectory into the calcaneocuboid joint. Calcaneus and cuboid labeled

Equipment needed:

- High-frequency linear array transducer
- 25G 1.5″ needle
- 0.5 mL of steroid preparation
- 1–3 mL local anesthetic

Morton's Neuroma

Morton's neuroma (interdigital neuroma) is a common cause of forefoot pain and paresthesia, especially in women. It is a nonneoplastic enlargement of the common plantar digital nerve due to trauma, nerve entrapment, endoneurium edema, axonal degeneration, and/or vascular proliferation [30, 39]. The most common site for a Morton's neuroma is the 3rd web space, followed by the 2nd. Mulder's sign, where the examiner places medial and lateral stress compressing the metatarsal heads, displacing a neuroma in the plantar direction, may elicit a palpable click or pain. Ultrasound is both sensitive and specific, diagnosing Morton's neuroma with 95–98 % accuracy [40, 41].

Scanning Techniques and Anatomy to Identify

Place the patient supine with the leg straight and the foot lying comfortably. Position the transducer in the coronal plane, transverse to the metatarsal heads. The neuroma appears as a hypoechoic mass, replacing the normal hyperechoic fat found in the interdigital web space. Masses greater than 5 mm are more likely to be symptomatic [40]. In the sagittal plane, identification of the common plantar digital nerve leading into the neuroma and non-compressibility of the mass both support the diagnosis of neuroma, rather than bursitis (Fig. 7.15) [30].

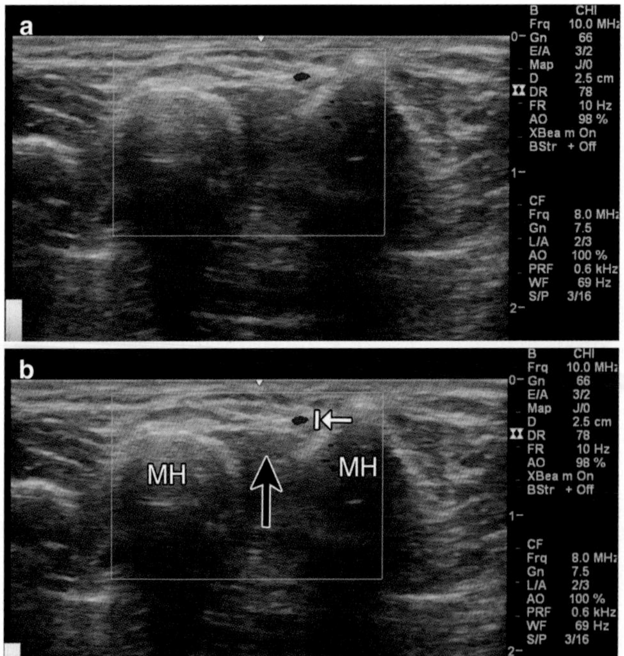

Fig. 7.15 (**a**) Coronal view of Morton's neuroma. (**b**) *Black arrow* indicates location of digital nerve. *White arrow with stop* indicates vasculature. *MH* metatarsal heads

Injection Technique: Out-of-Plane Coronal Approach

Patient positioning: Lay the patient supine with the knee flexed and the foot resting flat on the table.

Probe positioning: Place the probe transversely over the MTP joints. Visualize the neuroma in between the symptomatic MTP joints, and center it on the screen (Fig. 7.16a).

Markings: Identify small arteries.

Needle position: Enter the skin out-of-plane, advancing the needle posteriorly and inferiorly.

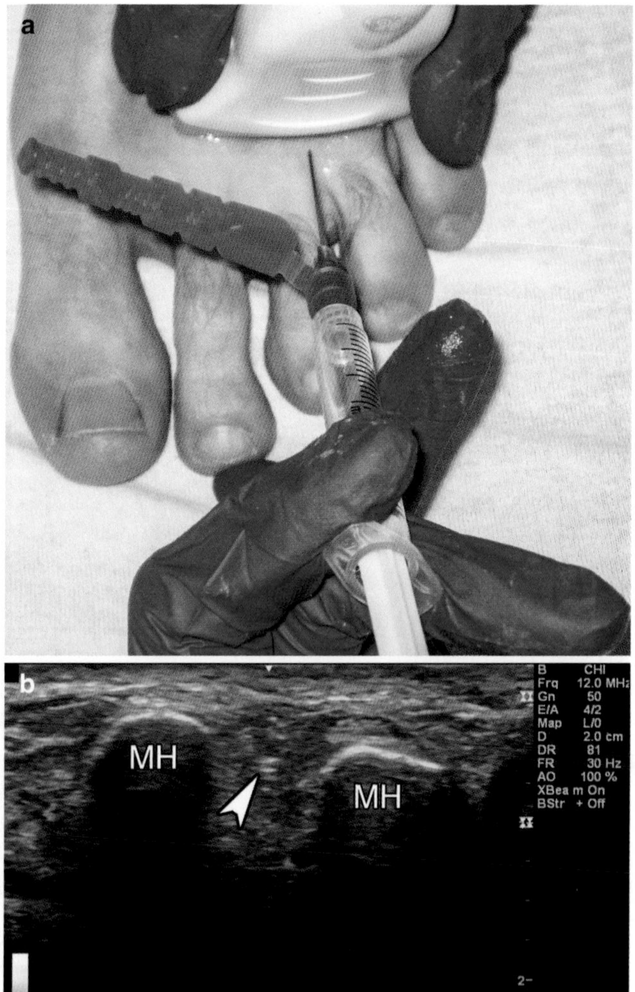

Fig. 7.16 (**a**) Example of coronal probe position over metatarsal heads with out-of-plane needle position. (**b**) Example of out-of-plane injection. *Arrowhead* indicates needle tip, *MH* metatarsal heads

Safety considerations: Advancing too deep can result in perforation of the sole of the foot.

Pearls:

- Power Doppler may be useful in differentiating between symptomatic and noninflamed interdigital neuromas [2].

Equipment needed:

- Medium-frequency linear array transducer (8–12 MHz)
- 22–25G 1.5″ needle
- 0.5 mL of steroid preparation
- 1–3 mL local anesthetic
- 3 mL alcohol or phenol

First Metatarsophalangeal Joint (MTP)

The first metatarsophalangeal (MTP) joint is a common site for forefoot pain. Differential includes gout, osteoarthritis, rheumatoid arthritis (RA), fracture, infection, turf toe, psoriatic arthritis, sesamoiditis, and EHL tendon rupture. Initial treatment includes orthotics with 1st MTP immobilization, rest, ice, compression, elevation (RICE), and activity modification. When pain persists, intra-articular injection of corticosteroid or hyaluronic acid may provide benefit (Table 7.4) [30, 43].

Table 7.4 Accuracy of first metatarsophalangeal joint (MTP) injections

Study – 1st MTP injection	Author	Accuracy (%)
Ultrasound guided (unblinded)	Reach et al. [2]	100
Ultrasound guided (unblinded)	Wempe et al. [42]	100

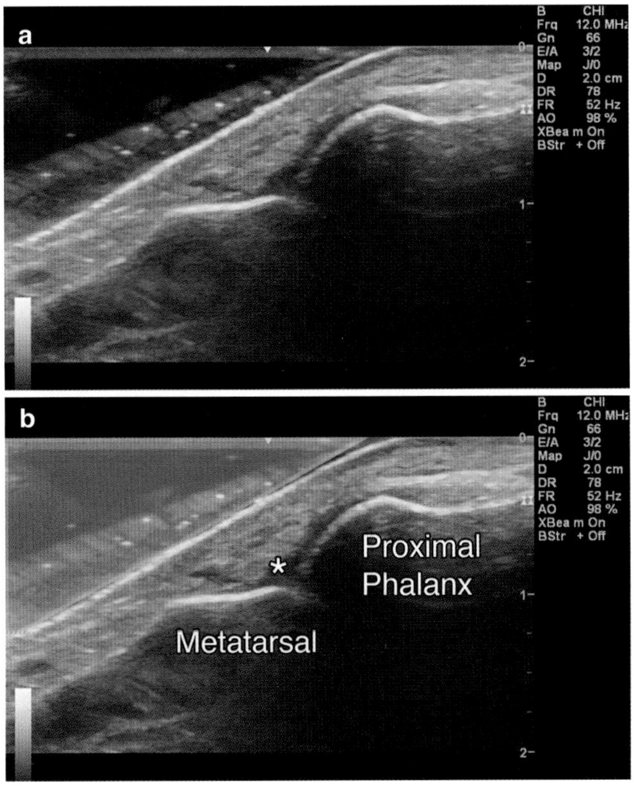

Fig. 7.17 (**a**) Sagittal gel standoff view over MTP joint. (**b**) Teal indicates gel. *Asterisk* indicates joint space. Metatarsal and proximal phalanx labeled

Scanning Technique and Anatomy to Identify

Begin by placing the transducer in the sagittal plane over the EHL tendon. Identify the distal phalanx, proximal phalanx, and 1st metatarsal. Slide the probe medially off of the tendon, and apply light traction and flexion to the toe, further opening up the joint space (Fig. 7.17).

Injection Technique: In-Plane Sagittal Approach

Patient positioning: Place the patient supine with knee flexed. Position the foot so that the forefoot is hanging off the edge, to facilitate manual traction.

Probe positioning: Place the probe in the sagittal plane, just medial to the EHL tendon (Fig. 7.18a).

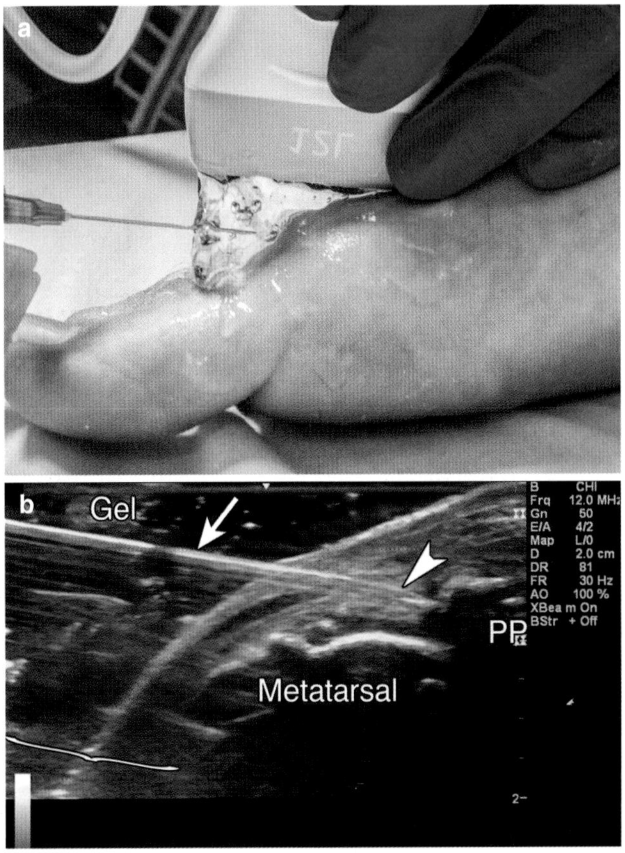

Fig. 7.18 (**a**) Example of sagittal probe position with gel standoff over first MTP joint with in-plane needle position. (**b**) Sagittal gel standoff view of first MTP with *arrowhead* indicating entry into joint. *Arrow* indicates needle. *Bracket* indicates needle reverberation. *PP* proximal phalanx. Metatarsal and gel labeled

Markings: None.

Needle position: Enter the skin in-plane with the transducer, advancing distal to proximal. Maintain a superficial trajectory and use gel standoff for better access.

Safety considerations: Avoid the EHL tendon.

Pearls:

- Applying axial traction may assist in opening up the joint.
- If gout is suspected, consider aspiration and lab work.
- Use a gel standoff to keep the needle parallel to the transducer and facilitate joint entry.

Equipment needed:

- High-frequency linear array transducer
- 25G 1.5″ needle
- 0.5 mL of steroid preparation
- 1–3 mL local anesthetic

Peroneal (Fibular) Tendon Sheath

The peroneus longus runs from the proximal fibula to the base of the first metatarsal and the peroneus brevis from the distal lateral fibula to the fifth metatarsal. Together, they dorsiflex (peroneus longus) and evert (peroneus brevis) the foot at the ankle. Injury to the tendons from repetitive eversion, trauma, or sudden dorsiflexion of the foot can lead to tenosynovitis, subluxation/dislocation, rupture, or chronic tendinopathy. Diagnosis is largely clinical but ultrasound is a useful and expedient alternative to MRI when imaging is indicated [44, 45]. Treatment begins with rest, immobilization, physical therapy, and anti-inflammatory medications. Persistent cases can be treated with injection therapy and surgery. Corticosteroid injections have proven to be useful but must be carefully performed given the close proximity to the sural nerve (Table 7.5) [45, 46].

Table 7.5 Accuracy of peroneal tendon sheath injection

Study – peroneal tendon sheath injection	Author	Accuracy (%)
Palpation	Muir et al. [46]	60
Ultrasound guided	Muir et al. [46]	100

Scanning Techniques and Anatomy to Identify

Lay the patient on their side with the lateral aspect of the affected ankle facing up. A rolled-up towel can be placed under the medial malleolus for comfort. Locate the lateral malleolus and position the transducer in the axial plane posterior to the fibula in the retromalleolar groove, approximately 3–4 cm proximal to the fibular tip. Starting superiorly, the peroneus brevis' muscle belly and tendon will be seen first. More inferiorly, approaching the fibular tip, the peroneus longus tendons may be identified [30, 47]. Follow the tendons in cross section along their course, wrapping around the malleolus. Visualize them just inferior and anterior to the medial malleolus in preparation for injection (Fig. 7.19).

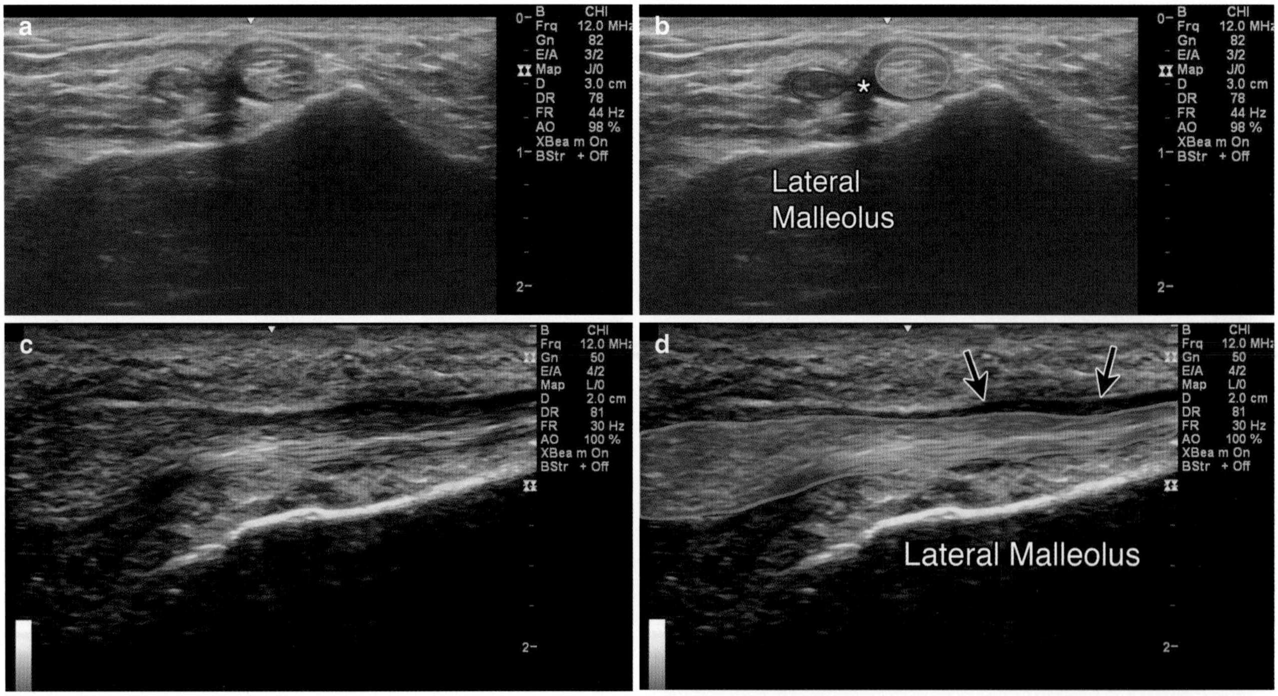

Fig. 7.19 (**a**) Short-axis view of peroneal tendons. (**b**) *Orange* indicates peroneusa brevis. *Asterisk* indicates tenosynovitis. *Purple* indicates peroneus longus. Lateral malleolus labeled. (**c**) Longitudinal view of the peroneus brevis tendon. (**d**) *Orange* indicates peroneus brevis tendon. *Arrows* indicate tenosynovitis. Lateral malleolus labeled

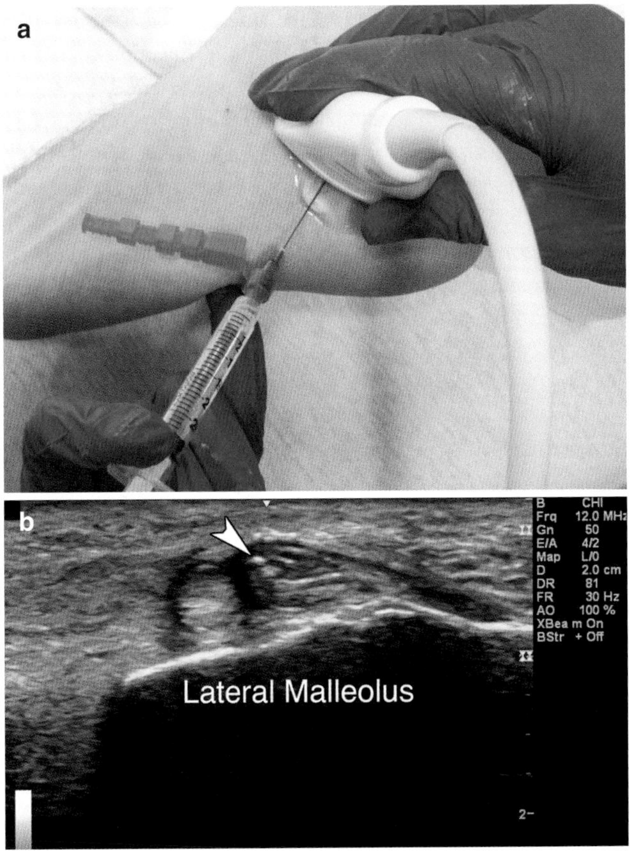

Fig. 7.20 (**a**) Example of short-axis probe position over peroneal tendons with out-of-plane needle position. (**b**) Example of out-of-plane injection. *Arrowhead* indicates needle tip. Lateral malleolus labeled

Injection Technique: Out-of-Plane Short-Axis Approach

Patient positioning: Lay the patient in on their side with the lateral aspect of the affected ankle facing up.

Probe positioning: The probe is placed inferior and anterior to the lateral malleolus, short axis to the tendons (Fig. 7.20a).

Markings:

Needle position: Enter the skin out-of-plane to the probe from either side of it, and advance to the tendon sheath.

Safety considerations: Look for and avoid the sural nerve, although it is not easily visualized.

Pearls:

- To assess for dynamic instability, place the transducer in the axial plane posterior to the distal fibula, and have the patient actively dorsiflex and evert the ankle [30].

Equipment needed:

- Medium-frequency linear array transducer (8–12 MHz)
- 25G 1.5″ needle
- 0.5 mL of steroid preparation
- 1–3 mL local anesthetic

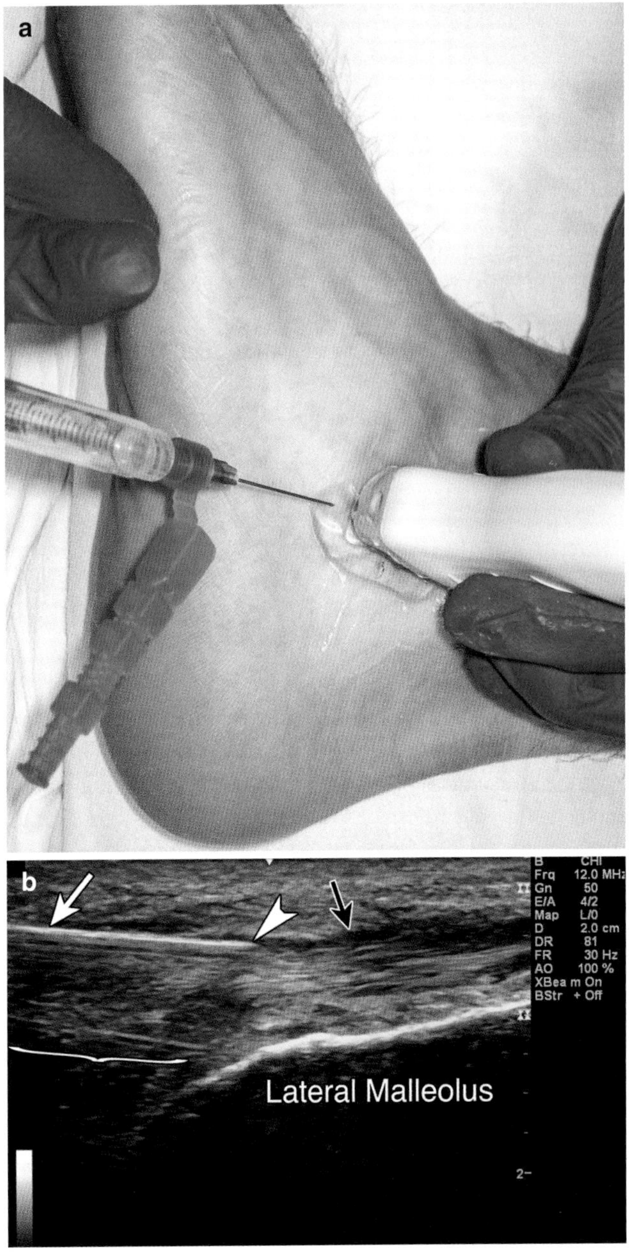

Fig. 7.21 (**a**) Example of longitudinal probe position over peroneal tendons with in-plane needle position. (**b**) Example of in-plane injection. *White arrowhead* indicates needle tip. *White arrow* indicates needle. *Bracket* indicates needle reverberation. *Black arrow* indicates fluid within tendon sheath. Lateral malleolus labeled

Injection Technique: In-Plane Longitudinal Approach

Patient positioning: Lay the patient in on their side with the lateral aspect of the affected ankle facing up.

Probe positioning: The probe is placed inferior and anterior to the lateral malleolus longitudinal to the peroneal tendons (Fig. 7.21a).

Markings:

Needle position: Enter the skin in-plane to the probe from either side of it and advance to the tendon sheath.

Safety considerations: Look for and avoid the sural nerve, although it is not easily visualized.

Pearls:

- To assess for dynamic instability, place the transducer in the axial plane posterior to the distal fibula, and have the patient actively dorsiflex and evert the ankle [30].

Equipment needed:

- Medium-frequency linear array transducer (8–12 MHz)
- 25G 1.5″ needle
- 0.5 mL of steroid preparation
- 1–3 mL local anesthetic

Plantar Fascia (Aponeurosis)

The plantar fascia arises proximally from the medial tuberosity of the calcaneus and attaches distally at the metatarsal heads of the proximal phalanges of the toes. It provides supports for the foot arch and acts as a shock absorber during weight-bearing activities. A 2003 Cochrane review by Crawford and Thomson described the condition as self-limiting, often resolving within a year's time regardless of treatment type [48]. According to another study by Tsai et al., 80–90 % of those affected respond to conservative treatment [49]. Patients who fail conservative measures may benefit from corticosteroid injections, PRP, or dry needling techniques. However, repeated steroid injections to this area can result in plantar fat pad atrophy or spontaneous plantar fascia rupture [26, 49, 50]. Palpation-guided injections are reported to have anywhere from 31 to 35 % treatment success rate [35]. Ultrasound guidance can decrease the risk of complication by guiding the needle along the plantar margin of the fascia and avoiding fat pad injection. In addition, response to injection therapy can be monitored by serial measurements of the plantar fascia [30].

Scanning Techniques and Anatomy to Identify

Lay the patient prone with their feet hanging off the table or at the end of the examination table with a pillow underneath. Place the transducer in the sagittal plane over the plantar aspect of foot at the level of the calcaneal insertion. Here, the width of the fascia may be measured along its whole course, noting areas of thickening. Normal plantar fascia appears echogenic and striated. Hypoechoic thickening (>4 mm) is an abnormal finding that is often seen at the proximal attachment of the fascia on the calcaneus [30, 33]. With the proximal attachment centered on the screen, rotate the probe 90° to visualize the attachment site in the coronal plane in preparation for injection (Fig. 7.22).

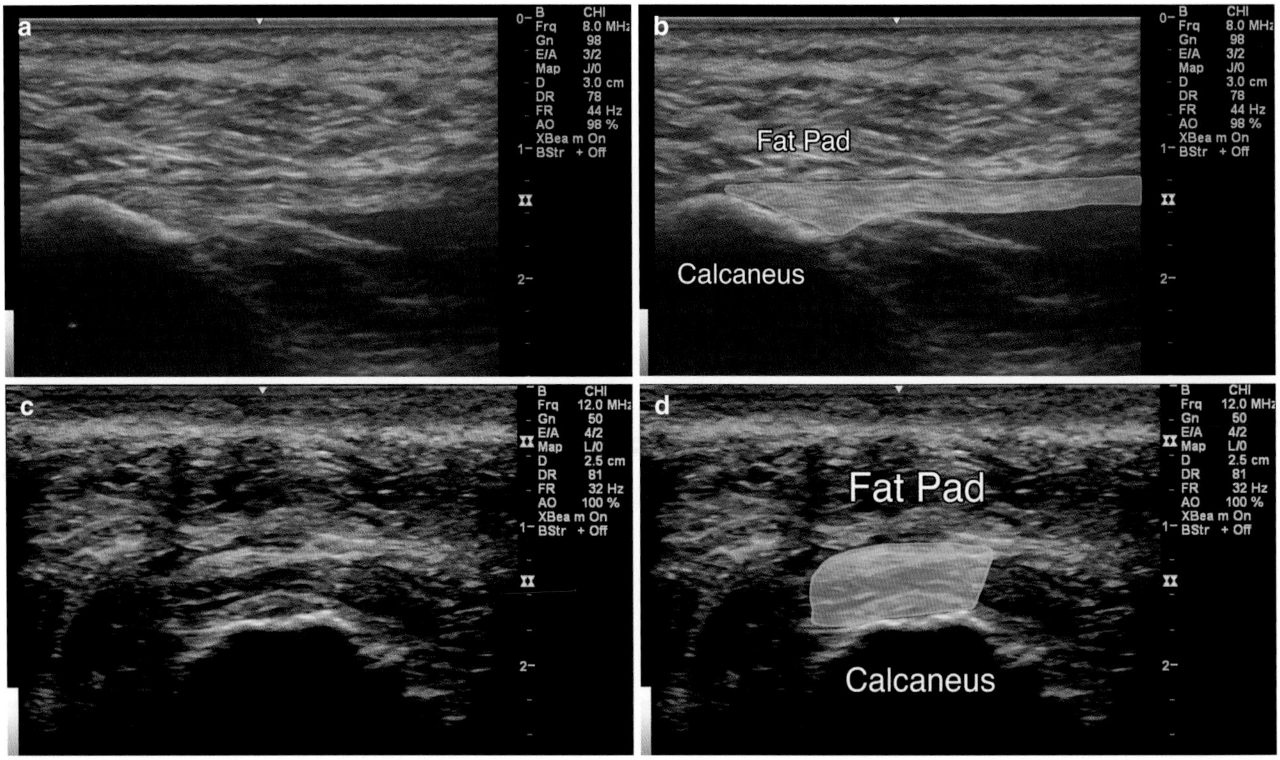

Fig. 7.22 (**a**) Sagittal view of plantar fascia. (**b**) *Green* indicates plantar fascia. Fat pad and calcaneus labeled. (**c**) Coronal view of plantar fascia. (**d**) *Green* indicates plantar fascia. Fat pad and calcaneus labeled

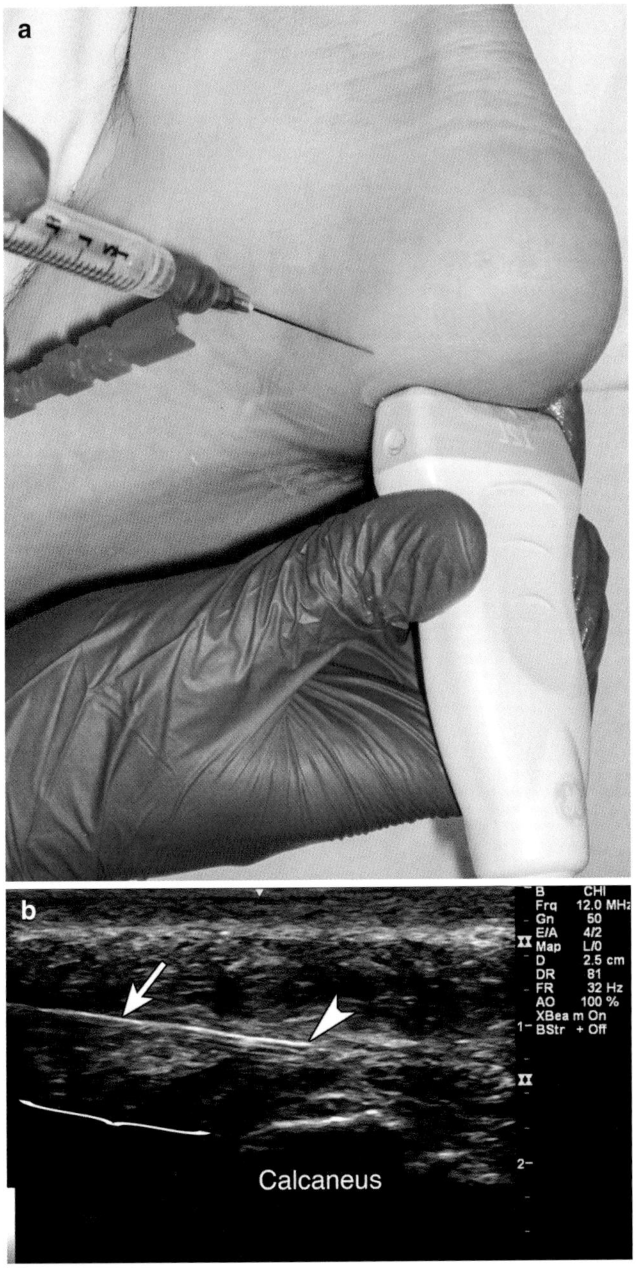

Fig. 7.23 (**a**) Example of coronal probe position over plantar fascia with in-plane needle position. (**b**) Example of in-plane injection. *Arrowhead* indicates needle tip. *Arrow* indicates needle. *Bracket* indicates needle reverberation. Calcaneus labeled

Injection Technique: In-Plane Axial Approach

Patient positioning: Lay the patient prone with the feet hanging over the edge of the table.

Probe positioning: Place the transducer longitudinally over the plantar aspect of foot at the level of the calcaneal insertion. Rotate the probe 90° to visualize the calcaneal attachment in the coronal plane (Fig. 7.23a).

Markings: None.

Needle position: Enter the skin from either the medial or lateral heel, in-plane with the transducer, and guide it to the plantar fascia. Switch to the sagittal plane to visualize the needle out-of-plane, and help guide it to areas of calcification, hypoechogenicity, or thickening. This can be facilitated with a "K" turn, retracting the needle and rotating radially to increase needle coverage without rebreaking skin.

Safety considerations: Avoid injecting the fat pad. When injecting within the fascia, use minimal volume to decrease the risk of rupture.

Pearls:

- With dynamic scanning, active ankle dorsiflexion may help to better visualize the plantar fascia margins.

Equipment needed:

- High-frequency linear array transducer
- 25G 1.5″ needle
- 0.5–1.0 mL of steroid preparation
- 1–3 mL local anesthetic

Tarsal Tunnel Syndrome

The tarsal tunnel is formed by the groove between the posterior calcaneus and medial malleolus. It wraps around the inferior malleolus, following the course of its overlying flexor retinaculum. It contains the tendons of the tibialis posterior, flexor digitorum longus, flexor hallucis longus, and the posterior tibial nerve, artery, and vein. Within the tunnel the posterior tibial nerve bifurcates into the medial and lateral plantar nerves, although this can occur proximal to the tunnel in 5 % of cases [43]. Before the bifurcation, also within the tunnel, the medial calcaneal nerve branches off from the posterior tibial nerve; however, it has been shown to arise from the lateral plantar nerve 25 % of the time [43]. It has also been shown to branch off earlier and bypass the tarsal tunnel superficial to the flexor retinaculum [30]. Ultrasound can be helpful in detecting soft tissue and osseous abnormalities within the tarsal tunnel [51] and is very useful in guiding injections to this crowded region.

Scanning Techniques and Anatomy to Identify

Position the patient on their side with the medial aspect of the affected ankle facing up. Place the probe in the axial plane just superior and posterior to the medial malleolus. From anterior to posterior, identify the tibialis posterior tendon; flexor digitorum tendon; posterior tibial artery, vein, and nerve; and lastly the flexor hallucis longus [34]. The overlying flexor retinaculum should appear hyperechoic and fibrillar. Slide the probe inferiorly and anteriorly following the course of the tunnel while rotating it accordingly to maintain cross-sectional views. Look for the bifurcation into

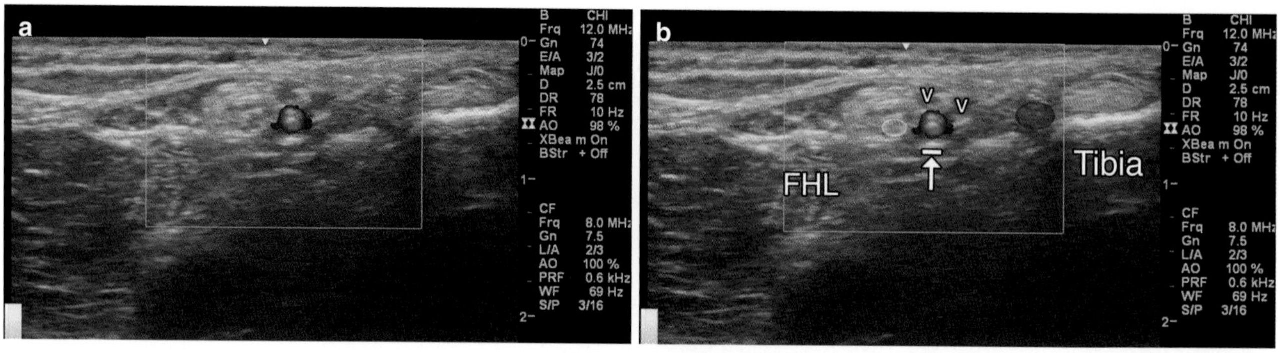

Fig. 7.24 (**a**) Axial view of tarsal tunnel with Doppler utilization. (**b**) *Orange* indicates tibialis posterior tendon. *Purple* indicates flexor digitorum longus. *Arrow with stop* indicates tibial artery adjacent to veins. *Yellow* indicates tibial nerve. *FHL* flexor hallucis longus

the plantar nerves, as well as the emergence of the medial calcaneal nerve. Find the level prior to the bifurcation where the flexor retinaculum is clearly visible, which generally occurs towards the proximal end of the tunnel. Use power Doppler to monitor the vascular distribution in preparation for injection (Fig. 7.24).

Injection Technique: Out-of-Plane Axial Approach

Patient positioning: Lay the patient in the lateral decubitus position with the medial aspect of the ankle facing upwards.

Probe positioning: Place the probe in the axial plane just superior and posterior to the medial malleolus. Slide the probe distally until the flexor retinaculum is clear. Try to stay proximal to the bifurcation of the posterior tibial nerve (Fig. 7.25a).

Markings:

Needle position: Enter the skin out-of-plane with the probe, from either proximal to distal or distal to proximal. Use power Doppler to plan the trajectory towards the nerve while avoiding the vascular structures.

Safety considerations: Avoid the posterior tibial artery and vein.

Pearls:

- Hydrodissection around the nerve is recommended to loosen any adhesions that may be present.

Equipment needed:

- High-frequency linear array transducer
- 25G 1.5″ needle
- 0.5 mL of steroid preparation
- 1–3 mL local anesthetic

Injection Technique: In-Plane Axial Approach

Patient positioning: Lay the patient in the lateral decubitus position with the medial aspect of the ankle facing upwards.

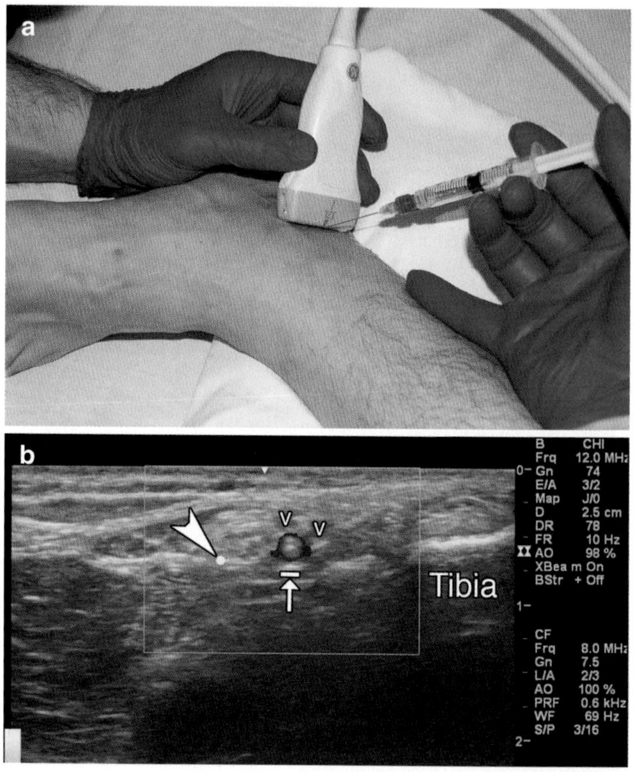

Fig. 7.25 (**a**) Example of axial probe position over tarsal tunnel with out-of-plane needle position. (**b**) Example of out-of-plane injection. *Arrowhead* indicates needle tip. *Arrow with stop* indicates tibial artery. Tibia labeled

Probe positioning: Place the probe in the axial plane just superior and posterior to the medial malleolus. Slide the probe distally until the flexor retinaculum is clear. Try to stay proximal to the bifurcation of the posterior tibial nerve (Fig. 7.26a).

Markings:

Needle position: Enter the skin in-plane with the probe, from anterior to posterior. Use power Doppler to plan the trajectory towards the nerve while avoiding the vascular structures.

Safety considerations: Avoid the posterior tibial artery and vein.

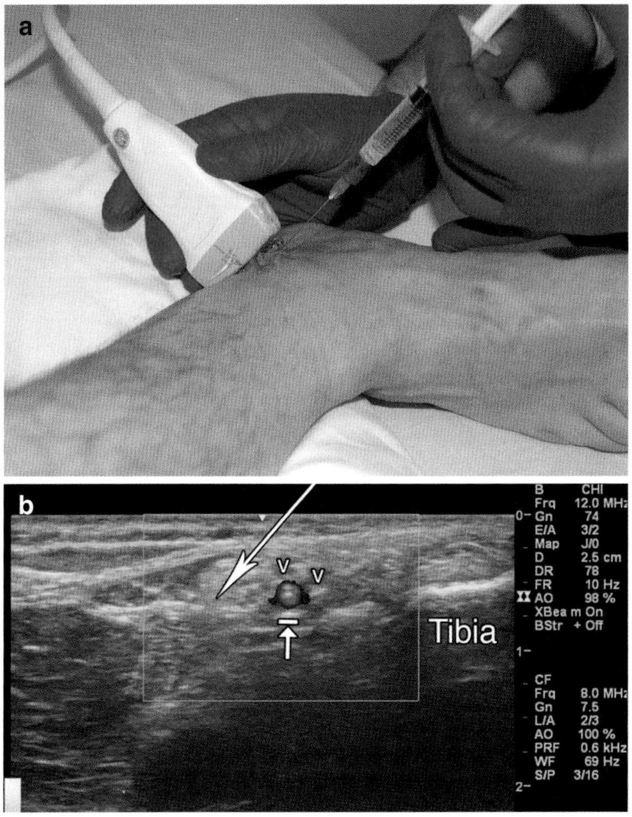

Fig. 7.26 (**a**) Example of axial probe position over tarsal tunnel with in-plane needle position. (**b**) Example of in-plane injection. *Arrow* indicates needle trajectory with gel standoff technique avoiding the medial tendons and vessels. *Arrow with stop* indicates tibial artery. Tibia labeled

Pearls:

- If the medial malleolus is prominent, it may interfere with the needle guidance. In this case rotate the probe so that its anterior edge is just above the malleolus, leaving a clear path.
- Hydrodissection around the nerve is recommended to loosen any adhesions that may be present.

Equipment needed:

- High-frequency linear array transducer
- 25G 1.5″ needle
- 0.5 mL of steroid preparation
- 1–3 mL local anesthetic

References

1. Wang S, Chhem RK, Cardinal E, Cho KH. Joint sonography. Radiol Clin North Am. 1999;37:653–68.
2. Reach J, Easle M, Bavornrit C, Nunley J. Accuracy of ultrasound guided injections in the foot and ankle. Foot Ankle Int. 2009;30(3):239–42.
3. Fessell DP, Jacobson JA, Craig J, et al. Using sonography to reveal and aspirate joint effusions. Am J Roentgenol. 2000;174:1353–62.
4. Wisniewski SJ, Smith J, Patterson DG, Carmichael SW, Pawlina W. Ultrasound-guided versus nonguided tibiotalar joint and sinus tarsi injections: a cadaveric study. PM R. 2010;2(4):277–81.
5. Kirk KL, Campbell JT, Guyton GP, Schon LC. Accuracy of posterior subtalar joint injection without fluoroscopy. Clin Orthop Relat Res. 2008;466:2856–60.
6. Fessell DP, van Holsbeeck M. Foot and ankle sonography. Radiol Clin North Am. 1999;37:831–58.
7. Nazarian LN, Rawool NM, Martin CE, et al. Synovial fluid in the hindfoot and ankle: detection of amount and distribution with ultrasound. Radiology. 1995;197:275–8.
8. Henari S, et al. Ultrasonography as a diagnostic tool in assessing deltoid ligament injury in supination external rotation fractures of the ankle. Orthopedics. 2011;34(10):639–43.
9. Milz P, Milz S, Putz R, Reiser M. 13 MHz high-frequency sonography of the lateral ankle joint ligaments and the tibiofibular syndesmosis in anatomic specimens. J Ultrasound Med. 1996;15(4):277–84.
10. Kraus T, Heidari N, Borbas P, Clement H, Grechenig W, Weinberg AM. Accuracy of anterolateral versus posterolateral subtalar injection. Arch Orthop Trauma Surg. 2011;131(6):759–63.
11. Smith J, Finnoff JT, Henning PT, Turner NS. Accuracy of sonographically guided posterior subtalar joint injections. J Ultrasound Med. 2009;28:1549–57.
12. Campbell DG, Menz A, Isaacs J. Dynamic ankle ultrasonography. A new imaging technique for acute ankle ligament injuries. Am J Sports Med. 1994;22(6):855–8.
13. Colville MR. Surgical treatment of the unstable ankle. J Am Acad Orthop Surg. 1998;6(6):368–77.
14. Stone DA, Abt JP, House AJ, Akins JS, Pederson JJ, Keenan KA, Lephart SM. Local anaesthetics use does not suppress muscle activity following an ankle injection. Knee Surg Sports Traumatol Arthrosc. 2013;21(6):1269–78 [Epub 2012; Apr 7:1–10].
15. Balduini FC, Vegso JJ, Torg JS, et al. Management and rehabilitation of ligamentous injuries to the ankle. Sports Med. 1987;4(5):364–80.
16. Schuberth JM, Collman DR, Rush SM, Ford LA. Deltoid ligament integrity in lateral malleolar fractures: a comparative analysis of arthroscopic and radiographic assessments. J Foot Ankle Surg. 2004;43(1):20–9.
17. Taser F, Shafiq Q, Ebraheim NA. Anatomy of lateral ankle ligaments and their relationship to bony landmarks. Surg Radiol Anat. 2006;28(4):391–7.
18. Siegler S, Block J, Schneck CD. The mechanical characteristics of the collateral ligaments of the human ankle joint. Foot Ankle. 1988;8(5):234–42.
19. Funder V, Jorgensen JP, Andersen A, et al. Ruptures of the lateral ligaments of the ankle. Clinical diagnosis. Acta Orthop Scand. 1982;53(6):997–1000.
20. Checa A, Chun W, Pappu R. Ultrasound-guided diagnostic and therapeutic approach to Retrocalcaneal Bursitis. J Rheumatol. 2011;38(2):391–2.
21. Peetrons P, Creteur V, Bacq C. Sonography of ankle ligaments. J Clin Ultrasound. 2004;32(9):491–9.
22. Mahlfeld K, Kayser R, Mahlfeld A, Grasshoff H, Franke J. Value of ultrasound in diagnosis of bursopathies in the area of the Achilles tendon. Ultraschall Med. 2001;22(2):87–90.
23. Chu NK, Lew HL, Chen CP. Ultrasound-guided injection treatment of retrocalcaneal bursitis. Am J Phys Med Rehabil. 2012;91(7):635–7.
24. Wijesekera NT, et al. Ultrasound guided treatments for chronic Achilles tendinopathy: an update and current status. Skeletal Radiol. 2010;39:425–34.
25. Mitchell AWM, Lee JC, Healy JC. The use of ultrasound in the assessment and treatment of Achilles tendinosis. J Bone Joint Surg Br. 2009;91(11):1405–9.

26. Acevedo JI, Beskin JL. Complications of plantar fascia rupture associated with corticosteroid injection. Foot Ankle Int. 1998;19: 91–7.
27. Gaweda K, et al. Treatment of Achilles tendinopathy with platelet rich plasma. Int J Sports Med. 2010;31:577–83.
28. Jacobsen JA. Fundamentals of musculoskeletal ultrasound. Philadelphia: Elsevier; 2007.
29. Daftary A, Ronald S. Sonographic evaluation and ultrasound-guided therapy of the Achilles tendon. Ultrasound Q. 2009;25(3): 103–10.
30. Park TA, Del Toro DR. The medial calcaneal nerve: anatomy and nerve conduction technique. Muscle Nerve. 1995;18:32–8.
31. Wiegerinck JI, et al. Injection techniques of platelet-rich plasma into and around the Achilles tendon: a cadaveric study. Am J Sports Med. 2011;39(8):1681–6.
32. Öhberg L, Alfredson H. Ultrasound guided sclerosis of neovessels in painful chronic Achilles tendinosis: pilot study of a new treatment. Br J Sports Med. 2002;36:173–5.
33. Chen CK, Lew HL, Chu NC. Ultrasound-guided diagnosis and treatment of plantar fasciitis. Am J Phys Med Rehabil. 2012;91(2): 182–4.
34. De Maeseneer M, Marcelis S, Jager T, et al. Sonography of the normal ankle: a target approach using skeletal reference points. AJR Am J Roentgenol. 2009;192:487–95.
35. Tsai WC, Hsu CC, Chen CP, Chen MJ, Yu TY, Chen YJ. Plantar fasciitis treated with local steroid injection: comparison between sonographic and palpation guidance. J Clin Ultrasound. 2006;34(1):12–6.
36. Richter M, Thermann H, Huefner T, et al. Chopart joint fracture-dislocation: initial open reduction provides better outcome than closed reduction. Foot Ankle Int. 2004;25:340–8.
37. van Dorp KB, de Vries MR, van der Elst M, Schepers T. Chopart joint injury: a study of outcome and morbidity. J Foot Ankle Surg. 2010;49(6):541–5.
38. Melao L, Canella C, Weber M, et al. Ligaments of the transverse tarsal joint complex: MRI-anatomic correlation in cadavers. AJR Am J Roentgenol. 2009;193:662–7.
39. Shapiro PP, Shapiro SL. Sonographic evaluation of interdigital neuromas. Foot Ankle Int. 1995;16:604–6.
40. Hughes RJ, Ali K, Jones H, Kendall S, Connell DA. Treatment of Morton's neuroma with alcohol injection under sonographic guidance: follow-up of 101 cases. AJR Am J Roentgenol. 2007;186: 1535–9.
41. Quinn TJ, Jacobson JA, Craig JG, van Holsbeeck MT. Sonography of Morton's neuromas. AJR Am J Roentgenol. 2000;174: 1723–8.
42. Wempe MK, Sellon JL, Sayeed YA, Smith J. Feasibility of first metatarsophalangeal joint injections for sesamoid disorders: a cadaveric investigation. PM R. 2012;6:1–5.
43. Havel PE, Ebraheim NA, Clark SE. Tibial branching in the tarsal tunnel. Foot Ankle. 1988;9:117–9.
44. Grant TH, Kelikian AS, Jereb SE, McCarthy RJ. Ultrasound diagnosis of peroneal tendon tears. A surgical correlation. J Bone Joint Surg Am. 2005;87(8):1788–94.
45. Karageanes SJ, Sharp K. Peroneal tendon sheath injuries and treatment and management. Wed Md. 2011. Available at: http://emedicine.medscape.com/article/91344-overview. Accessed on April, 2012.
46. Muir JJ, Curtiss HM, Hollman J, Smith J, Finnoff JT. The accuracy of ultrasound-guided and palpation-guided peroneal tendon sheath injections. Am J Phys Med Rehabil. 2011;90(7):564–71.
47. Sofka CM, et al. Sonographic evaluation and sonographic-guided therapeutic options of lateral ankle pain: peroneal tendon pathology associated with the presence of an os peroneum. HSS J. 2010;6: 177–81.
48. Crawford F, Thomson C. Interventions for treating plantar heel pain. Cochrane Database Syst Rev [Internet]. 2003 [cited 2013 Jan]. Available from: http://onlinelibrary.wiley.com/doi/10.1002/14651858.CD000416/abstract;jsessionid=F30B77D4AC98A79B9A0BD0DD497B0AA0.d03t04.
49. Tsai WC, Wang CL, Tang FT, Tsu T-C, Hsu K-H, Wong M-K. Treatment of proximal plantar fasciitis with ultrasound-guided steroid injection. Arch Phys Med Rehabil. 2000;81:1416–21.
50. Sellman JR. Plantar fascia rupture associated with corticosteroid injection. Foot Ankle Int. 1994;15:376–81.
51. Nagaoka M, Matsuzaki H. Ultrasonography in tarsal tunnel syndrome. J Ultrasound Med. 2005;24:1035–40.

Trigger Point Injections

8

Stephen Nickl and Lauren M. Terranova

Myofascial pain syndrome (MPS) as defined by Travell and Simons is characterized by trigger points (TrP), limited ROM of the affected muscle(s), and neurologic symptoms (autonomic, proprioceptive) [1, 2]. The diagnosis of MPS is based on the presence of 1 or more trigger points. Trigger points (TrP) can be latent or active [1]. Latent TrP are associated with stiffness and restricted ROM but no pain unless palpated. Active TrP produce a referred pain pattern specific to that muscle spontaneously and when the TrP is palpated. The physical findings for diagnosis of a myofascial trigger point are (1) palpation of a tender nodule in a taut band, (2) a referred pain pattern specific for the muscle, (3) a local twitch response (LTR) with snapping palpation or triggering with needle, and (4) restricted ROM [2].

Pathophysiology of Trigger Points

The pathophysiology behind the TrP is becoming clearer. Shah summarizes the current concept well stating that active TrP "are a source of ongoing peripheral nociception that may induce central sensitization." [3] In 1999, Simons presented the "integrated hypothesis" which involves (1) problems with biomechanics, (2) development of trigger points, and (3) sensitization of the spinal cord [4]. It states that trigger points are initiated by biomechanical factors, resulting in local muscle injury in the form of trigger points. These tender taut bands are associated with increased motor end plate activity and focal hypertonicity [5, 6]. This process leads to increased energy demand from the taut band producing "a local energy crisis." This energy crisis leads to ischemia and the release of noxious substances. It was not until Shah in 2005, using a microdialysis needle, revealed that substance P, calcitonin gene-related peptide (CGRP), bradykinin, 5-hydroxytryptophan (5-HT), norepinephrine, TNF-alpha, and interleukin-1beta were elevated in the active TrP of patients with MPS confirming Simons' "Integrated hypothesis." [7–9] Additionally, CGRP is specifically associated with increased end plate activity which supports studies conducted by Hubbard and Simons using electromyography [5, 6]. The sustained nociceptive activity caused by the trigger point leads to sensitization of the dorsal horn. This results in allodynia and hyperalgesia, the hallmarks of central sensitization [10, 11]. Wide dynamic range (WDR) neurons in the dorsal horn become sensitized which may explain the referred pain patterns, autonomic symptoms, and activation of the limbic system [11–13]. Woolf suggests that injury to any body part can lead to central sensitization [11]. The treatment should focus on treating the trigger point and turning off the nociceptive input. Many physicians feel that if the sources of the biomechanical maladaptations (i.e., spinal stenosis, radiculopathy, zygapophysial joint arthropathy, scoliosis, tendinopathy, osteoarthritis) are treated correctly, the trigger points will resolve. Simons and Travell, however, believe MPS is an entity within itself and specific to muscle.

Treatments for Myofascial Pain Syndrome

Over the years a variety of different methods have been used to treat trigger points, which can be broken down into four major subgroups: manual techniques, modalities, medications, and needle intervention. Manual techniques are used extensively by therapists, physiatrists, and osteopathic physicians. These techniques include the spray and stretch with ethyl chloride, post isometric relaxation (PIR) or muscle energy, strain-counterstrain, deep-stroking massage, and trigger point pressure release [1, 14, 15]. Modalities include the use of transcutaneous electrical nerve stimulator, ultrasound, and laser therapy as an adjunctive therapy in the treatment of MPS [16].

S. Nickl, DO (✉) • L.M. Terranova, MD, DO
Department of Rehabilitation Medicine,
Icahn School of Medicine at Mount Sinai,
New York, NY, USA
e-mail: snickl1372@gmail.com; terranova.lauren@gmail.com

D.A. Spinner et al. (eds.), *Atlas of Ultrasound Guided Musculoskeletal Injections*, Musculoskeletal Medicine,
DOI 10.1007/978-1-4614-8936-8_8, © Springer Science+Business Media, LLC 2014

Medications used to treat MPS include muscle relaxants, benzodiazepines, neuropathic agents, topical analgesics, and NSAIDS. Annaswamy in 2011 did a thorough literature review of the medications that are used to treat MPS [16]. The muscle relaxants cyclobenzaprine and tizanidine, though widely used, lack high-quality randomized controlled trials (RCT) to support their efficacy. Benzodiazepines, specifically clonazepam and diazepam, have RCT studies that strongly support their use [16]. Neuropathic agents include tricyclic antidepressants (TCAs) (amitriptyline) and anticonvulsants (gabapentin and pregabalin). There are two RCT trials that support the use of amitriptyline, but there are no RCT studies that support the use of gabapentin or pregabalin. Topical analgesics are widely used to treat generalized musculoskeletal pain. The most common analgesic medications (lidocaine, methyl salicylate, and diclofenac) all have at least 1 RCT that shows some support for their use in MPS. NSAIDs are common first-line agents used to treat musculoskeletal pain. Overall there is scarcity of any research about the efficacy of NSAIDs in MPS. In one RCT, ibuprofen proved to be beneficial in pain reduction in combination with diazepam when compared to diazepam alone [16].

Needle interventions include dry needling and wet needling, i.e., injection. Lewit was the first to document the "needle effect," which is the immediate analgesia after dry needling the TrP [17]. He also relates that the pain intensity produced by needling the TrP was directly related to the success of treatment and as a sign of precision. Hong had similar results but in addition he stated that "it is essential to elicit a local twitch response (LTR) during injection to obtain an immediately desirable effect." [18] Many high-quality RCT studies have found no significant difference between dry needling, injections with lidocaine, injection with normal saline, and injection with steroid, supporting the theory that needling of the trigger point alone is sufficient to reduce pain and increase ROM [16, 18–20]. Some authors still prefer to use lidocaine with TrP injections as it leads to less postinjection pain [2, 18]. After injection many clinicians will pepper the area "in a fanlike manner or in a full circle" to ensure the trigger is adequately deactivated [2]. To obtain a long-lasting effect, the patient may need several injections into the trigger point over a few weeks time [2]. The other major agent used for injection is botulinum toxin (BTX) which several studies have shown to be no more effective than bupivacaine, dry needling, or saline [19, 21, 22].

To avoid causing excessive trauma to the muscle, a 25 g needle is recommended for injections with lidocaine. To reach deep muscles like the quadratus lumborum, a 22 g spinal needle may be indicated. If dry needling, a solid bore needle would cause less trauma than a hypodermic one.

Ultrasound Identification of Trigger Points

A number of recent articles support the use of ultrasound (US) for guiding trigger point injections. The benefits include the following: (1) prevent complications by avoiding nerves, vessels, and viscera; (2) increase accuracy (and efficacy) of trigger point injections; and (3) aid in recognition and treatment of trigger points in deep muscles.

Botwin documented the use of ultrasound guidance for TrP injections in the cervicothoracic region to increase accuracy and to prevent complications, such as pneumothorax [23]. Rha demonstrated that ultrasound is useful in detecting local twitch response in deep back musculature, but they did not describe the appearance of the trigger point [24]. Sikdar and Ballyns documented that (1) TrP appeared as focal, hypoechoic regions on 2-D ultrasound, (2) TrP are firmer than the surrounding muscle with vibration sonoelastography, and (3) active TrP have a highly resistive vascular bed by Doppler [25–27]. Contrary to Sikdar and Ballyns' description of the TrP as hypoechoic, Shankar in a case report found that TrP in the trapezius and supraspinatus appeared as localized areas of hyperechogenicity [28]. Shankar postulates that the difference is secondary to the low-frequency, curved array transducer used by Sikdar in his studies, but Sikdar reports using a linear array transducer. Shanker reports that the earliest report of the TrP US appearance was by Gerwin in 1997, who described it as hyperechoic [29]. In a letter, Niraj describes trigger points as a "mixed echoic area" in the rectus abdominis [30]. It appears that the ultrasound appearance of trigger points is still under dispute.

The Ballyns study was conducted at the Rehabilitation Medicine Department of the National Institute of Health and Clinical Research Center and clearly has the strongest data. It has the largest sample size, utilized secondary imaging techniques to help quantify muscle (vibration sonography and Doppler), and used a pressure algometer to determine pain thresholds. Their description of TrP using 2-D gray scale ultrasonography is likely the most accurate. Nonetheless, even Ballyn when describing the appearance used the modifier "typically" in the description of the trigger point (Table 8.1). Some questions still need to be answered. Is the echogenic appearance of TrP a continuum? Is it related to the severity of the trigger point? Is it related to the specific muscle, i.e., trapezius or rectus abdominis? Is it related to the proximity of the trigger point to the myotendinous junction?

Trapezius Muscle

The trapezius muscle is composed of three main parts: upper, middle, and lower [31]. Each part has a different function and fiber direction. The trapezius is innervated by cranial nerve

Table 8.1 Ultrasound appearance of trigger points by study

Study	Sample size	Transducer/US system	TrP ultrasound appearance
Sikdar et al. [27]	9	Linear array12–5 MHz (Philip iU22 clinical US system with L12–5 transducer)	"Focal hypoechoic (darker) areas with heterogeneous echotexture"
Ballyns et al. [25]	44	Linear array12–5 MHz (Philip iU22 clinical US system with L12–5 transducer)	"Typically, trigger points appear as focal hypoechoic (darker) areas with a heterogeneous echo texture"
Niraj et al. [30]	10	High-resolution linear array 12–7 MHz (Sonosite S-Nerve US system)	"Mixed echoic area"

XI (accessory nerve) and by C2–C4 cervical nerves. The function of the upper trapezius is to rotate the clavicle at the sternoclavicular joint, move the scapula obliquely upward, and rotate the glenoid cavity inferiorly. The middle trapezius retracts the scapula medially. The lower trapezius stabilizes the scapula and moves it medially and downward. According to Travell and Simons, trigger points in the upper trapezius are activated by everyday activities that involve sustained elevation of the shoulders such as painting, playing a musical instrument, holding a telephone without elbow support, and typing on a computer without armrests [2]. Other events that can also lead to generation of trapezius trigger points include whiplash, tight bra straps, heavy over the shoulder bags, or trauma. Travell and Simmons identified six trigger points in the trapezius muscle [2]. Two are located in the upper part, two in the middle part, and two in the lower part. The trigger points in the superior part refer pain over the posterior aspect of the neck and along the temporal and periarticular areas. The trigger points in the middle trapezius refer pain along the paraspinal area. In the inferior trapezius, pain is referred over the mastoid, behind the neck, and between the scapula.

Scanning Techniques and Anatomy to Identify: Upper Trapezius

The superior fibers of the trapezius originate at the occipital bone and cervical spinous processes via the nuchal ligament and insert on the lateral third of the clavicle forming the anterior margin of the trapezius. The fibers of anterior margin of the trapezius run obliquely inferior and lateral towards the posterior border of the lateral third of the clavicle [31]. Deep to the anterior margin is the supraclavicular fossa. This region is dangerous to inject due to the presence of many important life-sustaining nerves, vessels, and viscera. In the supraclavicular fossa are the subclavian artery and vein, brachial plexus, phrenic nerve, and apex of the lung.

With the patient either seated or prone, identify the trigger point by palpation. Place the probe along the posterior portion of the upper trapezius. Scan over the trigger point and identify it by US. The most superficial layer of muscle is the trapezius. When injecting the superior trap, the trajectory of the needle is dependent on the location. If along the far lateral region, a posterior to anterior trajectory will avoid the supraclavicular fossa entirely. If injecting more medially, a flat medial to lateral trajectory will avoid all other structures unless a long needle is used. Use the Doppler to identify any veins or arteries. Ribs, clavicle, and scapula are easily identifiable as hyperechoic.

Scanning Techniques and Anatomy to Identify: Middle Trapezius

The middle fibers of the trapezius originate from the aponeurosis at the level of the T1–T4 spinous processes and insert onto the acromion and the scapular spine. The middle trapezius can be divided into the lateral (scapular) region and the medial (rhomboid) region.

The lateral region is defined by scapula being deep to the trapezius. With the ultrasound probe parallel and superior to the scapular spine, the layers of tissue from superficial to deep are skin/subcutaneous fat, trapezius muscle, supraspinatus muscle, and the blade of scapula. The only vessels and nerve to be concerned with are the suprascapular artery, vein, and nerve as they pass through the suprascapular notch. This region is safer for injection since the lung is protected by the scapula (Fig. 8.1).

The medial region lies between the medial border of the scapula and the T1–T4 spinous processes. With the ultrasound probe oriented either transverse or longitudinal to the fibers of the trapezius, the layers of tissue of superficial to deep are the subcutaneous fat, trapezius muscle, rhomboid minor or levator scapulae, serratus posterior superior, erector spinae muscles, and ribs. The spinal accessory nerve (SAN) runs deep to the trapezius but superficial to the rhomboids and levator scapulae. The SAN runs inferior parallel to the spinous processes and medial to the medial border of the scapula. The SAN can be identified by turning on the Doppler and locating the superior branch of the transverse cervical artery and veins which run adjacent to the SAN. The SAN is about 1 mm in diameter and is monofascicular by ultrasound [32]. Deep to the rhomboids and levator scapulae but superficial to the serratus posterior superior and erector spinae muscle run the dorsal scapular nerve and the deep branch of the transverse cervical artery (Dorsal scapular artery) along the medial border of the scapula. Risk of pneumothorax is small due to thickness of the musculature in this region. Nonetheless, the ribs are easily identified by US as hyperechoic.

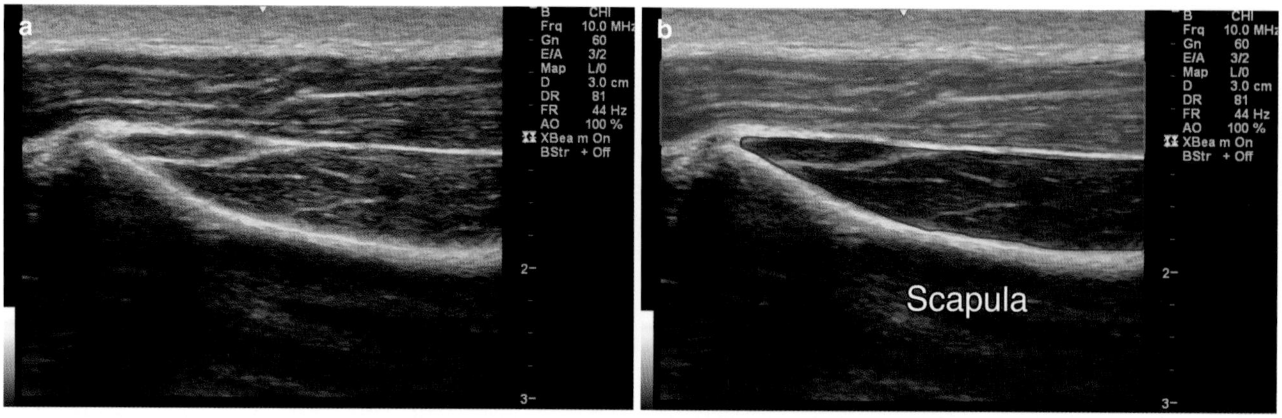

Fig. 8.1 (**a**) Coronal view of upper trapezius muscle. (**b**) *Orange* indicates trapezius muscle, *purple* indicates supraspinatus muscle, scapula labeled

Scanning Techniques and Anatomy to Identify: Lower Trapezius

The lower fibers of the trapezius originate from the T5 to T12 spinous processes and insert onto the inferior portion of scapular spine. Similar to the middle trapezius, the lower trapezius can be divided into a lateral and medial region.

The lateral region is defined by the presence of the scapula deep to all tissues. This region occupies a small area inferior to the scapular spine. Place the US probe parallel and inferior to the scapular spine. The layers of tissue from superficial to the deep are the subcutaneous fat, the trapezius, the infraspinatus, and the blade of the scapula. Again, much like the lateral region of the middle trapezius, this region is safe to inject, as there are no major nerves or vessels and the scapula protects the lung.

The medial region spans quite a distance from T5 to T12. In the majority of this region, the rhomboid major muscle lies deep to the trapezius except in the more inferior portion where the erector spinae or the latissimus dorsi may lie deep. The SAN and associated vessels are less easily identified, as this is where they terminate.

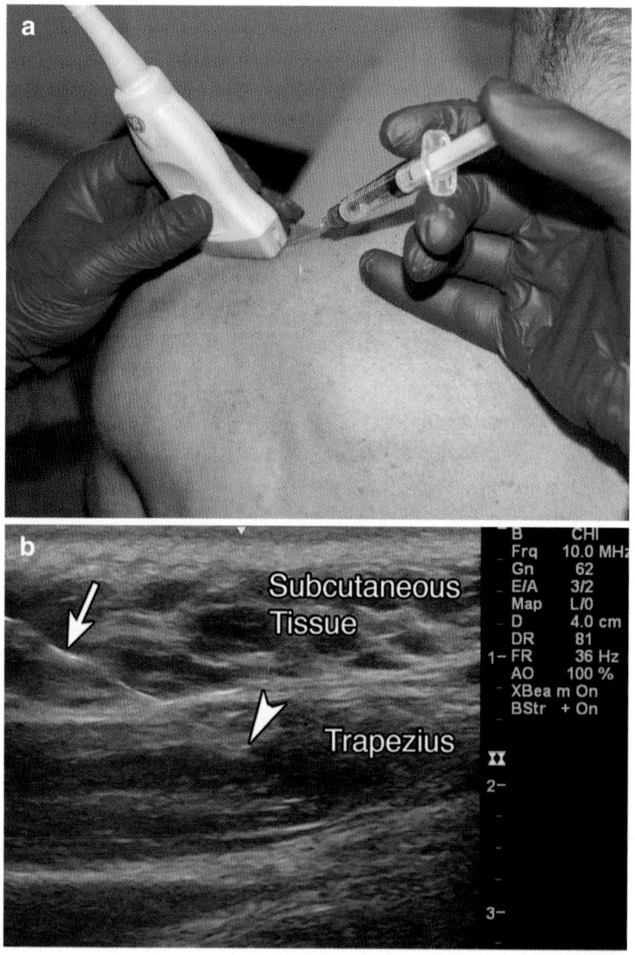

Fig. 8.2 (**a**) Example of coronal probe position over upper trapezius muscle with in-plane needle position. (**b**) Example of in-plane approach, *arrowhead* indicates needle tip, *arrow* indicates needle, subcutaneous tissue and trapezius labeled

Injection Technique: In-Plane Longitudinal Approach

Patient positioning: The patient should lie in the prone position for the lower and middle trapezius and either prone or seated for the upper trapezius.

Probe positioning: Place the probe over the trigger point either transverse or longitudinal to the muscle fibers (Fig. 8.2a).

Markings: When injecting the superior trapezius, use the color Doppler to identify the subclavian artery and vein in the supraclavicular fossa and the superficial branch of the transverse cervical artery, which lies in the fascia deep to the medial trapezius and superficial to all other musculature. The apex of the lung is approximately 2.5 cm above the medial third of the clavicle at the level of the anterior border of the SCM [31].

Needle position: The needle should be inserted parallel to the transducer for optimal visualization, with simultaneous injection of local anesthetic.

Safety considerations: There is a risk of the following: prolonged bleeding, infection, allergic reaction, increased pain and spasm, decreased functional scores, and pneumothorax.

Pearls:

- Avoid pneumothorax by identifying the hyperechoic ribs and pleura between the individual ribs.
- Use Doppler to identify vessels to avoid intravascular injection.
- If the taut band rolls under the needle, anchor the trigger point along its length with fingers or thumb to prevent rolling.
- If a referred pain pattern and local twitch response were elicited prior to injection, then once the needle enters the trigger point they should occur again.
- Postinjection it is important to have the patient actively stretch each muscle injected through its full range of motion.

Equipment needed:

- High-frequency linear array transducer (10 MHz+)
- 25G 1.5″ needle
- 1–3 ml local anesthetic

Scalenus Anterior

The muscles that lie directly lateral to the cervical vertebral column are the scalenes. In total there are four scalenus muscles: anterior, medius, posterior, and minimus. Trigger points in the scalenes can cause shoulder, back, or arm pain. These trigger points can be activated by pulling, lifting, coughing, musculoskeletal asymmetry, or anything that causes a disturbance in gait [4]. Contraction of the anterior and middle scalene elevates the first rib and flexes the head ipsilaterally. Activation of the posterior scalene elevates the second rib and flexes the neck ipsilaterally. These muscles also assist during respiration. They are innervated by branches off of the anterior cervical rami (C2–C8). Trigger points of the scalenes refer pain to the anterior chest, the ipsilateral upper limb, and the medial border of the scapula [4].

Scanning Techniques and Anatomy to Identify

Scalenus anterior is formed by multiple musculotendinous fascicles that originate from the anterior tubercles of the transverse processes of C3 to C6 and blend together and insert onto the scalene tubercle of the 1st rib. Place the patient supine with his neck supported and head rotated to the contralateral side about 20°. Place the transducer axially, along the posterior margin of the SCM about midway between the mastoid process and clavicle. The anterior scalene is the muscular belly just posterior to the SCM. Medial to the anterior scalene is the carotid space including the internal jugular vein, common carotid artery, and vagus nerve. At this level the carotid space lies deep to the SCM and thus easily avoided. Anterior to the scalene is the phrenic nerve, and posterior is the brachial plexus and subclavian artery and vein (Fig. 8.3).

Injection Technique: In-Plane Axial Approach

Patient positioning: Place the patient supine with his neck supported and head rotated to the contralateral side about 20°.

Probe positioning: Place the probe in the axial plane along the posterior margin of the sternocleidomastoid muscle (Fig. 8.4a).

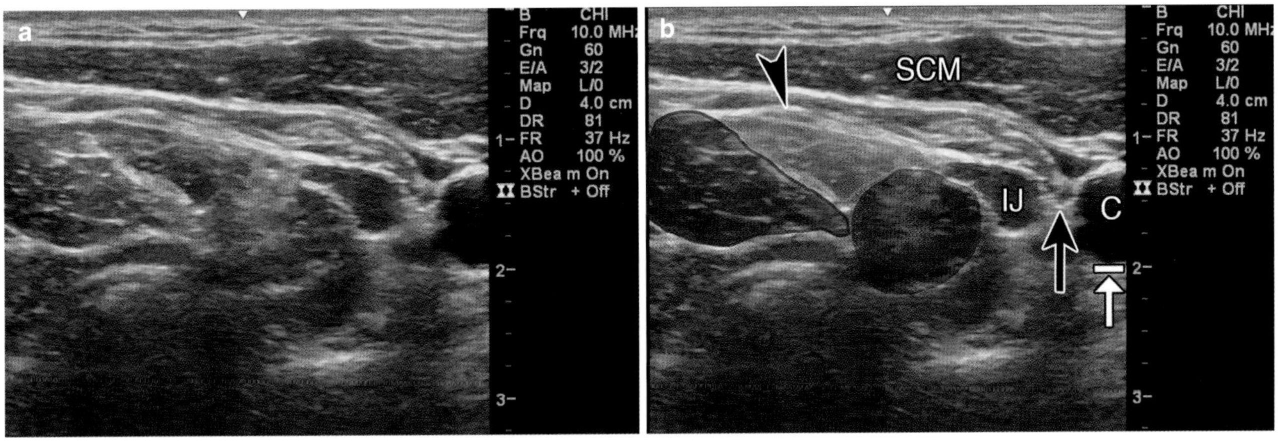

Fig. 8.3 (**a**) Axial view of scalene muscles. (**b**) *Purple* indicates posterior scalene, orange indicates middle scalene, *magenta* indicates anterior scalene, *black arrow* indicates vagus nerve, *black arrowhead* indicates phrenic nerve, *SCM* sternocleidomastoid muscle, *IJ* internal jugular vein, *C* carotid artery, *white arrow with stop* also indicates carotid artery

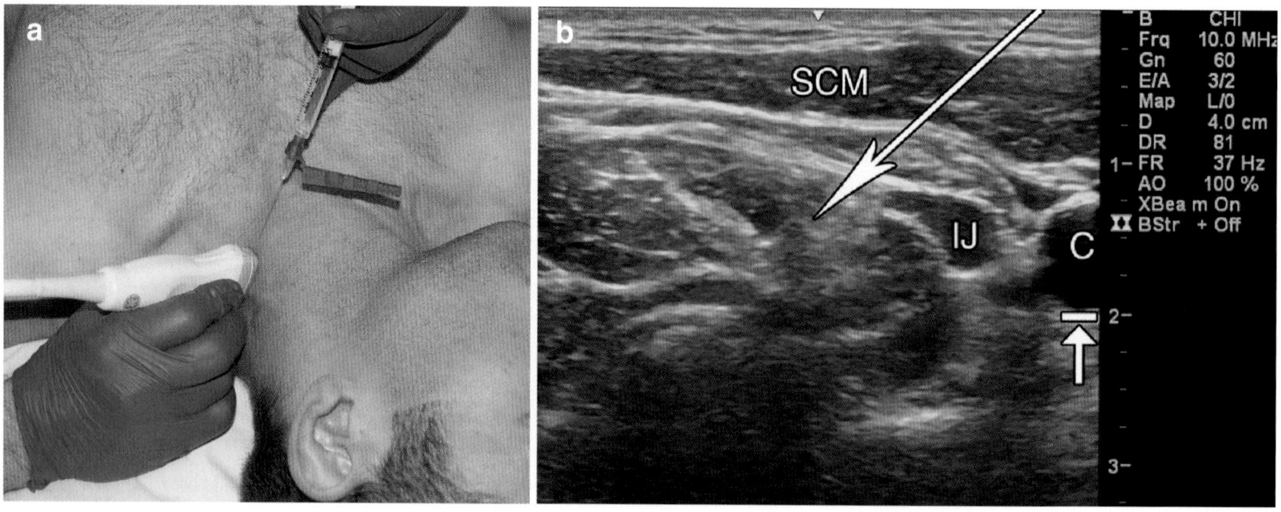

Fig. 8.4 (a) Example of probe position over the anterior scalene. (b) Example of in-plane axial approach, *long white arrow* indicates trajectory into the anterior scalene, *SCM* sternocleidomastoid muscle, *C* carotid artery, *IJ* internal jugular vein, *arrow with stop* also indicating carotid artery

Markings: Use color Doppler to identify the internal carotid, internal jugular, subclavian artery/vein, and external carotid artery.

Needle position: The needle should be inserted parallel to the transducer for optimal visualization, with simultaneous injection of local anesthetic.

Safety considerations:

- Brachial plexus palsy: Torriani in 2009 reported 33 % incidence of brachial plexus palsy while performing US-guided anterior scalene injections with bupivacaine for thoracic outlet syndrome management [33]. In a similar study with botulinum toxin, Torriani (2010) reported no incidence of brachial plexus palsy [34]. As this evidence suggests, to avoid unintended nerve blocks in this region, it is best to use botulinum toxin.
- Phrenic nerve palsy: The incidence of phrenic nerve palsy for interscalene block is reported as high as 100 % in several studies [35]. Using high-resolution ultrasonography, Kessler reports that the phrenic nerve is monofascicular with a mean diameter of 0.76 mm and was identifiable in 93.5 % of 23 volunteers [36].

Pearls:

- Injections of the anterior scalene should be performed with botulinum toxin since injections with local anesthetic are likely to lead to temporary brachial plexus or phrenic nerve palsy.
- The phrenic nerve runs directly superficial to the scalenes and can be identified by ultrasound.
- Use Doppler to identify the internal carotid, internal jugular, external jugular, and associated branches to these vessels.
- If the taut band rolls under the needle, anchor the trigger point along its length with fingers or thumb to prevent rolling.
- If a referred pain pattern and local twitch response were elicited prior to injection, then once the needle enters the trigger point they should occur again.
- Postinjection it is important to have the patient actively stretch each muscle injected through its full range of motion.

Equipment needed:

- High-frequency linear array transducer (10 MHz+)
- 25 gauge, 1.5″ needle
- 1–3 ml of local anesthetic or botulinum toxin preparation

Sternocleidomastoid Muscle (SCM)

The SCM can be divided into a sternal and clavicular division. Both divisions have their own function and referred pain patterns. Patients with a trigger point in the sternal division may complain of pain over their eye or face, whereas patients with a clavicular division trigger point may report pain over their ear or forehead [4]. In addition, trigger points in the SCM are associated with autonomic symptoms [4]. Sternal division trigger points may be associated with lacrimation of the eye. Activation of clavicular division trigger points may cause the patient to feel dizzy. The SCM is innervated by the accessory nerve (cranial nerve XI) and by the C1–C2 branches of the cervical plexus. When bilateral SCM muscles are activated, the head is extended. Unilateral contraction of the SCM muscle will cause the head to side bend ipsilaterally and rotate the head to the contralateral side [31].

Scanning Techniques and Anatomy to Identify

The SCM forms the anterior border of the posterior cervical triangle and posterior border of the anterior cervical triangle.

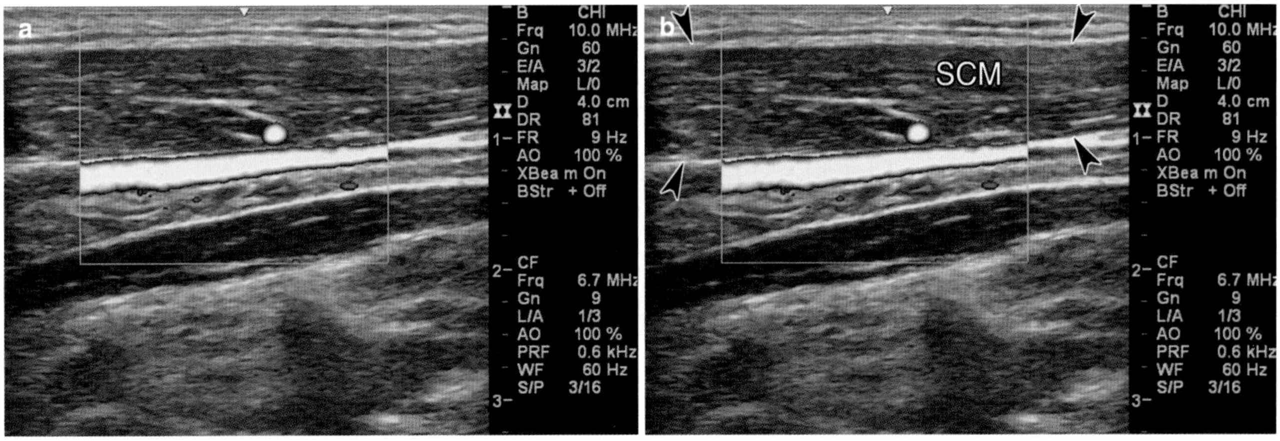

Fig. 8.5 (**a**) Coronal view of sternocleidomastoid with Doppler. (**b**) SCM sternocleidomastoid muscle, *black arrowheads* outline SCM, Doppler showing carotid artery running just deep to the SCM

The SCM descends from the mastoid process and attaches inferiorly by two heads. The sternal head inserts at the manubrium and lies superficial to the clavicular head. The clavicular head inserts along the medial third of the clavicle. It lays superficial to all muscles in the anterior neck except for the platysma. Deep to the SCM nearly along its entire length is the carotid space which houses the common carotid artery, internal jugular vein, and vagus nerve. Cranial nerves IX, X, XI, and XII traverse the superior carotid space. Place the probe over the trigger point in a plane longitudinal to the SCM. Scan along its length to identify and avoid the structures above (Fig. 8.5).

Injection Technique: In-Plane Coronal Approach

Patient positioning: Place the patient in a supine position with the head rotated to the contralateral side.

Probe positioning: Place the probe longitudinal to the fibers of the SCM (Fig. 8.6a).

Markings: Use the color Doppler to identify the common carotid artery and internal jugular vein.

Needle position: The needle should be inserted parallel to the transducer for optimal visualization, with simultaneous injection of local anesthetic.

Safety considerations: Dysphagia is a significant side effect associated with SCM injection with botulinum toxin performed blind or by EMG guidance. Hong demonstrated that using EMG guidance alone resulted in a 34.7 % incidence rate, but when EMG guidance was used in conjunction with US guidance, the incidence of dysphagia was reduced to zero [37].

Pearls:

- The SCM is quite superficial and the needle should be carefully advanced as to avoid injuring deep structures.
- Use the color Doppler to identify and avoid injection into the carotid space.

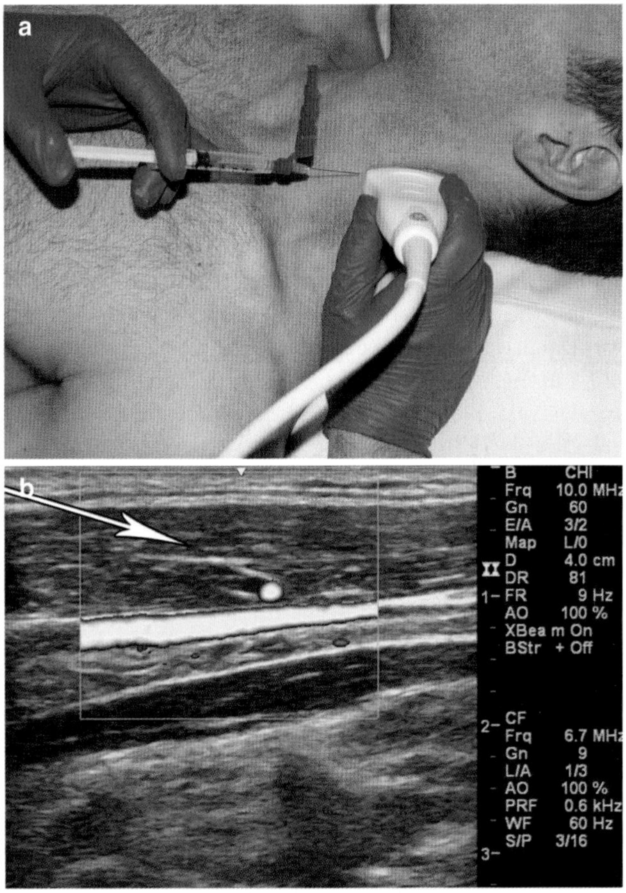

Fig. 8.6 (**a**) Example of coronal probe position over the SCM. (**b**) Example of in-plane coronal approach, *white arrow* indicates trajectory into sternocleidomastoid muscle, Doppler deep to SCM highlights carotid artery

- If the taut band rolls under the needle, anchor the trigger point along its length with fingers or thumb to prevent rolling.
- If a referred pain pattern and local twitch response were elicited prior to injection, then once the needle enters the trigger point, they should occur again.

- Postinjection it is important to have the patient actively stretch each muscle injected through its full range of motion.
  Equipment needed:
- High-frequency linear array transducer (10 MHz+)
- 25 gauge, 1.5″ needle
- 1–3 ml of local anesthetic

Levator Scapulae (LS)

The levator scapulae are a common source of myofascial pain with a referred pain pattern over the base of the neck [4]. The levator scapulae rotate the glenoid cavity inferiorly and elevate and retract the scapula [4, 31]. They attach to the transverse processes of the atlas and axis, and to the posterior tubercles of C3 and C4 [31]. The levator scapulae fibers descend and attach to the scapula at the superior medial border. The LS is innervated by the dorsal scapular nerve and directly by the cervical nerve roots of C3 and C4.

Scanning Techniques and Anatomy to Identify

Orient the probe along the trapezius between the occiput and the superior angle of the scapula. Aim the probe anterior. From superficial to deep lie the subcutaneous tissue, the trapezius, and the levator scapulae. Deep (anterior) to the levator scapulae are the scalenes superiorly and the posterior ribs of T1 through T3. Medial to the levator scapulae are splenius cervicis and splenius capitis (Fig. 8.7).

Injection Technique: In-Plane Sagittal Approach

Patient positioning: Patient should lay in the prone position.

Probe positioning: Place the probe longitudinally over the levator scapula as described above in the scanning techniques (Fig. 8.8a).

Markings: Use color Doppler to identify the superficial branch of the transverse cervical artery, which runs deep to the trapezius but superficial to the levator scapulae. Along with this artery runs the spinal accessory nerve (SAN).

Needle position: The needle should be inserted parallel to the transducer for optimal needle visualization with simultaneous injection of local anesthetic.

Safety considerations: If injecting close to the insertion at the scapula, beware of lung apex.

Pearls:

- Identify the SAN which runs deep to the trap and superficial to the levator scapulae to avoid injury.
- If the taut band rolls under the needle, anchor the trigger point along its length with fingers or thumb to prevent rolling.
- If a referred pain pattern and local twitch response were elicited prior to injection, then once the needle enters the trigger point, they should occur again.
- Postinjection it is important to have the patient actively stretch each muscle injected through its full range of motion.
  Equipment needed:
- High-frequency linear array transducer (10 MHz+)
- 25 gauge, 1.5″ needle
- 1–3 ml of local anesthetic

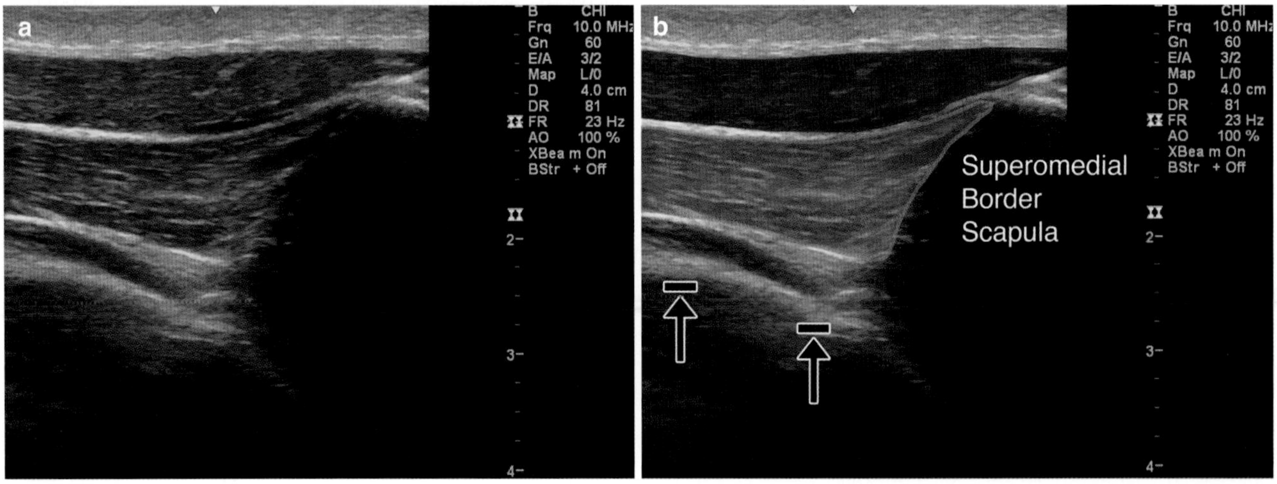

Fig. 8.7 (**a**) Sagittal view of levator scapula. (**b**) *Purple* indicates trapezius, *orange* indicates levator scapula, *black arrows* with stops indicate rib, superomedial border scapula labeled

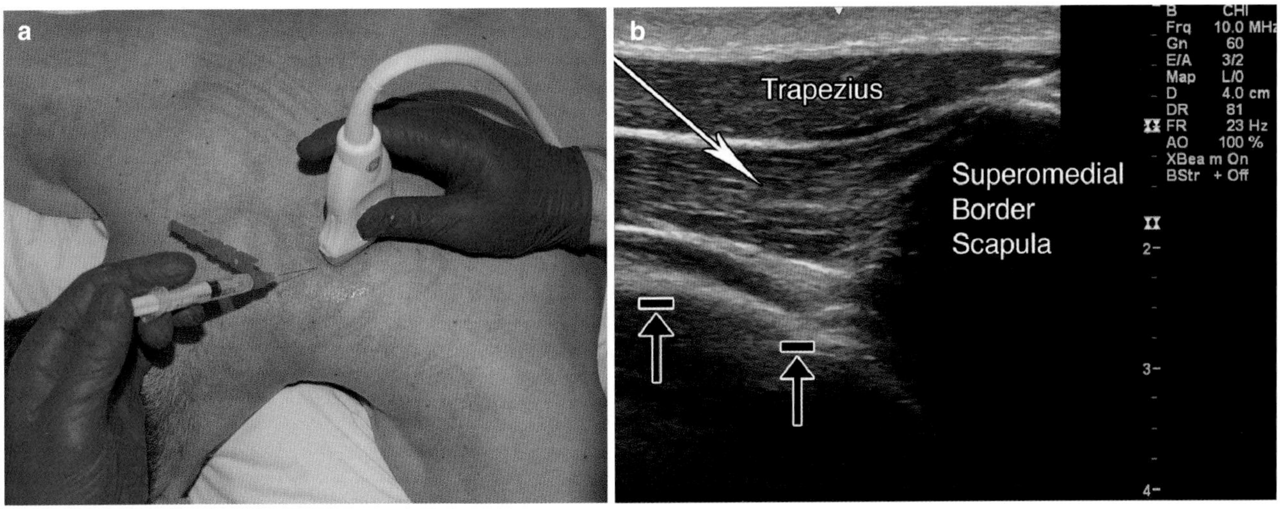

Fig. 8.8 (**a**) Example of sagittal probe position over the levator scapula. (**b**) Example of in-plane sagittal approach, *white arrow* indicates needle trajectory, *black arrows with stops* indicate rib, trapezius and superomedial border scapula labeled

Rhomboids

The rhomboid major and minor muscles run parallel to each other and descend from the upper thoracic vertebrae to the medial border of the scapula. Rhomboid minor is a small muscle that runs from the ligamentum nuchae and the spinous processes of C7 and T1 to the medial end of the spine of the scapula [31]. Rhomboid major is a larger sheetlike muscle that extends from the spinous processes and supraspinatus ligaments of T2–T5 to the medial border of the scapula inferior to the spine of the scapula [31]. Both muscles are innervated by the dorsal scapular nerve. The rhomboids refer pain to the medial border of the scapula and are activated by the constant stretch from protracted shoulders.

Scanning Techniques and Anatomy to Identify

With the ultrasound probe oriented transverse to the fibers of the rhomboid major (sagittal), the layers of tissue from superficial to deep are subcutaneous fat, trapezius muscle, rhomboid major, erector spinae muscles (medial), and ribs. Deep to the rhomboids and levator scapulae but superficial to the serratus posterior superior and erector spinae muscle run the dorsal scapular nerve and the deep branch of the transverse cervical artery (Dorsal scapular artery) along the medial border of the scapula. Turn the probe longitudinal to the rhomboids with the lateral edge of the ultrasound probe on the medial scapula to attain an axial view (Fig. 8.9).

Injection Techniques: In-Plane Axial Approach

Patient positioning: Patient seated or prone.

Probe positioning: Place probe in the axial plane over the rhomboids (Fig. 8.10a).

Markings: Use color Doppler to identify the dorsal scapular artery.

Needle position: The needle should be inserted parallel to the transducer from medial to lateral for optimal needle visualization with simultaneous injection of local anesthetic.

Safety considerations: There is a risk of the following: prolonged bleeding, infection, allergic reaction, increased pain and decreased functional scores, and pneumothorax.

Pearls:

- Identify the ribs and underlying lungs prior to injection to help avoid placing the needle too deep.
- If the taut band rolls under the needle, anchor the trigger point along its length with fingers or thumb to prevent rolling.
- If a referred pain pattern and local twitch response were elicited prior to injection, then once the needle enters the trigger point, they should occur again.
- Postinjection it is important to have the patient actively stretch each muscle injected through its full range of motion.

Equipment needed:

- High-frequency linear array transducer (10 MHz+)
- 25 gauge, 1.5″ needle
- 1–3 ml of local anesthetic

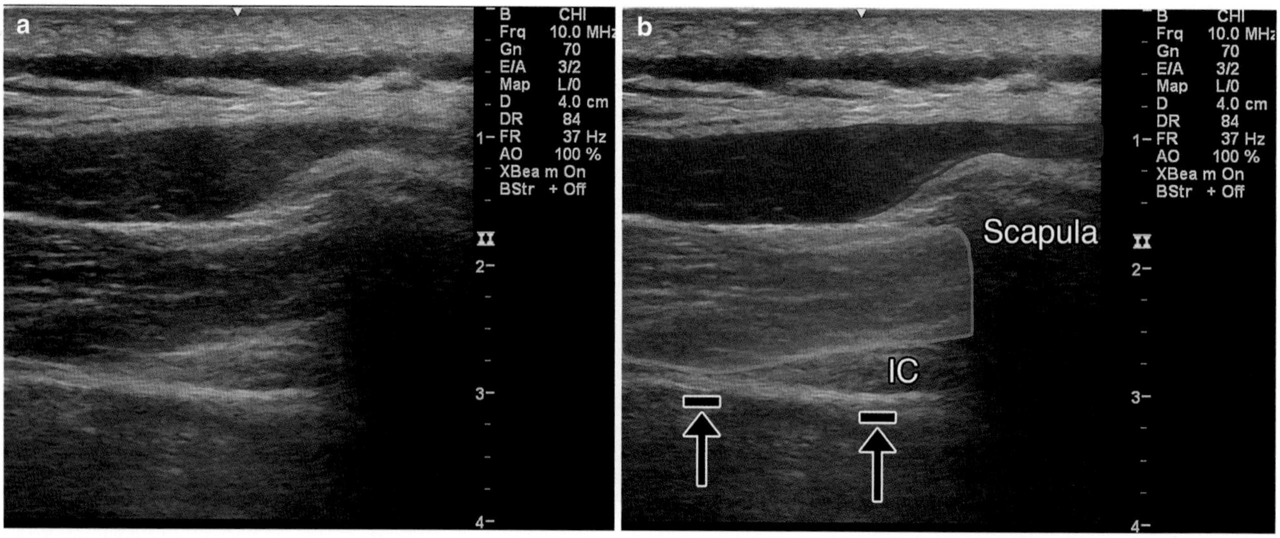

Fig. 8.9 (**a**) Axial view of rhomboids. (**b**) *Purple* indicates trapezius, *orange* indicates rhomboids, *IC* indicates intercostal muscle, *black arrows* with stops indicate pleura, scapula labeled

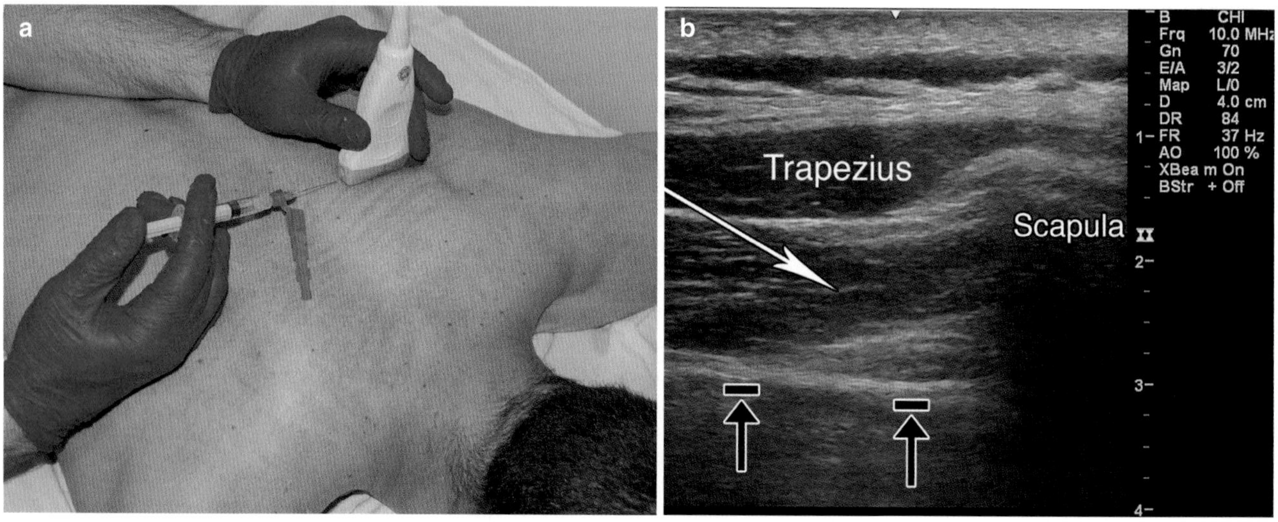

Fig. 8.10 (**a**) Example of axial probe position over rhomboids. (**b**) Example of in-plane axial approach, *white arrow* indicates needle trajectory into rhomboids, *black arrows* with stops indicate pleura, trapezius and scapula labeled

References

1. Simons DG, Travell JG. Myofascial origins of low back pain. Parts 1, 2, 3. Postgrad Med. 1983;73:66–108.
2. Travell J, Simons DG. Myofascial pain and dysfunction: the trigger point manual, vol. 1. Baltimore: Williams & Wilkins; 1983.
3. Shah JP, Heimur J. New frontiers in the pathophysiology of myofascial pain. Pain Pract. 2012;22(2):26–33.
4. Simons DG, Travell JG, Simons LS. Travell & Simons' myofascial pain and dysfunction: the trigger point manual, vol. 1. 2nd ed. Baltimore: Williams & Wilkins; 1999.
5. Hubbard DR, Berkoff GM. Myofascial trigger points show spontaneous needle activity. Spine. 1993;18:1803–7.
6. Simons DG, Hong CZ, Simons LS. Endplate potentials are common to midfiber myofascial trigger points. Am J Phys Med Rehabil. 2002;81(3):212–22.
7. Shah JP, Phillips TM, Danoff JV, Gerber LH. An in vivo microanalytical technique for measuring the local biochemical milieu of human skeletal muscle. J Appl Physiol. 2005;99:1977–84.
8. Shah JP, Danoff JV, Desai M, et al. Biochemicals associated with pain and inflammation are elevated in sites near to and remote from active myofascial trigger points. Arch Phys Med Rehabil. 2008;89:16–23.
9. Shah JP, Gilliams EA. Uncovering the biochemical milieu of myofascial trigger points using in-vivo microdialysis: an application of muscle pain concepts to myofascial pain syndrome. J Bodyw Mov Ther. 2008;12(4):371–84.
10. Mense S. How do muscle lesions such as latent and active trigger points influence central nociceptive neurons? J Musculoskelet Pain. 2010;18(4):348–53.
11. Woolf CJ. Central sensitization: implications for the diagnosis and treatment of pain. Pain. 2011;152(3 Suppl):S2–15.

12. Niddam DM, Chan RC, Lee SH, Yeh TC, Hsieh JC. Central modulation of pain evoked from myofascial trigger point. Clin J Pain. 2007;23:440–8.
13. McPartland JM. Travell trigger points: molecular and osteopathic perspectives. J Am Osteopath Assoc. 2004;104:244–9.
14. Jones LH. Strain and counterstrain. Colorado Springs: The American Academy of Osteopathy; 1981.
15. Kuchera WA, Kuchera ML. Foundations for osteopathic medicine. 2nd ed. Philadelphia: Lippincott Williams & Wilkins; 2003.
16. Annaswamy TM, De Luigi AJ, O'Neill BJ, et al. Emerging concepts in the treatment of myofascial pain: a review of medications, modalities, and needle-based interventions. PM R. 2001;3:940–61.
17. Lewit K. The needle effect in the relief of myofascial pain. Pain. 1979;6(1):83–90.
18. Hong CZ. Lidocaine injection versus dry needling to myofascial trigger point. The importance of the local twitch response. Am J Phys Med Rehabil. 1994;73(4):256–63.
19. Kamanli A, Kaya A, Ardicoglu O, et al. Comparison of lidocaine injection, botulinum toxin injection, and dry needling to trigger points in myofascial pain syndrome. Rheumatol Int. 2005;25:604–11.
20. Cummings TM, White AR. Needling therapies in the management of myofascial trigger point pain: a systematic review. Arch Phys Med Rehabil. 2001;82:986–92.
21. Ferrante FM, Bean L, Rothrock R, King L. Evidence against trigger point injection techniques for the treatment of cervicothoracic myofascial pain with botulinum toxin type A. Anesthesiology. 2005;103:377–83.
22. Graboski CL, Gray DS, Burnham RS. Botulinum toxin A vs bupivacaine trigger point injections for the treatment of myofascial pain syndrome: a randomized double blind crossover study. Pain. 2005;118:170–5.
23. Botwin KP, Sharma K, Saliba R, Patel BC. Ultrasound-guided trigger point injections in the cervicothoracic musculature: a new and unreported technique. Pain Physician. 2008;11:885–9.
24. Rha D, Shin JC, Kim YK, Jung JH, Kim YU, Lee SC. Detecting local twitch responses of myofascial trigger points in the lower-back muscles using ultrasonography. Arch Phys Med Rehabil. 2011;92:1576–80.
25. Ballyns JJ, Shah JP, Hammond J, Gebreab T, Gerber LH, Sikdar S. Objective sonographic measures for characterizing myofascial trigger points associated with cervical pain. J Ultrasound Med. 2011;30:1331–40.
26. Sikdar S, Ortiz R, Gebreab T, Gerber LH, Shah JP. Understanding the vascular environment of myofascial trigger points using ultrasonic imaging and computational modeling. Conf Proc IEEE Eng Med Biol Soc. 2010;2010:5302–5.
27. Sikdar S, Shah JP, Gebreab T, Yen RH, Gilliams E, Danoff J, Gerber LH. Novel applications of ultrasound technology to visualize and characterize myofascial trigger points and surrounding soft tissue. Arch Phys Med Rehabil. 2009;90:1829–38.
28. Shankar Hartharan H, Reddy S. Two- and three-dimensional ultrasound imaging to facilitate detection and targeting of taut bands in myofascial pain syndrome. Pain Med. 2012;13:971–5.
29. Gerwin RD, Duranleau D. Ultrasound identification of the myofascial trigger point [Letter]. Muscle Nerve. 1997;20(6):767–8.
30. Niraj G, Collett BJ, Bone M. Ultrasound-guided trigger point injection: first description of changes visible on ultrasound scanning in the muscle containing the trigger point. Br J Anaesth. 2011;107(3):474–5.
31. Standring S. Gray's anatomy: the anatomical basis of clinical practice. 40th ed. Edinburgh: Churchill-Livingstone, Elsevier; 2008.
32. Kessler J, Gray AT. Course of the spinal accessory nerve relative to the brachial plexus. Reg Anesth Pain Med. 2007;32(2):174–6.
33. Torriani M, Gupta R, Donahue DM. Sonographically guided anesthetic injection of anterior scalene muscle for investigation of neurogenic thoracic outlet syndrome. Skeletal Radiol. 2009;38:1083–7.
34. Torriani M, Gupta R, Donahue DM. Botulinum toxin injection in neurogenic thoracic outlet syndrome: results and experience using a ultrasound-guided approach. Skeletal Radiol. 2010;39:973–80.
35. Urmey WF, Talts KH, Sharrock NE. One hundred percent incidence of hemidiaphragmatic paresis associated with interscalene brachial plexus anesthesia as diagnosed by ultrasonography. Anesth Analg. 1991;72(4):498–503.
36. Kessler J, Schafhalter-Zoppoth I, Gray AT. An ultrasound study of the phrenic nerve in the posterior cervical triangle: implications for the interscalene brachial plexus block. Reg Anesth Pain Med. 2008;33(6):545–50.
37. Hong JS, Sathe GG, Niyonkuru C, Munin MC. Elimination of dysphagia using ultrasound guidance for botulinum toxin injections in cervical dystonia. Muscle Nerve. 2012;46:535–9.

Neuromuscular/Chemodenervation

9

Sarah Khan, Emerald Lin, and Jonathan S. Kirschner

Spasticity is a velocity-dependent increase in a muscle's resistance to passive range of motion and is caused by the loss of supraspinal inhibition of the muscle stretch reflex. Spasticity can be both functionally useful and functionally detrimental. Therefore, how we manage and treat it can have a significant impact on the lives of patients with upper motor neuron disorders such as stroke, traumatic or anoxic brain injury, and spinal cord injury. Dystonia is a neurological movement disorder characterized by involuntary motor contractions resulting in abnormal posturing and twisting motions. Both spasticity and dystonia often result in major impairments with activities of daily living, ambulation, and independence while causing pain and discomfort. Severe cases of spasticity leave patients vulnerable to contractures and skin breakdown.

Chemodenervation with botulinum toxin for focal spasticity and focal dystonia is an effective treatment for improving functional independence. It is often used in conjunction with other agents and therapy, or after failed attempts with other treatments. Outcome measures must include active vs. passive function, and the physician must consider the patient and family's expectations of function. Muscles must be selected to take advantage of functional spasticity, such as by avoiding antigravity muscles that should not be weakened.

Botulinum toxin injections have commonly been performed with the use of electromyography (EMG) and electrical stimulation (E-stim) to target specific muscles to improve accuracy. EMG guidance uses a needle electrode inserted into the muscle to record its electrical activity. Increased auditory feedback indicates increased motor unit firing of a spastic muscle. Electrical stimulation guidance utilizes electrical current through a needle probe inserted into the targeted muscle to cause it to contract.

In recent years, the use of ultrasound for the imaging of musculoskeletal conditions has become more common. Ultrasound technology allows the physician to directly visualize and diagnose pathologic structures and take advantage of the dynamic ability of ultrasound to aid in accurately targeting interventional injection sites. Cadaver studies involving ultrasound injections to joints and tendons have been shown to have greater accuracy compared to blind injection procedures [1–3].

The accuracy rates using anatomical landmarks and palpation are usually accurate for larger and more superficial muscles, but decline for deeper and smaller muscles [4, 5]. EMG guidance is the current gold standard for chemodenervation injections. Ultrasound may prove to be beneficial as a supplemental modality for accurately targeting individual muscles or muscle regions for which EMG or E-stim guidance was used initially but was unsuccessful in achieving optimal results. Ultrasound-guided chemodenervation injections may be valuable for targeting deeper muscles, such as the tibialis posterior; muscles that are difficult to target using anatomical landmarks, such as the individual muscle bellies of the flexor digitorum superficialis (FDS); or muscles that are near vital vascular structures, such as those targeted for cervical dystonia. Furthermore, patients with spasticity or those who are postsurgical tend to have a different anatomy than the "normal" patient. Another potential novel use for ultrasound in chemodenervation is the identification and injection of muscle regions that are not typically injected with EMG or E-stim alone given the difficulty and risk of the injection without visual guidance, such as using an anterior approach to inject the tibialis posterior and a dorsal approach to inject the iliopsoas muscle.

S. Khan, DO (✉)
Brain Injury Unit, Department of Rehabilitation Medicine, Hofstra Medical School, North Shore Long Island Jewish Glen Cove Hospital, Glen Cove, NY, USA
e-mail: sarahkhan1981@gmail.com, dr.s.khan22@gmail.com

E. Lin, MD
Kessler Institute for Rehabilitation, West Orange, NJ, USA
e-mail: lin.emerald@gmail.com

J.S. Kirschner, MD, FAAPMR, RMSK
Interventional Spine and Sports Medicine Division, Department of Rehabilitation Medicine, Icahn School of Medicine at Mount Sinai, New York, NY, USA
e-mail: jonathan.kirschner@mountsinai.org

D.A. Spinner et al. (eds.), *Atlas of Ultrasound Guided Musculoskeletal Injections*, Musculoskeletal Medicine,
DOI 10.1007/978-1-4614-8936-8_9,

Table 9.1 Common spasticity patterns [6]

Pattern	Etiology
Flexor synergy with hemiparesis	CVA, traumatic or nontraumatic brain injury, cerebral palsy
Crouch gait	Cerebral palsy
Torticollis	Prematurity, cervical dystonia
Scissoring gait	Cerebral palsy

Prior to initiating treatment with botulinum toxin, it is important to take a thorough history to determine the most appropriate treatment, beginning with the diagnosis causing the patient's spasticity, severity of symptoms, and what treatments have been tried thus far. It is also important to discuss with the patient and family, as appropriate, their functional goals, expectations, and ability to adhere to treatments. A complete physical exam assessing joint range of motion and clinical assessment of tone using an assessment tool such as the Modified Ashworth Scale or Tardieu Scale is important to document at every exam to assess the efficacy of treatment. It is important to assess static tone (at rest) and dynamic tone, as well as examine the patient's gait and transfers. Table 9.1 shows common spasticity patterns that may be observed in patients.

A comprehensive approach considering treatment options including stretching, ROM, splinting, orthotics, medications, chemodenervation injections, chemoneurolysis, intrathecal baclofen, and surgical correction should be taken. A thorough assessment of spasticity is necessary to determine the best treatment combination that fits the patient's needs and goals. Spasticity due to spinal cord injury and multiple sclerosis tends to be more generalized, and therefore oral medications and intrathecal baclofen are usually the best treatment options combined with a therapy program. For patients with focal spasticity resulting from stroke or traumatic brain injury, botulinum toxin injections or chemoneurolysis procedures tend to be the treatment of choice, combined with therapy. Oral medications may be helpful but often are limited due to cognitive side effects. For more severe spasticity, intrathecal baclofen therapy may be more effective.

If chemodenervation with botulinum toxin is used for treatment, it is important to make sure the patient has not had botulinum toxin injections to other muscle sites within the past 3 months to avoid the risk of antibody formation. Patients that have developed antibodies to botulinum toxin A may be treated with botulinum toxin B. Risks and benefits of the procedure should be thoroughly discussed with the patient and/or caregiver as well as realistic goals for treatment. It is imperative to consider the patient's functional goals when prescribing botulinum toxin. The effect of the toxin injection is to decrease spastic tone to improve pain or improve range of motion to allow for proper hygiene or to improve function. It is important to explain to the patient and caregivers that botulinum toxin does not increase strength as a result of the toxin itself. Decreasing the patient's spasticity may secondarily improve the patient's voluntary control over movement in antagonistic muscles (for patients that have or are recovering voluntary muscle control) as this would reduce or eliminate the barrier that spasticity imposes on voluntary movement. The physician should also be aware that the patient may have functional benefit as a result of their tone (e.g., stability in ambulation or when dressing) and that weakening certain muscles with botulinum toxin would result in a loss of function for the patient.

Botulinum toxin A and botulinum toxin B are used clinically for treatment of spasticity. There are three different formulations of botulinum toxin A available in the USA. They include onabotulinumtoxin A (Botox), abobotulinumtoxin A (Dysport), and incobotulinumtoxin A (Xeomin). Botulinum toxin B is known as rimabotulinumtoxin B (Myobloc). Table 9.2 includes details regarding the ingredients, mechanism of action, FDA and off-label indications and side effects of each of these botulinum toxin formulations. There is a lack of standardization of botulinum dosage between these agents, and the concentration of injections to different muscles often varies. When initiating treatment, start at the lowest dose and titrate up to minimize adverse reactions (see Table 9.2).

Onabotulinum toxin A is the oldest formulation and most commonly used by practitioners. Table 10.3 shows muscles commonly treated with Onabotulinum toxin A and typical dosages used for injection into specific muscles. Do not exceed 400 units of botulinum toxin A at an initial treatment session and do not inject greater than 50 units per injection site [10]. For children, the maximum recommended dosage per treatment session is 12 units/kg or 400 units, whichever is lowest [11]. FDA approval for botulinum toxin is limited to five muscles for upper extremity spasticity in adults: the biceps brachii, flexor carpi radialis (FCR), flexor carpi ulnaris (FCU), flexor digitorum sublimis (FDS), and flexor digitorum profundus (FDP). Use in other muscles and use for pediatric patients remain off-label at this time, but is commonly used by many practitioners (see Table 9.3).

Forearm Flexor Spasticity: Clenched Fist/Thumb in Palm

Commonly targeted forearm muscles for upper extremity spasticity are wrist flexors, finger flexors, and pronators. The wrist flexors include the flexor carpi radialis and flexor carpi ulnaris. The finger flexors include the flexor digitorum superficialis which flexes the proximal interphalanges and the flexor digitorum profundus, which flexes the distal interphalanges. The flexor pollicis longus flexes the interphalangeal joint of the thumb. Pronator teres and pronator quadratus are responsible for forearm pronation.

Henzel et al. compared the ultrasound localization of forearm flexor muscles to anatomical landmarks described

Table 9.2 Chemodenervation agents [7]

	Botulinum toxin A			Botulinum toxin B
	Botox	Xeomin	Dysport	
	Onabotulinumtoxin A	Incobotulinumtoxin A	Abobotulinumtoxin A	Rimabotulinumtoxin B
Derivative/ ingredients	Neurotoxin from Clostridium botulinum, human albumin	Neurotoxin from Clostridium botulinum	Neurotoxin from Clostridium botulinum	Neurotoxin from Clostridium botulinum, contains human albumin
Mechanism of action	Prevents ACh release from presynaptic membrane—SNAP 25 "Rule of 3s"—3 days to begin to see effect, 3 weeks to see maximal effects, 3 months to wear off (these are generalized)	Prevents ACh release from presynaptic membrane—SNAP 25	Prevents ACh release from presynaptic membrane—SNAP 25	Prevents ACh release from presynaptic membrane—VAMP/ synaptobrevin
FDA indications	Cervical dystonia, blepharospasm, overactive bladder UE spasticity in Biceps, FCR, FCU, FDS, FDP	Cervical dystonia, blepharospasm	Cervical dystonia	Cervical dystonia
Off-label use	Spasticity from stroke, MS, Parkinson's disease, CP, SCI, TBI Focal dystonias	Spasticity from stroke, MS, TBI, CP, SCI, headache	Spasticity from stroke, TBI, CP, MS, SCI	Spasticity associated with cerebral palsy, chronic anal fissure Sialorrhea associated with ALS or Parkinson's disease
Additional benefits		Made without binding proteins, theoretically decreasing the formation of antibodies, formation of which theoretically decreases therapeutic response [8] Does not need refrigeration until reconstitution—good in severe weather conditions/blackouts		
Side effect/pitfalls	All botulinum toxin type A has similar side effect profiles, including the following: weakness, flu-like syndrome Botulism: Loss of strength and muscle weakness all over the body i.e. distal spread Double vision Blurred vision and drooping eyelids Hoarseness or change or loss of voice Trouble saying words clearly Loss of bladder control Trouble breathing Trouble swallowing/dysphagia Symptoms can happen hours to weeks after an injection Collateral sprouting at 3 months → decreased effect Possible formation of antibodies	Same	Same	Headache, dry mouth, dysphagia, dyspepsia, injection site pain, flu-like symptoms Peripheral motor neuropathic diseases (e.g., ALS, motor neuropathy) Neuromuscular junctional disorders (e.g., myasthenia gravis, Lambert-Eaton syndrome) Increased risk for severe dysphagia and respiratory compromise in pts. with neuromuscular disorders Risk of respiratory compromise and death esp. in children treated off-label for cerebral palsy-associated spasticity

(continued)

Table 9.2 (continued)

	Botulinum toxin A			Botulinum toxin B
	Botox	Xeomin	Dysport	
	Onabotulinumtoxin A	Incobotulinumtoxin A	Abobotulinumtoxin A	Rimabotulinumtoxin B
Dosage	Maximal initial dose: 400 units dosage is made to be 1:1 to Botox	For cervical dystonia: 120 units per treatment session	Recommended initial dose: 500 units, for both toxin-naïve and previously treated patients	Prior botulinum toxin injection: 2,500–5,000 units IM, divided among affected muscles
	In children, weight based:	Median doses injected during double-blind phase 3 study:	Dose modifications in 250-unit increments	Naive: Administer lower dose for initial treatment
	12 units/kg	SCM—25 units	Initial dose by muscle (median):	
		Splenius capitis/ semispinalis capitis—48 units	SCM—125	
		Trapezius—25 units	Splenius capitis—200	
		Levator scapulae—25 units	Trapezius—103	
		Scalenus (medius and anterior)—20 units [9]	Levator scapulae—105	
			Scalenus (medius and anterior)—116	
			Semispinalis capitis—132	
			Longissimus—150	

by Delagi for the flexor carpi radialis, pronator teres, and flexor pollicis longus, and the landmark mapping technique for the flexor digitorum superficialis developed by Bickerton [11, 13]. This study showed that ultrasound localization of the muscle bellies of certain forearm muscles, in particular the pronator teres, the flexor pollicis longus, the flexor carpi radialis, and the flexor digitorum superficialis to the 3rd or ring finger, was distinctly different from the points localized via surface landmarks or mapping. In a study by Munin, the mapping technique for the flexor digitorum superficialis muscle described by Bickerton was demonstrated to be feasible and effective to accurately target this muscle's individual muscle bellies [14]. The mapping technique is time intensive, however taking 10 min in this study. The use of ultrasound would allow the identification of the muscle within several seconds to a few minutes, depending on the operator's experience. Also, limitation in limb range of motion and positioning, as well as muscle atrophy and fibrosis, may interfere with anatomical mapping. Ultrasound identification of target muscles would likely be beneficial in these situations (Table 9.4).

Scanning Technique and Anatomy to Identify

Position the arm in external rotation with forearm supinated. If this position is not possible due to spasticity, abduct and internally rotate the arm and pronate as much as possible. Begin scanning over the medial epicondyle in the longitudinal plane where the flexor tendon attachments will be identified. The transducer can then be rotated 90° into the transverse (axial) plane. Move the probe distally to the proximal third of the forearm where the pronator teres, flexor carpi radialis, and flexor digitorum profundus can be visualized. The pronator teres is the most lateral (radial) muscle, and the flexor carpi radialis and the palmaris longus are just medial to this muscle in the superficial compartment. In this same transverse view, the flexor digitorum profundus is visualized deep to these muscles. Moving the transducer more medial (ulnar) and slightly more distal, the flexor carpi ulnaris is identified along the medial ulna. The flexor digitorum superficialis (FDS) 2 and 3 are scanned at the midpoint of the forearm, and the bellies of the FDS 4 and 5 are visualized as the transducer is moved more medial. The flexor pollicis longus muscle is seen just lateral and superficial to the FDS 2 and 3 (Fig. 9.1).

Injection Techniques: In-Plane Axial Approach

Patient positioning: Seated comfortably and placed in a position with the forearm extended and supinated, preferably on a flat surface, with access to the anterior forearm.

Table 9.3 Spasticity testing and suggested dosing [7, 12]

Spastic clinical pattern	Muscles involved	Range of motion testing	Botox (units) (suggested dosage for normal size adult)	Dysport (units) (suggested dosage for adult)
Hip flexion	Iliopsoas	Thomas test: positive if cannot keep opposite leg extended	Iliacus: 50–100	Iliacus: 200–400
Crouched gait	Rectus femoris	Hip extension ROM	Psoas: 50–150 Rectus femoris: 75–150	
Adducted hip Scissoring gait	Hip adductors: adductor brevis, adductor longus, adductor magnus gracilis (knee flexion and hip adduction)	Hip abduction normal ROM 40° from midline	Adductor brevis: 50–100 Adductor longus: 50–100 Adductor magnus:50–100 Gracilis: 50–100	Adductor longus: 500–750 Adductor magnus: 500–750
Knee flexion	Medial hamstrings: semimembranosus, semitendinosus Lateral hamstrings: biceps femoris	Popliteal angle or supine knee extension	Medial: 50–150 Lateral: 50–200	Medial: 150–400 Lateral: 150–400
Extended or stiff knee	Quadriceps: rectus femoris, vastus lateralis, vastus medialis, vastus intermedius	Ely's test: positive if unable to flex heel to buttock, hip rises in prone position	Rectus femoris: 75–200 Vasti: 25–50 each	Vastus lateralis: 150 Vastus medialis: 150
Equinovarus foot	Medial and lateral gastrocnemius, soleus, tibialis posterior	Gastrocnemius: ankle dorsiflexion with knee extended Soleus: ankle dorsiflexion with knee flexed Tibialis posterior: ankle eversion	Gastrocnemius: Medial: 25–75 Lateral: 25–75 Soleus: 50–200 Tibialis posterior: 25–150	Medial: 150–400 Lateral: 150–400
Toe curling	Flexor digitorum longus or brevis	Toe extension	50	100
Adducted/internally rotated shoulder	Pectoralis major Latissimus dorsi Teres major Subscapularis	Shoulder abduction Shoulder external rotation	PM: 60–140 LD: 80–160 TM: 25–50 SS: 25–50	PM: 150–300 LD: 150–300 TM: 100 SS: 100–150
Flexed elbow	Brachioradialis Brachialis Biceps Pronator teres: proximal portion	Elbow extension ROM BR: elbow flexion in neutral position Brach: elbow flexion in pronated position Bic: elbow flexion in supinated position	Brachioradialis: 40–80 Brachialis: 30–60 Biceps: 60–120 Pronator teres: 25–50	Brachioradialis: 100–150 Brachialis: 150–200 Biceps: 200–300 Pronator teres: 100–200
Pronated forearm	Pronator teres Pronator quadratus	Forearm supination ROM	Pronator teres: 25–50 Pronator quadratus: 20–40	Pronator teres: 100–200 Pronator quadratus: 100–200
Flexed wrist	Flexor carpi radialis Flexor carpi ulnaris Extrinsic finger flexors	Wrist extension ROM	FCR: 40–70 FCU: 20–40 Ext FF: 40–80	FCR: 100–200 FCU: 100–150 Ext FF: 100–150
Clenched fist	Flexor digitorum superficialis Flexor digitorum profundus	FDS: Proximal interphalangeal extension FDP: Distal interphalangeal extension	FDS: 20–80 FDS: 20–80	FDS: 100–200 FDP: 100–200
Thumb in palm	Flexor pollicis longus Flexor pollicis brevis Adductor pollicis	Thumb extension	FPL: 20–30 FPB: 10–20 AP: 10–20	FPL: 100–150 FPB: 50–100 AP: 50–100

Probe positioning: Place the transducer on the anterior forearm in the axial plane over the largest area of the muscle belly (Fig. 9.2a).

Markings: Identify the brachial artery and median or ulnar nerves.

Needle position: Insert the needle adjacent to the probe from either the medial or lateral side, depending on the muscles of interest. Inserting the needle along the rounded sides of the forearm maintains the ability to stay parallel to the transducer for optimal visualization.

Safety considerations: Utilize Doppler to avoid injury to the radial or ulnar artery/vein. Avoid the median or ulnar nerve (see elbow chapter for locations of these nerves).

Pearls:

- Isolate the individual components of the FDS or FDP by flexing at the PIP or DIP of the desired finger.
- May consider applying topical lidocaine cream or cold vaporant spray to injection site prior to procedure.
- If you use a longer needle, you can redirect to the different targets without having to repuncture the skin.

Equipment needed:

- Linear array transducer with a frequency (10+ MHz)
- Preparation of botulinum toxin
- 24+ gauge, Teflon-coated, injectable EMG/stimulator needle, 2.5″–3″
- EMG or nerve stimulator for additional guidance

Table 9.4 Muscles targeted for clenched fist/thumb in palm

Pronator teres
Flexor carpi radialis
Flexor carpi ulnaris
Palmaris longus
Flexor digitorum profundus
Flexor digitorum superficialis
Flexor pollicis longus

Iliopsoas Spasticity: Crouched Gait

The iliopsoas muscle is the primary hip flexor. It originates from the lateral vertebral bodies of T12 to L5 and inserts on the lesser trochanter of the femur. Spasticity of this muscle typically presents as hip and knee flexion, and internal rotation and adduction of the hip, known as "crouched gait."

Two techniques for ultrasound-guided injections of the iliopsoas muscle have been described. The first technique described uses an anterolateral approach angled 45° medially from the anterior superior iliac spine and swept through a 30° arc proximally and medially [15]. This approach carries a high risk of perforation of the bowel, external iliac vasculature, ureters, and femoral nerve compared to alternative approaches. This approach also appears to be more challenging and have more risk of perforation in larger adults compared to the pediatric population in this study. Westhoff describes the injection of the muscle via an anterior approach under the ilioinguinal ligament [16]. All 13 pediatric patients were noted to experience improvement in tone or range of motion, and no complications from the procedure were observed. However, this approach delivers botulinum toxin primarily to the iliacus portion of the iliopsoas, and not the psoas muscle. The anterior approach to the iliopsoas muscle using EMG localization is typically accurate, and the use of ultrasound does not confer additional benefit.

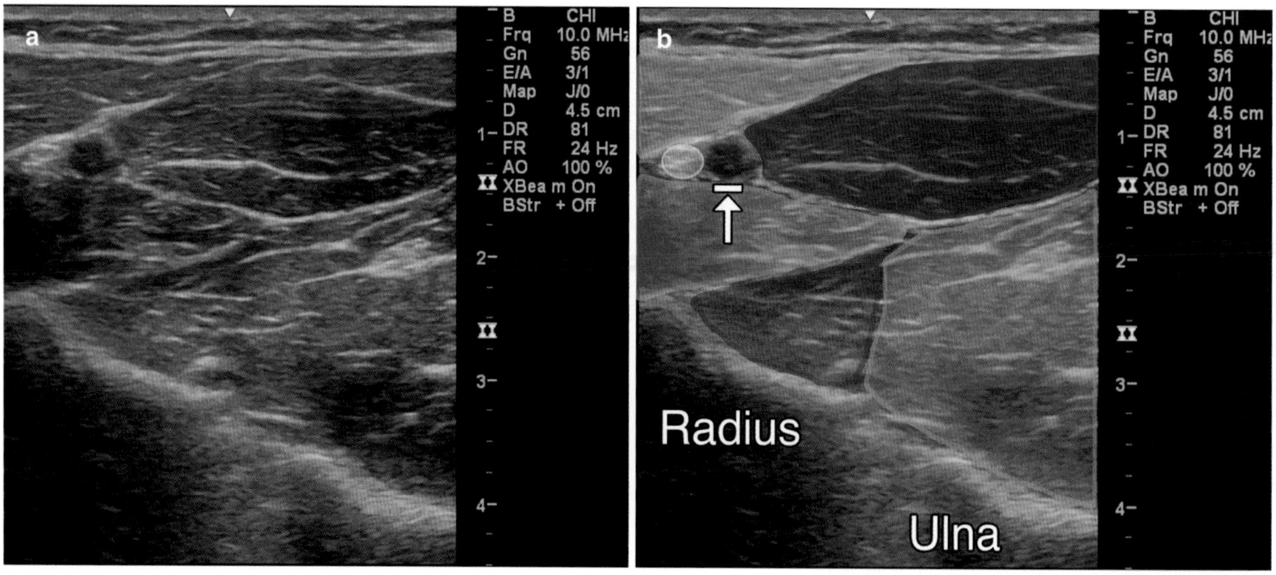

Fig. 9.1 (**a**) Transverse (axial) view of the anterior forearm. (**b**) *Green* indicates brachioradialis, *purple* indicates flexor carpi radialis, *teal* indicates pronator teres, *magenta* indicates flexor pollicis longus, *orange* indicates flexor digitorum profundus, *yellow* indicates radial nerve, *arrow with stop* indicates radial artery

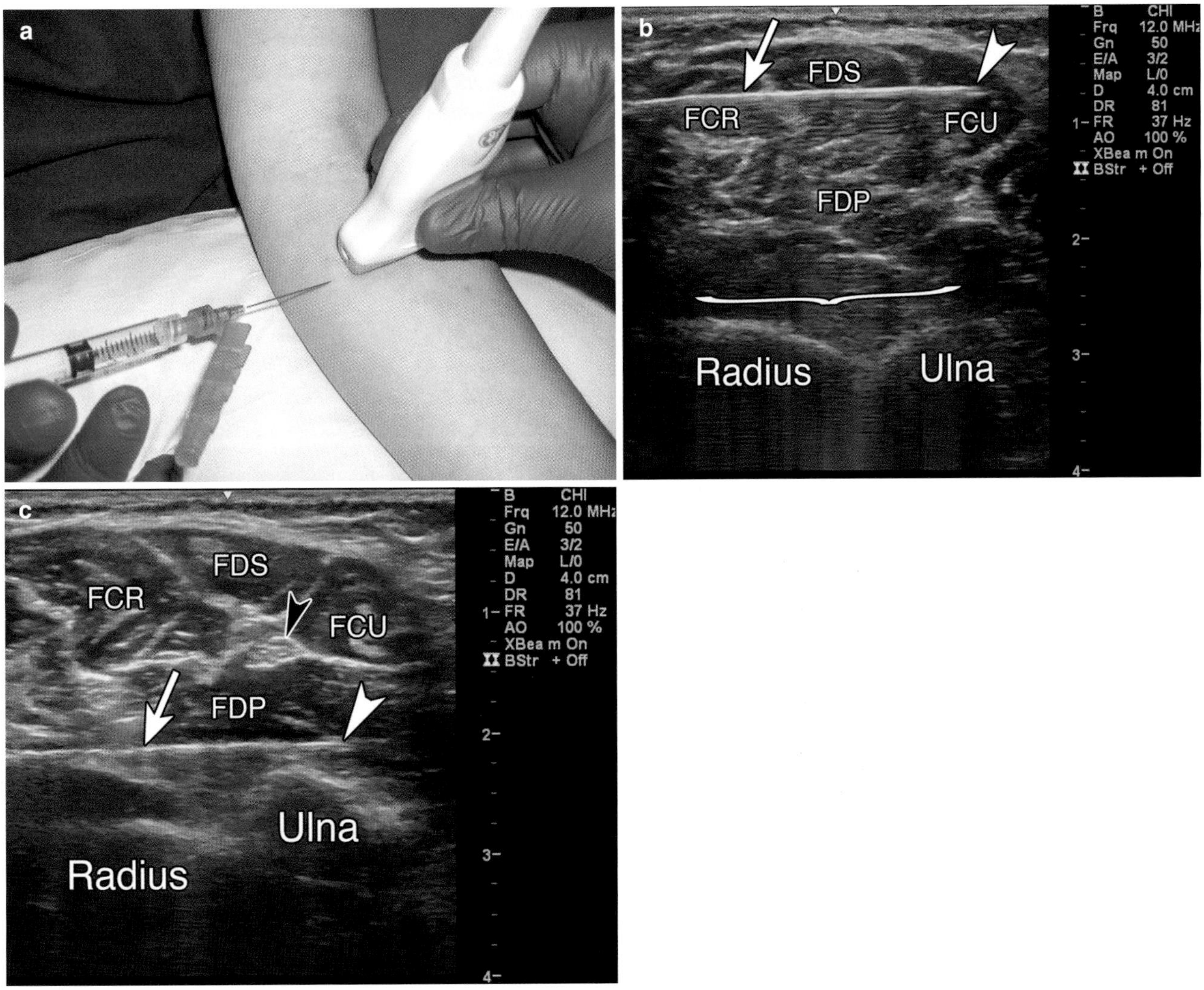

Fig. 9.2 (**a**) Example of axial probe position over proximal anterior forearm. (**b**) *Arrowhead* indicates needle tip in flexor carpi ulnaris, *arrow* indicates needle, *bracket* indicates needle reverberation, radius and ulna labeled, *FCR* flexor carpi radialis, *FDS* flexor digitorum superficialis, *FCU* flexor carpi ulnaris, *FDP* flexor digitorum profundus. (**c**) *White arrowhead* indicates needle tip in FDP, *white arrow* indicates needle, *black arrowhead* indicates ulnar nerve

When reviewing studies on motor end plate locations, the anterior injection approach to the iliopsoas delivers botulinum toxin into a region of the muscle distal to the primary motor end plate zone. Van Campenhout found that the proximal and distal limits of the motor end plate zone for the psoas muscle were located 30–70 % of the distance between the twelfth thoracic vertebrae and the inguinal ligament [17, 18]. Therefore, the dorsal approach is suggested to be an effective injection approach to deliver the botulinum toxin close to the primary motor end plates.

Ward described a blind technique using a dorsal approach to target the psoas by inserting the needle through the erector spinae at L2, L3, and L4 with a slight lateral approach to move just past the lateral border of the transverse processes. The needle is then advanced 1–1.5 cm to reach the psoas muscle [19]. The concern with a blind or EMG-guided technique using this approach is that there is little certainty that the needle has been inserted the correct depth to assure its placement in the psoas muscle. In order for a safe injection via the dorsal approach, visual guidance with ultrasound combined with auditory guidance from EMG is preferred. Takai found ultrasound to be reliable for determining the thickness and the cross-sectional area of the psoas muscle using a dorsal approach [20].

Spinner, Khan, and Kirschner recently demonstrated that ultrasound guidance combined with EMG guidance to inject the psoas muscle via a dorsal approach is feasible (in publication). In this approach, the psoas muscle is visualized in cross section adjacent to the L3 vertebra, and an in-plane technique is used to guide the needle into the muscle. The accuracy was confirmed by EMG. The combined ultrasound and EMG-guided dorsal approach to chemodenervation of the psoas muscle may prove useful as an alternative for the treatment of hip flexion spasticity for patients in which the traditional anterior approach to the injection has shown suboptimal results.

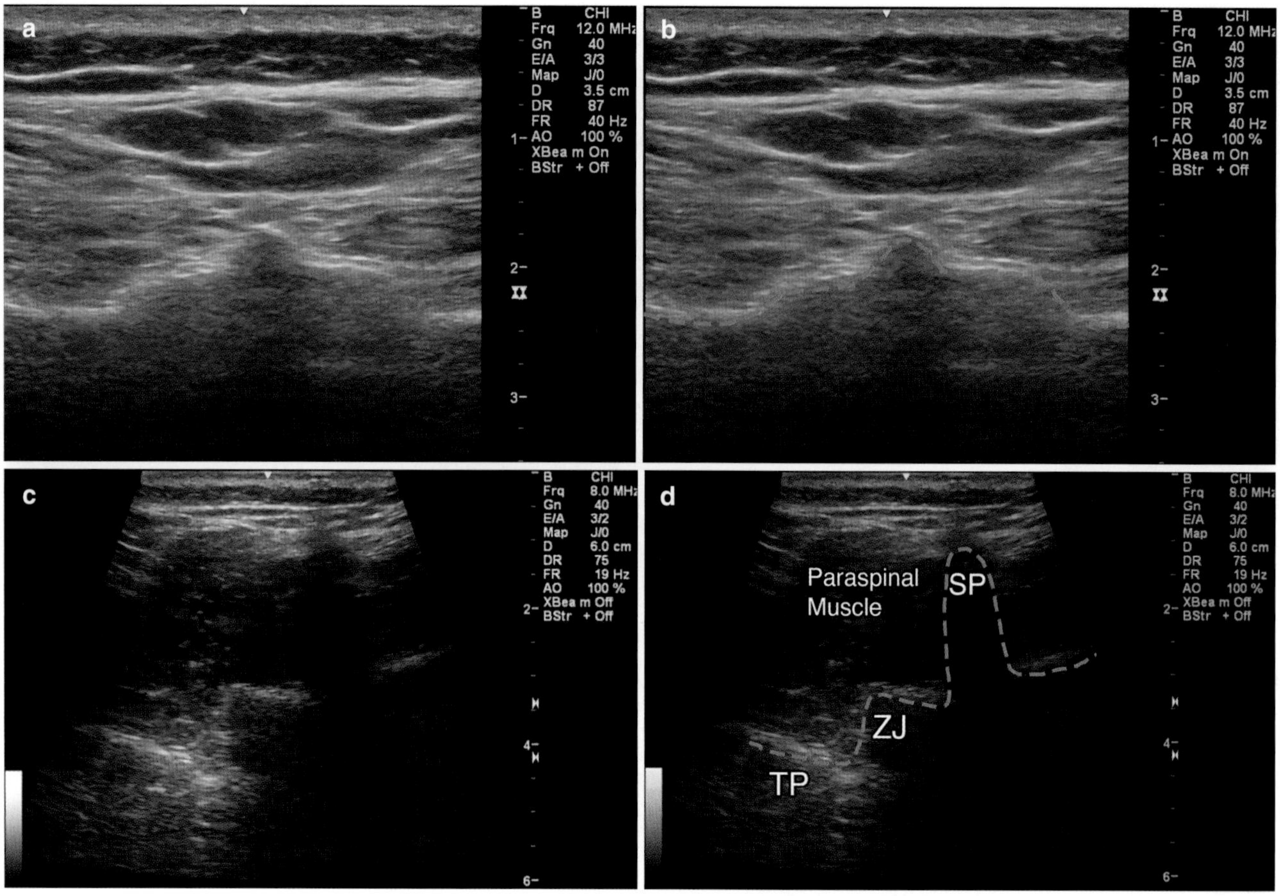

Fig. 9.3 (**a**) Axial view over sacrum. (**b**) *Orange dashed line* outlining hyperechoic bony cortex of sacrum. (**c**) Axial view over L5 vertebra. (**d**) *Orange dashed line* outlining bony anatomy of L5 vertebra, *SP* spinous process, *ZJ* zygapophyseal joint, *TP* transverse process, paraspinal muscle labeled

Scanning Techniques and Anatomy to Identify

The psoas muscle originates off the transverse processes of T12–L5. Begin scanning in an axial plane over the top of the sacrum where you will identify the hyperechoic dorsal bony surface. Slowly scan in this same plane cephalad until you identify a hypoechoic break between the sacrum and L5 spinous process. Slightly cephalad is the bony spinous process of L5. Continue scanning cephalad while counting levels until you reach L3. At this location, follow the hyperechoic bone down the laminae to the facet joints and then continue laterally until the hyperechoic tips of the transverse processes are seen (triple crown sign). The psoas muscle can be visualized in cross section laterally off of the transverse process (Fig. 9.3).

Injection Technique: Dorsal In-Plane Axial Approach

Patient positioning: Position prone or in the lateral recumbent position if hip flexion contracture or spasticity does not allow for prone lying.

Probe positioning: Place the transducer in the axial plane at the level of L3 centered over the psoas muscle belly (Fig. 9.4a).

Markings: Mark the spinal levels.

Needle position: Insert the needle in-plane from medial to lateral.

Safety considerations: Avoid the kidney by not injecting from the L1 to L2 level. Avoid bowel puncture by measuring depth and keeping the needle visualized throughout the entire course.

Pearls:

- Passive ranging of the hip may be used to help identify the psoas muscle.
- The depth of the psoas can be measured prior to injection and correlated with the needle selection to help prevent passing the needle too deep.

Equipment needed:

- Curvilinear or linear array transducer with a frequency between 8 and 3 MHz
- 24+ gauge, Teflon-coated, injectable EMG/stimulator needle, 2.5″–3″
- EMG or nerve stimulator for additional guidance

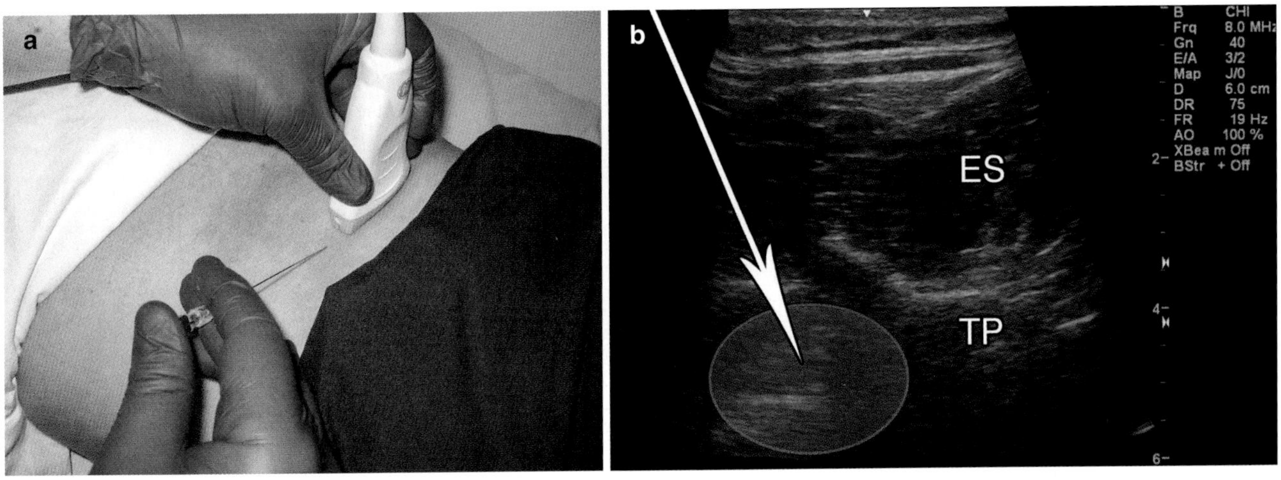

Fig. 9.4 (**a**) Example of axial probe position over L3 vertebra. (**b**) Example of in-plane axial approach, *white arrow* indicates needle trajectory, *TP* transverse process, *ES* erector spinae

Tibialis Posterior Spasticity: Ankle Inversion or Equinovarus

The tibialis posterior originates from the interosseus membrane, proximal tibia, and fibula, and inserts on the navicular, cuneiform, cuboid, and second to fourth metatarsal bones of the foot. Activation of this muscle causes plantar flexion and inversion of the foot. Spasticity of the tibialis posterior muscle may result in an equinovarus deformity. Its location deep in the posterior lower leg makes this a more challenging muscle to target for electrodiagnosis and chemodenervation injections. The accuracy of using anatomical landmarks and palpation to target this muscle has been shown to be about 11 % [5].

Two techniques have been described for a tibialis posterior injection. For the posterior-medial approach is, the practitioner inserts the needle just posterior to the medial tibia at the midpoint of the lower leg, about halfway between the tibial tuberosity and the medial malleolus. Using ultrasound, Won et al. [21] assessed the safety window and depth for EMG needle insertion into the tibialis posterior muscle using a posterior-medial approach into the upper 1/3 distal border compared to the midpoint of the distance between the tibial tubercle and the bimalleolar line. The safety window was defined as the distance between the tibia and neurovascular bundle, and the depth was defined as the distance between the skin and tibialis posterior muscle. Compression of the medial calf was used to decrease the depth necessary to reach the desired muscle. The safety window was significantly greater at the midpoint compared to the upper 1/3 (1.47 cm vs. 1.16 cm, respectively), and the depth was significantly less at the midpoint in relation to the upper 1/3 (2.31 cm vs. 2.52 cm, respectively). Needle insertion in the posterior-medial approach is medial to the tibia and the neurovascular bundle (which is located just posterior to the tibialis posterior muscle). The needle is inserted through the medial gastrocnemius and flexor digitorum longus to reach the tibialis posterior. Compression widens the flexor digitorum longus and displaces the neurovascular border laterally, improving the safety window and decreasing needle depth. An anatomical study of cadavers performed by Oddy et al. determined that the motor point of the tibialis posterior is located in an area 22 % of the distance of a reference line from the fibular head and proximal medial tibia to the intermalleolar line [22]. Therefore, chemodenervation to the distal limit of the upper 1/3 of the tibialis posterior may theoretically provide better results due to proximity to the motor points.

The anterior approach between the tibia and fibula traverses through the tibialis anterior muscle and the interosseous membrane to reach the tibialis posterior muscle in the upper 1/3 segment, with the tibial neurovascular bundle located lateral to the targeted muscle. The safety window in the posterior-medial approach with compression is greater, and the depth is less than the anterior approach. Studies involving MRI and ultrasound of the tibialis posterior examining the posterior and anterior approach have shown that the safety window for needle insertion is greatest using an anterior approach in the proximal 1/3 of the tibia [23, 24].

Scanning Technique and Anatomy to Identify

Posterior-Medial Approach: Position the patient prone with the ankle off the end of the examining table. Begin scanning transversely with ultrasound probe at the midpoint of the lower leg, about halfway between the tibial tuberosity and the medial malleolus. The tibialis posterior muscle lays deep to the gastrocnemius and flexor digitorum longus muscles. Try to identify the posterior tibial artery, vein, and tibial nerve located lateral and just superficial to the tibialis posterior muscle.

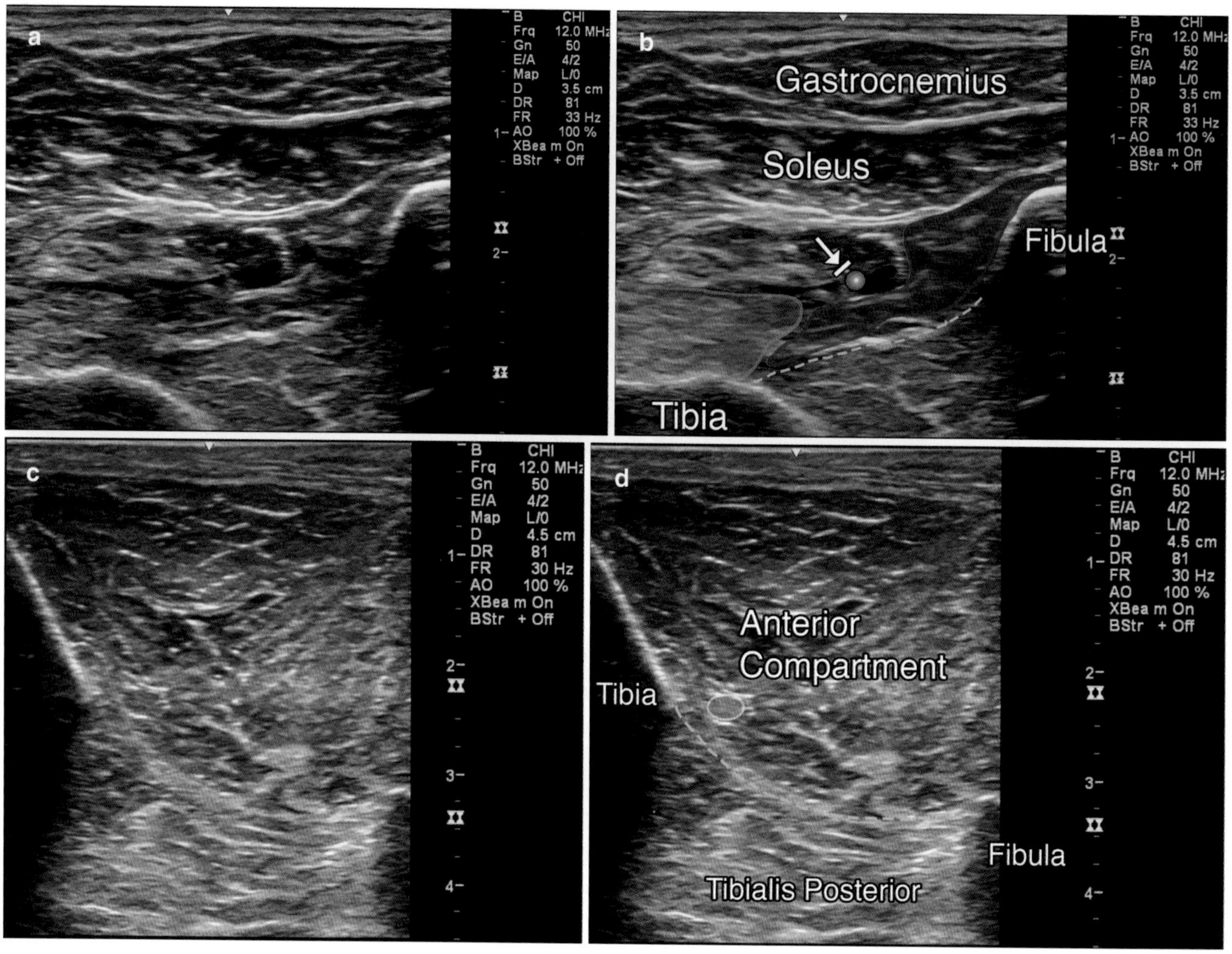

Fig. 9.5 (**a**) Posterior transverse (axial) view of tibialis posterior muscle. (**b**) *Purple* indicates tibialis posterior, *orange* indicates flexor digitorum longus, *arrow with stop* indicates posterior tibial artery, soleus, gastrocnemius, fibula, and tibia labeled. (**c**) Anterior transverse (axial) view of tibialis posterior muscle. (**d**) *Yellow* indicates deep fibular (peroneal) nerve, *green dashed line* indicates interosseous membrane, anterior compartment, tibialis posterior, tibia, and fibula labeled

Anterior Approach: Position the patient supine. Place the ultrasound probe axially along the proximal 1/3 of the anterior lower leg between the tibia and fibula. The tibialis posterior muscle lies deep to the interosseous membrane and the more superficial tibialis anterior muscle. Try to identify the anterior tibial artery and vein and deep fibular nerve, which lay medial to the fibula and along the lateral border of the interosseous membrane (Fig. 9.5).

Injection Techniques: Posteromedial In-Plane Axial Approach

Patient positioning: Prone with lower extremities in neutral position and the ankles extended over the end of table.

Probe positioning: Place the transducer transversely along the medial calf at the approximate midpoint of the distance from the tibial tubercle and the malleoli. Apply compression to increase the safety window (causing widening of the flexor digitorum longus resulting in lateral displacement of the neurovascular bundle) (Fig. 9.6a).

Markings: Identify the neurovascular bundle, consisting of the posterior tibial artery, vein, and tibial nerve, located lateral and just superficial to the tibialis posterior muscle. The tibia is located medially and the fibula deep to the tibialis posterior.

Needle position: Insert the needle from medial to lateral in-plane with the probe traversing through the medial gastrocnemius and flexor digitorum longus.

Safety considerations: Utilize Doppler to identify the tibial artery and vein. Compression with the probe will help displace the neurovascular bundle to increase the safety window.

Pearls:

- Passive ankle inversion may be used to help identify the tibialis posterior muscle.

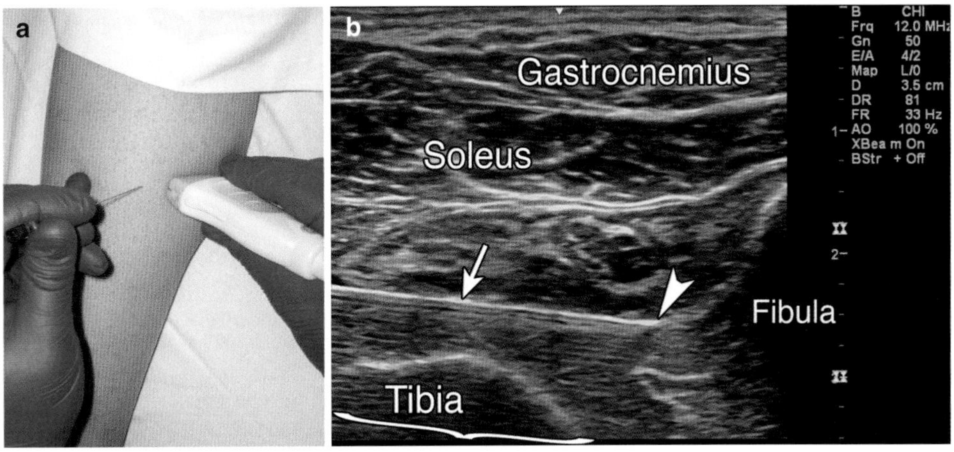

Fig. 9.6 (**a**) Example of axial probe position over dorsal calf. (**b**) Example of in-plane axial approach, *white arrow* indicates needle, *arrowhead* indicates needle tip, *brackets* indicate reverberation, gastrocnemius, soleus, tibia, and fibula labeled

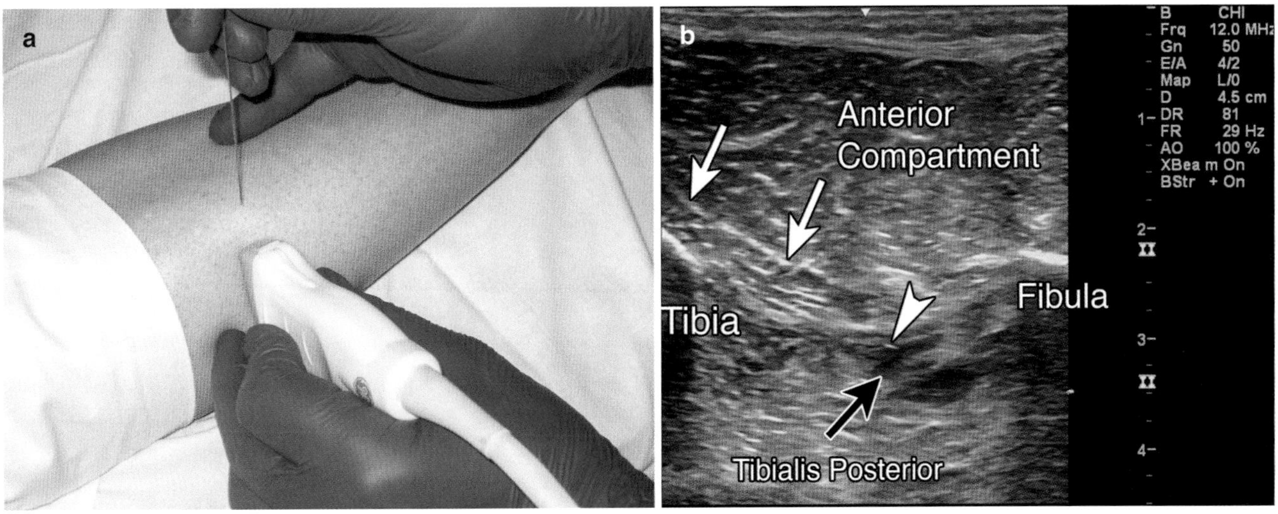

Fig. 9.7 (**a**) Example of axial probe position over anterior compartment lower leg. (**b**) *White arrows* indicate needle, *white arrowhead* indicates needle tip, *black arrow* indicates anechoic injectate filling tibialis posterior, anterior compartment, tibialis posterior, tibia, and fibula labeled

Injection Techniques: Anterior In-Plane Axial Approach

Patient positioning: Supine with the affected lower extremity in slight internal rotation.

Probe positioning: Place the transducer along the anterior leg in the axial plane lateral to the tibia at the approximate border of the proximal 1/3 and middle 1/3 of the distance from the tibial tubercle to the malleoli (Fig. 9.7a).

Markings: Identify the interosseous membrane between the tibia and fibula. The tibialis posterior lies deep to the interosseous membrane. The anterior tibial neurovascular bundle is found lateral and just superficial.

Needle position: Insert the needle lateral to the tibia, in-plane, through the anterior tibialis muscle and interosseous membrane.

Safety considerations: Avoid the neurovascular bundle, consisting of the anterior tibial artery and vein and deep fibular nerve, which lie medial to the fibula along the lateral border of the interosseous membrane. Utilize Doppler to identify the anterior tibial artery and vein.

Pearls:

- Given the depth of the injection, the needle tip will not be visualized as it traverses through the deep portion of the tibialis anterior and through the interosseus membrane to the tibialis posterior.
- The deflection of the interosseus membrane on the ultrasound screen will indicate the needle is traversing through this area.
- An EMG needle may be used to provide auditory feedback indicating its position in the tibialis posterior muscle after the needle pierces through the interosseus membrane.
- The anterior approach is useful if you want to minimize number of needle "sticks" for the patient who also needs a tibialis anterior injection.

Equipment needed:

- Linear array transducer with a frequency 8+ MHz
- Preparation of botulinum toxin

- 24+ gauge, Teflon-coated, injectable EMG/stimulator needle, 2.5″–3″
- EMG or nerve stimulator for additional guidance

Cervical Dystonia: Abnormal Neck Posture

Idiopathic cervical dystonia (CD) is a commonly occurring adult-onset focal dystonia characterized by abnormal neck posture, neck pain, and muscle hypertrophy. Botulinum toxin is the first-line treatment for this condition and is known to provide sufficient relief of symptoms in more than 85 % of patients [25]. A good response relies on proper selection of muscles and appropriate medication dosages. Traditionally, injections are guided by palpation or EMG guidance. However, these methods are not foolproof, especially for deeply located muscles. Both botulinum toxin A (Botox, Disport, Xeomin) and B (Neurobloc, Myobloc) are deemed safe and effective treatment for cervical dystonia.

The most common types of CD are torticollis (head turned) and laterocollis (head and neck tilt). Other types include retrocollis (head and neck extension), anterocollis (head and neck flexion), or a combination of these types. Many studies have attempted to classify patterns by analysis of muscles involved and usually rely on the Tsui score or the Toronto Western Spasmodic Torticollis Rating Scale (TWSTRS) [26]. For example, Hefter et al. selected one of 12 injection protocols they created based on a combination of the following: the presence or absence of shoulder elevation, tremor, sternocleidomastoid muscle hypertrophy (graded), and contralateral or ipsilateral movement direction [27]. Their muscles of choice to inject included the following: sternocleidomastoid (SCM), levator scapula and/or scalenes, and splenius capitis and/or trapezius and/or semispinalis. Lee et al. selected 14 patients with idiopathic CD and used ultrasound and PET/CT to select muscles for botulinum injection. They then used EMG to guide their injections, except for eight patients with muscles that extended beyond the reach of the EMG needle. For the remaining muscles, sonographic guidance was performed in six patients by a musculoskeletal radiologist. In another study using CT guidance, 13 botulinum injections were performed into specifically chosen muscles of eight patients. The most common site was the obliquus capitis inferior muscle, followed by the longus colli muscles. Other muscles included the obliquus capitis superior, scalenes anterior, scalenes posterior, and levator scapulae. All injections were deemed successful with a decrease in pain and improvement in neck movement, whether by ultrasound guidance or CT guidance [28] (see Tables 9.5, 9.6, and 9.7).

Table 9.5 Cervical Dystonia Rating Systems

Tsui score [26]	Toronto Western Spasmodic Torticollis Rating Scale [29]
(A) Amplitude of sustained movements:	I. Torticollis Severity Scale
Rotation	A. Maximal excursion
Tilt Anterocollis/retrocollis Combined score = A	1. Rotation (turn: right or left)
(B) Duration of sustained movements (C) Shoulder elevation (D) Tremor severity:	2. Laterocollis (tilt: right or left, exclude shoulder elevation)
Duration Severity × duration = D	3. Anterocollis/retrocollis (a or b)
Total score = [(A) × (B)] + (C) + (D)	4. Lateral shift
	5. Sagittal shift
	B. Duration factor
	C. Effect of sensory tricks
	D. Shoulder elevation/anterior displacement
	E. ROM
	F. Time
	Disability scale
	A. Work
	B. ADLs
	C. Driving
	D. Reading
	E. TV
	F. Activities outside the home
	Pain
	A. Severity
	B. Duration
	C. Disability due to pain

Please see Tsui scale and TWSTRS scoring documents for details

Scanning Technique and Anatomy to Identify

Injections are usually given into the sternocleidomastoid, anterior/posterior scalenes, splenius capitis, levator scapulae, scalene, and/or the trapezius muscles. (Please see trigger point chapter for injection techniques.)

Pearls:

- Contralateral splenius group is major head rotator, not sternocleidomastoid (SCM).
- SCM is actually an extensor and contralateral rotator.
- Longissimus colli: Long and thin muscle; therefore, this muscle has a long moment arm.
- Levator scapulae are perpendicular to SCM.
- Scalenes attach up to C2.
- *Remember scalenes are used in respiration.

Equipment needed:

- Linear array transducer with a frequency of 10+ MHz
- Preparation of botulinum toxin

Table 9.6 Imaging-guided BTX injection [28]

Torticollis pattern type	Target	Botulinum toxin A (Botox) dose (IU)	Guidance
RC, right	Right OCI	40	Sonography
RC, right; LC, left; AC	Right OCI	40, 50	Sonography
RC, right; LC, right[a]	Right OCI	90	Sonography
RC, right; LC, right[a]	Right OCI, left OCS	30, 20	Sonography
RC, right; LC, left	Right OCI	55	Sonography
RC, right; AC	Right OCI	30	Sonography

RC rotatory torticollis, *LC* lateral torticollis, *OCI* obliquus capitis inferior, *AC* anterior torticollis, *Lc* longus colli, *OCS* obliquus capitis superior, *ScA* scalenus anterior, *ScP* scalenus posterior

[a]LC, right indicates that head was tilted to right side and neck was titled to left side relative to trunk

Table 9.7 Cervical rotators

Contralateral rotators	Ipsilateral rotators
Upper trapezius	Splenius capitis to cervicis
Levator scapulae (rotation) [31]	Levator scapulae (tilt)
Splenius group	Inferior oblique
SCM	

- 24+ gauge, Teflon-coated, injectable EMG/stimulator needle, 2.5″–3″
- EMG or nerve stimulator for additional guidance

Salivary Gland Injections: Sialorrhea and Chronic Aspiration

The salivary glands produce approximately 1–1.5 L of saliva daily in adults and about 0.75–0.9 L in children. Salivary contribution comes mainly from the submandibular gland (65 %), as well as the parotid (20 %), sublingual (7–8 %), and minor glands (7–8 %) [30]. The parotid is mainly responsible for salivation in response to smell and taste. The submandibular is located between the anterior and posterior belly of the digastric muscles under the mandible. The parotid is located midway between the external auditory canal and angle of the mandible.

Children develop neuromotor control of the oral cavity between 18 and 24 months of age, so drooling is normal in infants and toddlers. The presence of drooling over age 4 is considered pathological. Drooling tends to be due to oromotor dysfunction rather than overproduction of saliva in neurological conditions, such as stroke, Parkinson's disease, ALS, and cerebral palsy. Anterior drooling presents only as external drooling around the mouth and chin, and may be very socially uncomfortable for the patient as well as lead to sores around the mouth and chin. Patients with posterior drooling often have choking and develop chronic aspiration and pneumonia that many times leads to frequent hospitalizations.

Botulinum toxin is used as a treatment to control sialorrhea due to its inhibition of presynaptic acetylcholine in the parasympathetically innervated salivary glands. The effect of botulinum toxin injection into the salivary glands typically lasts for 6 months, compared to approximately 3 months for muscles [32]. There is no consensus regarding which glands are the best to inject and how many injections are recommended for optimal treatment effect. Many prefer to only inject the submandibular glands, as these glands are responsible for the majority of saliva production throughout the day, and therefore not interfere with the parotid glands which are active mainly with stimulation from food. Some studies have showed good results with injection of both sets of glands. Based on current literature, it has been recommended to limit initial botulinum toxin injections to the submandibular glands, especially for fasting patients [33]. Combined parotid and submandibular gland injections have been suggested for patients with more severe swallowing issues or aspiration or patients that have failed response to submandibular gland injections alone [34].

Tables 9.8 and 9.9 provide an overview of procedural specifications and summary of several studies examining ultrasound guidance for salivary gland injections. There was one randomized clinical trial by Dogu et al. that compared ultrasound-guided vs. blind injections [39]. Two 15 unit botulinum toxin A doses were injected into each parotid gland in patients with Parkinson's disease. The study demonstrated significant improvement in objective saliva measures at 1 week postinjection for the ultrasound-guided group and superior improvement at weeks 4 and 12 postinjection compared to the blinded injection group. Subjective reduction in saliva was significantly improved in both the ultrasound-guided injection and blind injection group with greater reduction in the ultrasound group.

Ultrasound guidance for salivary gland injections is useful to avoid vascular or nerve injury during neurotoxin injection procedure. Eid noted an anatomical variant of the arterial supply in the submandibular gland that would come in close proximity to the safety zone described for blind injections

Table 9.8 Procedural specifications of ultrasound-guided salivary gland injections

Study	Glands injected	Neurotoxin used	Dosing used	Volume	# of participants	# of injections per gland
Breheret et al. [35]	Submandibular and parotid	Botox	Submandibular: 20 units each Parotid: 30 units each	100 units/2 mL = 5 units/0.1 mL	70 pts. with neuromusc. d/o incl. ALS, PD, and CP	Submandibular: 1 injection Parotid: 2 injections (15 units each)
Norgarden (2011) [32]	Submandibular and parotid	Botox	25 units	0.8 mL/gland	6 children with CP	1 injection/gland
Guidubaldi (2011) [52]	Submandibular and parotid	Botulinum toxin A (Dysport) vs. botulinum toxin B (Neurobloc)	Dysport: Parotid—100 units Submandibular—25 units Neurobloc: Parotid—1,000 units Submandibular—250 unit	Dysport: 25 units/0.1 mL Neurobloc: 250 units/0.1 mL	14 pts. with ALS or PD	Parotid: 2 injections Submandibular: 1 injection
Moller et al. (2011) [36]	Submandibular and parotid	Botulinum toxin A (Botox)	Parotid: 25–40 units Submandibular: 15–30 units	--Did not specify--	15 pts. with ALS or PD	-Did not specify more than 1 inj/gland-
Wu et al. (2011) [37]	Submandibular and parotid	Botulinum toxin A (Botox)	30 units < 15 kg, 40 units: 15–25 kg, 50 units >25 kg. Max. dose for each submandibular gland was 10 units No more than 50 units total dose	10 units/0.1 mL	20 children with CP	1 injection/gland
Khan et al. (2011) [38]	Submandibular and parotid	Botulinum toxin A (Botox)	5 units/kg	Small volume of 0.25–0.50 mL/gland	45 children with neurological impairments	1 injection/gland
Scheffer (2010) [34]	Submandibular	Botox	15 units/gland—pts <15 kg 20 units/gland—pts 15–25 kg 25 units/gland—pts > 25 kg	–	131 children with CP or another nonprogressive neurological disorder	3 injections/gland
Erasmus et al. (2010) [40]	Submandibular	Botulinum toxin A (Botox)	30–50 units total dose	--Did not specify--	15 pts. with CP	-Did not specify more than 1 inj/gland-
Sriskandan et al. (2009) [41]	Submandibular	Botulinum toxin A (Botox)	20–25 units	--Did not specify--	4 pts. With CP	-Did not specify more than 1 inj/gland-
Pena (2009) [33]	Submandibular—only in fasting pts Submandibular and parotid—non-fasting pts.	Botulinum toxin A (Botox)	1 unit/kg/gland—9–40 units/gland Max. dosage 100 units	10 units/0.1 mL	36 children with neurological disorders	-Did not specify more than 1 inj/gland-
Marina et al. (2008) [42]	Submandibular and parotid	Botulinum toxin A (Botox)	25 units/gland	1.25 U/0.1–10 U/0.1 ml	20 pts: 14 CP, 4 PD, 1 anoxic encephalopathy, and 1 CVA	1 injection/gland
Reid et al. (2008) [43]	Submandibular and parotid	Botox	25 units/gland	1 mL/gland	24 treatment vs. 24 control	1 injection/gland
Wilken et al. (2008) [44]	Submandibular and parotid	Botulinum toxin A (Botox) vs. botulinum toxin B (Neurobloc)	Parotid: Botox 25–35 MU, Neurobloc 30–40 unit/kg Submandibular: Botox 15 MU, Neurobloc 20 units/kg	Botox: 100 unit/2 mL Botulinum toxin B: prepackaged in 1–1.5 mL solution	30 children with CP	Parotid: 2 injections Submandibular: 1 injection

Gerlinger et al. (2007) [45]	Submandibular and parotid	Botulinum toxin A	30–50 units/treatment	-Not specified-	21 children	2–3 injections/gland
Shetty et al. (2006) [46]	Submandibular only: 7pts Submandibular and parotid: 1 pt.	Botulinum toxin A (Botox)	Submandibular: 15 units each Parotid: 7.5 units	5 units/0.2 mL	8 adult pts. with dx incl. head and neck carcinoma, neurodegenerative diseases, quadriplegia, and idiopathic salivation	-Did not specify more than 1 inj/gland-
Hassin-Baer et al. (2005) [47]	Parotid	Botulinum toxin A (Botox)	First 4 pts: 5 units (up to 25 kg) or 10 units (above 25 kg)/gland. Booster injection (equal to the initial dose) given after a month if suboptimal response. After treatment of the first four patients noted these doses were inadequate; dose was increased to 10 units/gland for remaining pts.	100 units/2 mL	9 children: 6 with CP, 1 post-herpes encephalitis, 1 bilateral opercular syndrome, 1 metachromatic leukodystrophy, and 1 Rett's syndrome	1 injection/gland
Dogu (2004) [39]	Parotid	Botulinum toxin A (Botox)	30 units total into each gland	-Not specified-	15 pts. with PD	Two 15 unit injections into each parotid
Jongerius et al. (2004) [49]	Submandibular	Botulinum toxin A (Botox)	15 units/gland—pts <15 kg 20 units/gland—pts 15–25 kg 25 units/gland—pts>25 kg	-Not specified-	45 children with CP	At least 3 injections/gland

Table 9.9 Summary of studies involving ultrasound-guided salivary gland injections

Study	Design	Outcome measures	Results	Adverse effects
Pediatric studies				
Wu (2011) [37]	Randomized, DB, PC. 20 pts. randomized to exp. Grp ($n=10$) receiving Botox and control grp receiving NS via US guidance into salivary glands	Baseline, 1 and 3 month assessment—subjective drooling scale, salivary flow rate, and oral health (salivary composition and bacterial count)	Salivary flow rate: significant decrease in exp. grp vs. control at 1 and 3 month Subjective drooling: no significant difference in exp. vs. control grp at 1 and 3 month Oral health: no significant difference betw. salivary composition and bacterial colony count	None
Khan (2011) [38]	Retrospective medical chart review of neurologically impaired children who received botulinum toxin injections ($n=45$)	Duration of effect, saliva consistency, caregiver willingness to repeat treatment, caregiver satisfaction with treatment, and visual analogue scale of the child's quality of life after treatment	Mean *duration of effect* was 4.6 month. (range, 1–24 months) *Saliva consistency*: thicker saliva after the injection (47 %); both thick and foamy saliva (7 %) *Caregiver satisf. and QoL*: 80 % improved, 13 % no change, 7 % worse	1, aspiration pneumonia; 4, difficulty swallowing; 3, speech impairment; 2, pain 24 complications reported: 17 minor, 7 major; girls were 6.3 times more likely to experience late-onset complications than boys
Norgarden (2011) [32]	Crossed double-blind design was planned. Group (A1): injections to both the parotid and submandibular glands, group (B1): injections to the submandibular glands only	Objective: cotton roll saturation 3 min Subjective: VAS	Reduction of observed drooling in 3, while 4 patients reported subjective improvement 5 pts. completed A1 and 1 completed B1	4 pts. with increased dental plaques, 1 pt. with dysphagia, and 1 pt. with dysarthria × 2 months. Study terminated prior to completion due to adverse effects
Scheffer (2010) [34]	Prospective cohort study of 131 pts. With CP or other neurological disorder	Direct observational drooling quotient (DQ) and subjective VAS scores	46.6 % of pts. showed good response, DQ: mean reduction from baseline of 29–15 after 2 months and 19 after 8 months. Mean VAS score decreased from 80 at baseline to 53 after 2 months and increased to 66 after 8 months	Thickened saliva 41 %, temporary swallowing difficulty 3 %, xerostomia 1.7 %
Erasmus (2010) [40]	Prospective clinical trial of 15 pts. with CP.	Drooling intensity (DQ) and salivary flow rate at baseline and at 2, 4, 8, 16, and 24 weeks	Flow rates: significant differences point up to 16 week postinjection, except for at 4 week, which did not reach statistical significance Drooling quotient: statistically significant at 2, 4, 8, and 24 weeks	Swallowing and chewing problems: 7 pts Thickened saliva: 9 pts.
Sriskandan (2009) [43]	Prospective study of 4 pts. with CP with drooling	Questionnaire-based assessment of the severity and incidence of drooling at baseline and 3 mo	All showed significant improvement in severity of drooling	Difficulty in retaining prosthetic orbital globes in 1 pt.
Pena (2009) [33]	A 3-year retrospective review of 220 US-guided salivary gland injections in 36 patients	Mean pretreatment analysis period was 48 months, and the mean follow-up period was 21 months Anterior drooling: # of bibs and/or need for suctioning Posterior drooling: gagging, coughing, or suctioning frequency	Posterior drooling grp: 88 % improvement Anterior drooling grp: 66 % improvement Total # of hospital admissions for respiratory illness decreased by 56.4 %	one episode of self-limited oral bleeding
Reid (2008) [43]	Randomized controlled trial with parallel group design of 24 pts. with CP	Subjective: drooling impact scale at baseline and monthly postinjection up to 6 months	Max. response was at 1 month—highly significant difference in the mean scores between exp. and control groups. This difference remained significant at 6 months	Difficulty swallowing, choking, and deterioration of speech in 1 pt. for few days postinjection, 1 pt. with chest infection, and 1 pt. with 1st seizure
Wilken (2008) [44]	Randomized clinical trial in 30 pts. with neurological disorders comparing BoNT-A vs. BoNT-B	Subjective: Teacher Drooling Scale (TDS) at baseline and 4 week postinjection	Treatment successful in 83 % of pts. after 1st injection. Only 50 % pt. continued treatment. No significant difference between BoNT-A and BoNT-B	Viscous saliva: 5 children Unilateral parotitis: 1 case

Gerlinger (2007) [45]	Prospective study of 21 pts: 17 with CP and 4 with meningoencephalitis	Saliva volume (U/ml) over five minutes, concentrations of amylase (U/ml) and immunoglobulin (Ig) A, protein content (mg/ml), and electrolyte content	20 pts. responded well with decrease in saliva volume lasting 3–4 month, and increase in amylase and protein content. 1 pt. showed no change in salivation severity	None
Hassin-Baer (2005) [47]	Prospective clinical trial of 9 pts. with dx incl. CP, post-herpes encephalitis, bilateral opercular syndrome, metachromatic leukodystrophy, and Rett's syndrome	Objective: 2-min roll saturation test Subjective: severity and frequency of drooling scale	7/9 improved in objective measures, 3/9 improvement in subjective measures of drooling severity and frequency	None
Jongerius (2004) [49]	Controlled, open-label, clinical trial of 45 pts. with CP comparing BoNT injections vs. scopolamine	Objective: drooling quotient (DQ) Subjective: VAS at baseline, during, and after scopolamine washout and 2, 4, 8, 16, and 24 weeks post-BoNT injection	Both BoNT injections and scopolamine showed significant improvement in drooling, but scopolamine demonstrated more frequent and serious side effects	Scopolamine: 82.2 % of cases Most common: xerostomia (66.7 %), restlessness (35.6 %), somnolence (35.6 %), blurred vision due to pupillary dilation, and confusion (20 %) BoNT: 2 pts, flu-like symptoms, and 3 pts, swallowing difficulty
Pediatric and adult studies				
Breheret (2011) [35]	Retrospective study of 111 ultrasound-guided botulinum toxin injections on 70 pts. with dx incl. ALS, PD, and CP—study compared multiple dosing protocols	Telephone interview 6–8 weeks postinjection: subjective questionnaire of quality of life	Most effective protocol: 20 units of botulinum toxin into each submaxillary gland and 30 units of toxin into each parotid gland	No major complications Minor complications incl. swollen glands, thickened saliva, and pain during injection
Marina (2008) [42]	Prospective clinical trial of 20 pts. (mean age 15y) dx included CP, PD, hypoxic encephalopathy, and CVA	Dribbling rating score, dribbling frequency score, dribbling severity score, the number of towel changes in 24 h, and the visual analogue score at baseline, 2, 8, and 12 week postinjection	All patients/caregivers reported significant symptom improvement in dribbling: 8 pts, marked improvement; 10, moderate improvement; and 2, slight improvement	None
Adult studies				
Guidubaldi (2011) [52]	Prospective, randomized, crossover, double-blind trial comparing both BoNT-A and BoNT-B consecutively in 14 pts. with ALS or PD	Objective: cotton roll wt. Subjective: drooling severity scale, drooling frequency scale, adapted drool rating scale, VAS, and clinical global impression assessed at baseline, 1 and 4 week after injection, and every 4 weeks thereafter until drooling returned to baseline	No difference in objective or subjective improvement in BoNT-A and BoNT-B, but there was a significantly shorter latency in onset of BoNT-B compared to BoNT-A	
Moller (2011) [36]	Prospective clinical trial of 15 pts: 12 with ALS, 3 with PD	Subjective ratings of drooling, and objective measurement of saliva flow at baseline and every 2 weeks for up to 8 weeks	Max. reductions during the observation period were 40 % for drooling and 30 % for flow. Both significantly reduced 2 week after treatment. Further improvement in subjective report at 4 week, flow rates returned to baseline at 4 week, then decreased again at 8 week	None
Shetty (2006) [46]	Prospective clinical trial of 8 pts. with dx incl. neurological diseases, idiopathic salivation, and cancer	Subjective assessment of drooling severity and VAS scale at baseline, 6 weeks, and 6 months	Decreased salivation noted avg. of 5 days postinjection, 7 pts. reported significant reduction in salivation at 6 week and 5 pts. at 6 month., 1 pt. with PD had no significant benefit	Postinjection site pain in 1 pt
Dogu (2004) [39]	Randomized clinical trial of effectiveness of US-guided vs. "blind" injections in 15 pts. with PD	Objective saliva measurement: baseline, 1st, 4th, and 12th week postinjection Subjective: VAS daily × 1 week after treatment	Significant improvement of objective measures in exp. vs. control grp, both grps showed significant improvement in subjective measures	2 pt. in exp. grp. with mild dry mouth × 1 month

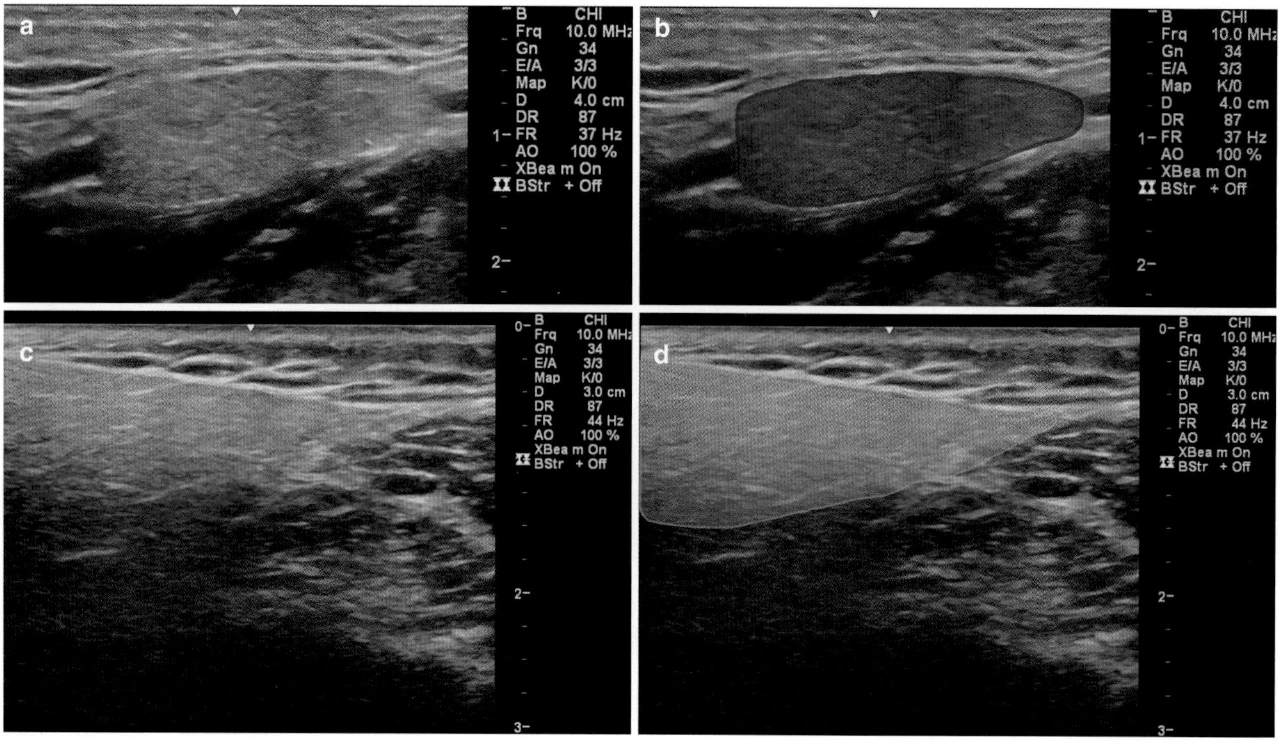

Fig. 9.8 (**a**) Transverse view of submandibular gland. (**b**) *Purple* indicates submandibular gland. (**c**) Transverse view of parotid gland. (**d**) *Orange* indicates parotid gland

[48]. When performing injections to the parotid gland, there is potential for injury to the facial nerve. The facial nerve exits the skull through the stylomastoid foramen and passes through the large parotid gland where the nerve divides into its branches. In order to protect the facial nerve from damage and prevent a facial droop as a complication of the neurotoxin injection, it has been recommended that E-stimulation be used to identify the nerve and target the injection away from the nerve branches [50].

Scanning Technique and Anatomy to Identify

Submandibular Gland: Place the patient supine with the head slightly extended and rotated away for better access to the gland. Position the transducer medial to the angle of the mandible. The gland is hypoechoic compared to surrounding tissues. Examine in both longitudinal and transverse planes.

Parotid Gland: Place the patient supine with slight rotation away. Place the transducer between the anterior ear and the angle of the mandible. The gland is hypoechoic and will appear more attenuative than the submandibular gland due its fat content (Fig. 9.8).

Injection Techniques: In-Plane Axial Approach (Submandibular)

Patient positioning: Lay the patient supine with the head in slight extension and rotation away.

Probe positioning: Center the probe over under the mandible over the submandibular gland (Fig. 9.9a).

Markings: The submandibular gland is located between the anterior and posterior belly of the digastric muscle under the mandible [51].

Needle position: Insert the needle in-plane using an axial approach aiming at the center of the gland.

Injection Techniques: Out-of-Plane Axial Approach (Parotid)

Patient positioning: Lay the patient supine with the head in slight extension and rotation away.

Probe positioning: Center the probe anterior to the ear over the parotid gland (Fig. 9.10a).

Markings: The parotid gland is localized midway between the external auditory canal and angle of the mandible [51].

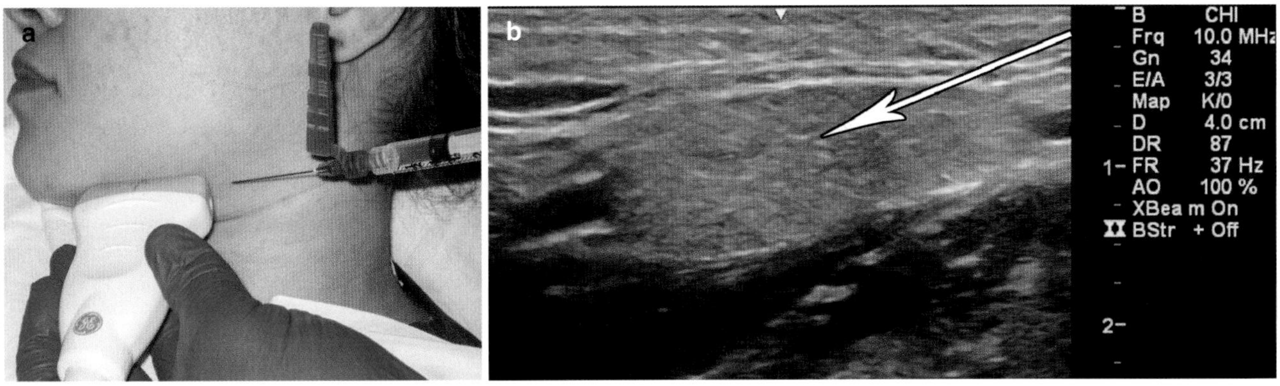

Fig. 9.9 (**a**) Example of axial probe position over submandibular gland. (**b**) *White arrow* indicates trajectory of needle into center of gland

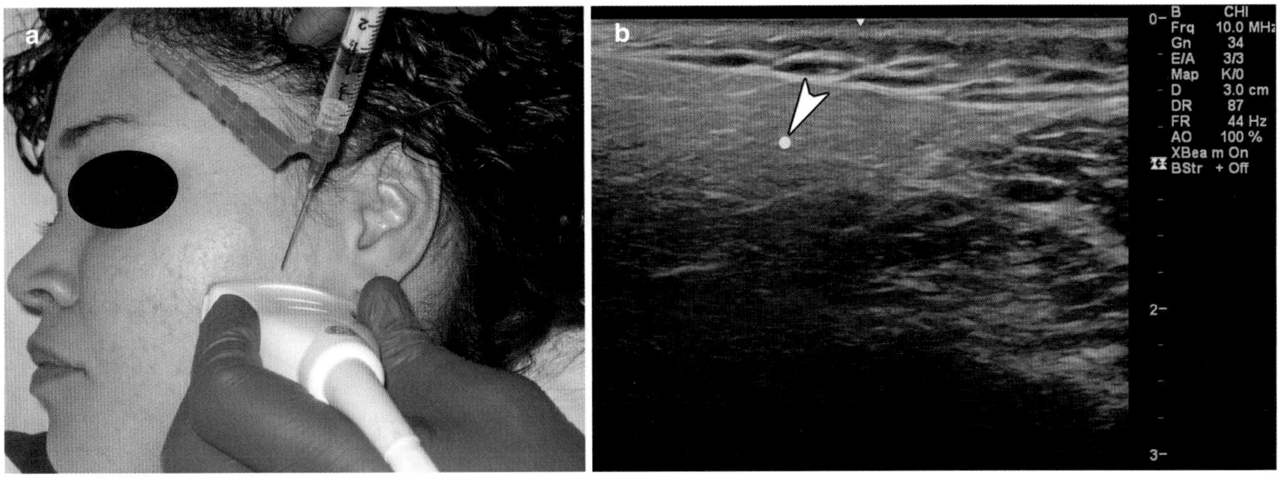

Fig. 9.10 (**a**) Example of probe position over parotid gland. (**b**) *White arrowhead* indicates needle tip centered in the parotid gland

Needle position: Insert the needle out-of-plane aiming at the center of the gland.

Safety considerations: Use small volumes to reduce risk of diffusion into surrounding pharyngeal and cervical muscles and soft tissues leading to dysphagia or dysarthria. Potential adverse effects reported in literature include the following: dysphagia, dysarthria, increase in viscoelasticity of saliva affecting swallowing function, increase in dental plaques (as saliva has a natural cleaning effect), swollen glands and pain during injection, dry mouth, infection, and bleeding [8, 50, 51].

Pearls:

- Consider use of topical lidocaine cream to preinjection sites for adults and older children to decrease pain.
- For young children, consider using conscious sedation during procedure.
- Extending neck may help target the submandibular glands.
- Advise patient or caregivers to only consume mashed or melted food for first week postinjection.

Equipment needed:

- High-frequency linear array transducer 7.5–15 MHz
- 25 gauge 1.5″ needle
- Botulinum toxin preparation
- Consider topical lidocaine cream to injection site prior to procedure

References

1. Curtiss HM, Finnoff JT, Peck E, Hollman J, Muir J, Smith J. Accuracy of ultrasound-guided and palpation-guided knee injections by an experienced and less-experienced injector using a superolateral approach: a cadaveric study. PM R. 2011;3(6):507–15.
2. Sabeti-Aschraf M, Lemmerhofer B, Lang S, Schmidt M, Funovics PT, Ziai P, Frenzel S, Kolb A, Graf A, Schueller-Weidekamm C. Ultrasound guidance improves the accuracy of the acromioclavicular joint infiltration: a prospective randomized study. Knee Surg Sports Traumatol Arthrosc. 2011;19(2):292–5.

3. Wisniewski SJ, Smith J, Patterson DG, Carmichael SW, Pawlina W. Ultrasound-guided versus nonguided tibiotalar joint and sinus tarsi injections: a cadaveric study. PM R. 2010;2(4):277–81.
4. Haig AJ, Goodmurphy CW, Harris AR, Ruiz AP, Etemad J. The accuracy of needle placement in lower-limb muscles: a blinded study. Arch Phys Med Rehabil. 2003;84(6):877–82.
5. Chin TY, Nattrass GR, Selber P, Graham HK. Accuracy of intramuscular injection of botulinum toxin A in juvenile cerebral palsy: a comparison between manual needle placement and placement guided by electrical stimulation. J Pediatr Orthop. 2005;25(3):286–91.
6. Lim ECH, Seet RCS. Botulinum toxin: description of injection techniques and examination of controversies surrounding toxin diffusion. Acta Neurol Scand. 2008;117(2):73–84.
7. Gooch JL, Patton CP. Combining botulinum toxin and phenol to manage spasticity in children. Arch Phys Med Rehabil. 2004;85(7):1121–4.
8. Stengel G, Bee EK. Antibody-induced secondary treatment failure in a patient treated with botulinum toxin type A for glabellar frown lines. Clin Interv Aging. 2011;6:281–4. doi:10.2147/CIA.S18997. Epub 2011 Nov 9.
9. LLC. Xeomin [package insert]. Greensboro: Merz Pharmaceuticals; 2011.
10. Lim EC, Seet RC. Use of botulinum toxin in the neurology clinic. Nat Rev Neurol. 2010;6(11):624–36.
11. Henzel MK, Munin MC, Niyonkuru C, Skidmore ER, Weber DJ, Zafonte RD. Comparison of surface and ultrasound localization to identify forearm flexor muscles for botulinum toxin injections. PM R. 2010;2(7):642–6.
12. Mayer NH, Esquenazi A. Managing upper motor neuron muscle overactivity. In: Zasler ND, Katz DI, Zafonte RD, editors. Brain injury medicine. 2nd ed. New York: Demos Medical Publishing; 2013. p. 821–49.
13. Bickerton LE, Agur AM, Ashby P. Flexor digitorum superficialis: locations of individual muscle bellies for botulinum toxin injections. Muscle Nerve. 1997;20(8):1041–3.
14. Munin MC, Navalgund BK, Levitt DA, Breisinger TP, Zafonte RD. Novel approach to the application of botulinum toxin to the flexor digitorum superficialis muscle in acquired brain injury. Brain Inj. 2004;18(4):403–7.
15. Willenborg MJ, Shilt JS, Smith BP, Estrada RL, Castle JA, Koman LA. Technique for iliopsoas ultrasound-guided active electromyography-directed botulinum a toxin injection in cerebral palsy. J Pediatr Orthop. 2002;22(2):165–8.
16. Westhoff B, Seller K, Wild A, Jaeger M, Krauspe R. Ultrasound-guided botulinum toxin injection technique for the iliopsoas muscle. Dev Med Child Neurol. 2003;45(12):829–32.
17. Van Campenhout A, Hubens G, Fagard K, Molenaers G. Localization of motor nerve branches of the human psoas muscle. Muscle Nerve. 2010;42(2):202–7.
18. Van Campenhout A, Molenaers G. Localization of the motor endplate zone in human skeletal muscles of the lower limb: anatomical guidelines for injection with botulinum toxin. Dev Med Child Neurol. 2011;53(2):108–19.
19. Ward AB. Botulinum toxin type A treatment of hip and thigh spasticity: a technique for injection of psoas major muscle. Eur J Neurol. 1999;6 suppl 4:S91–3.
20. Takai Y, Katsumata Y, Kawakami Y, Kanehisa H, Fukunaga T. Ultrasound method for estimating the cross sectional area of the psoas major muscle. Med Sci Sports Exerc. 2011;43(10):2000–4.
21. Won SJ, Kim JY, Yoon JS, Kim SJ. Ultrasonographic evaluation of needle electromyography insertion into the tibialis posterior using a posterior approach. Arch Phys Med Rehabil. 2011;92(11):1921–3.
22. Oddy MJ, Brown C, Mistry R, Eastwood DM. Botulinum toxin injection site localization for the tibialis posterior muscle. J Pediatr Orthop B. 2006;15(6):414–7.
23. Yang SN, Lee SH, Kwon HK. Needle electrode insertion into the tibialis posterior: a comparison of the anterior and posterior approaches. Arch Phys Med Rehabil. 2008;89(9):1816–8.
24. Rha DW, Im SH, Lee SC, Kim SK. Needle insertion into the tibialis posterior: ultrasonographic evaluation of an anterior approach. Arch Phys Med Rehabil. 2010;91(2):283–7.
25. Simpson DM, Blitzer A, Brashear A, et al. Assessment: botulinum neurotoxin for the treatment of movement disorders (an evidence-based review). Neurology. 2008;70(19):1699–706.
26. Tsui JC, Jon Stoessl A, Eisen A, Calne S, Calne D. Double-blind study of botulinum toxin in spasmodic torticollis. The Lancet. 1986;328(8501):245–7.
27. Hefter HKA, Müngersdorf M, Paus S, Stenner A, Jost W, Dysport Cervical Dystonia Study Group. A botulinum toxin A treatment algorithm for de novo management of torticollis and laterocollis. BMJ Open. 2011;1(2):e000196.
28. Lee IH, Yoon YC, Sung DH, Kwon JW, Jung JY. Initial experience with imaging-guided intramuscular botulinum toxin injection in patients with idiopathic cervical dystonia. AJR Am J Roentgenol. 2009;192(4):996–1001.
29. Consky ES, Lang AE. Clinical assessments of patients with cervical dystonia. In: Jankovic J, Hallett M, editors. Therapy with botulinum toxin. New York: Marcel Dekker, Inc; 1994. p. 211–37.
30. Kim H, Lee Y, Weiner D, Kaye R, Cahill AM, Yudkoff M. Botulinum toxin type a injections to salivary glands: combination with single event multilevel chemoneurolysis in 2 children with severe spastic quadriplegic cerebral palsy. Arch Phys Med Rehabil. 2006;87(1):141–4.
31. Walker FO. Botulinum toxin therapy for cervical dystonia. Phys Med Rehabil Clin N Am. 2003;14(4):749–66.
32. Nordgarden H, Osterhus I, Moystad A, et al. Drooling: are botulinum toxin injections into the major salivary glands a good treatment option? J Child Neurol. 2011;27:458–64.
33. Pena AH, Cahill AM, Gonzalez L, Baskin KM, Kim H, Towbin RB. Botulinum toxin A injection of salivary glands in children with drooling and chronic aspiration. J Vasc Interv Radiol. 2009;20(3):368–73.
34. Scheffer AR, Erasmus C, van Hulst K, van Limbeek J, Jongerius PH, van den Hoogen FJ. Efficacy and duration of botulinum toxin treatment for drooling in 131 children. Arch Otolaryngol Head Neck Surg. 2010;136(9):873–7.
35. Breheret R, Bizon A, Jeufroy C, Laccourreye L. Ultrasound-guided botulinum toxin injections for treatment of drooling. Eur Ann Otorhinolaryngol Head Neck Dis. 2011;128(5):224–9.
36. Moller E, Karlsborg M, Bardow A, Lykkeaa J, Nissen FH, Bakke M. Treatment of severe drooling with botulinum toxin in amyotrophic lateral sclerosis and Parkinson's disease: efficacy and possible mechanisms. Acta Odontol Scand. 2011;69(3):151–7.
37. Wu KP, Ke JY, Chen CY, Chen CL, Chou MY, Pei YC. Botulinum toxin type A on oral health in treating sialorrhea in children with cerebral palsy: a randomized, double-blind, placebo-controlled study. J Child Neurol. 2011;26(7):838–43.
38. Khan WU, Campisi P, Nadarajah S, et al. Botulinum toxin A for treatment of sialorrhea in children: an effective, minimally invasive approach. Arch Otolaryngol Head Neck Surg. 2011;137(4):339–44.
39. Dogu O, Apaydin D, Sevim S, Talas DU, Aral M. Ultrasound-guided versus 'blind' intraparotid injections of botulinum toxin-A for the treatment of sialorrhoea in patients with Parkinson's disease. Clin Neurol Neurosurg. 2004;106(2):93–6.
40. Erasmus CE, Van Hulst K, Van Den Hoogen FJ, et al. Thickened saliva after effective management of drooling with botulinum toxin A. Dev Med Child Neurol. 2010;52(6):e114–8.
41. Sriskandan N, Moody A, Howlett DC. Ultrasound-guided submandibular gland injection of botulinum toxin for hypersalivation in cerebral palsy. Br J Oral Maxillofac Surg. 2010;48(1):58–60.

42. Marina MB, Sani A, Hamzaini AH, Hamidon BB. Ultrasound-guided botulinum toxin A injection: an alternative treatment for dribbling. J Laryngol Otol. 2008;122(6):609–14.
43. Reid SM, Johnstone BR, Westbury C, Rawicki B, Reddihough DS. Randomized trial of botulinum toxin injections into the salivary glands to reduce drooling in children with neurological disorders. Dev Med Child Neurol. 2008;50(2):123–8.
44. Wilken B, Aslami B, Backes H. Successful treatment of drooling in children with neurological disorders with botulinum toxin A or B. Neuropediatrics. 2008;39(4):200–4.
45. Gerlinger I, Szalai G, Hollody K, Nemeth A. Ultrasound-guided, intraglandular injection of botulinum toxin A in children suffering from excessive salivation. J Laryngol Otol. 2007;121(10):947–51.
46. Shetty S, Dawes P, Ruske D, Al-qudah M, Lyons B. Botulinum toxin type-A (Botox-A) injections for treatment of sialorrhoea in adults: a New Zealand study. N Z Med J. 2006;119(1240):U2129.
47. Hassin-Baer S, Scheuer E, Buchman AS, Jacobson I, Ben-Zeev B. Botulinum toxin injections for children with excessive drooling. J Child Neurol. 2005;20(2):120–3.
48. Eid N, Ito Y, Otsuki Y. Submandibular gland botulinum toxin injections for drooling: the safe and risky zones. Surg Radiol Anat. 2011;33(5):465–6.
49. Jongerius PH, van den Hoogen FJ, van Limbeek J, Gabreels FJ, van Hulst K, Rotteveel JJ. Effect of botulinum toxin in the treatment of drooling: a controlled clinical trial. Pediatrics. 2004;114(3):620–7.
50. Lee JH, Lee BN, Kwon SO, Chung RH, Han SH. Anatomical localization of submandibular gland for botulinum toxin injection. Surg Radiol Anat. 2010;32(10):945–9.
51. Esquenazi A. Botulinum toxin in the treatment of lower limb spasticity. In: Brashear A, Elovic E, editors. Spasticity diagnosis and management. New York: Demos Medical Publishing; 2011. p. 119–29.
52. Guidubaldi A, Fasano A, Ialongo T, Piano C, Pompili M, Mascianà R, Siciliani L, Sabatelli M, Bentivoglio AR. Botulinum toxin A versus B in sialorrhea: a prospective, randomized, double-blind, crossover pilot study in patients with amyotrophic lateral sclerosis or Parkinson's disease. Mov Disord. 2011;26(2):313–9. doi:10.1002/mds.23473. Epub 2011 Jan 21.

Spine

10

David A. Spinner

Ultrasound is limited in its ability to image through bone, which is why most spinal injections are performed with fluoroscopic guidance. Ultrasound has several advantages, however. Ultrasound can be helpful to visualize superficial cervical structures and help to avoid critical blood vessels. Nerves can be seen on ultrasound but not on fluoroscopy. Ultrasound may be used to facilitate needle placement and can be combined with fluoroscopy to confirm contrast patterns. This can improve speed, safety, and the accuracy of an injection while decreasing radiation exposure. It should be noted that these are more advanced injections and should be performed after sufficient practice and supervision.

Cervical Spinal Nerves

Cervical radiculitis from herniated discs or spinal stenosis is a very common cause of neck and arm pain, numbness, and weakness [1]. Injections to treat cervical radiculitis are typically performed with fluoroscopy. However, in a randomized, blinded, controlled study by Jee et al., there were no differences in treatment effect and outcomes in an ultrasound-guided versus fluoroscopy-guided transforaminal block in the lower cervical spine [2] (Table 10.1). Ultrasound guidance enables visualization of critical blood vessels prior to the placement of a needle preventing inadvertent puncture [3]. Huntoon found that 20 % of dissected cervical foramina contained either the deep or ascending cervical artery within 2 mm of the directed needle target for a standard fluoroscopic approach. These arteries were found to enter the posterior foramen 33 % of the time [4]. Hoeft et al. found that radicular artery branches from the ascending or deep cervical arteries traverse the foramen as they cross medially [5]. Narouze et al. found in a small study of ten patients undergoing ultrasound-guided cervical nerve root injections that two patients had arteries in the posterior aspect of the foramen and one patient had a posteriorly located arterial supply that coursed medially into the foramen [6]. Serious complications from cervical transforaminal injections have been reported including stroke, paralysis, and death [7–9]. Ultrasound using Doppler mode allows the identification of critical vessels located near the intervertebral foramen or needle pathway and aids in avoiding inadvertent vascular injury, which is the leading cause of reported complication from cervical transforaminal injections [2].

Scanning Technique and Anatomy to Identify

The patient should lay in a lateral decubitus position with the affected side towards the ceiling or supine with the head rotated away from the affected side. The transducer is placed transversely, short axis to the C7 level. At this level, identify the prominent posterior tubercle and rudimentary anterior tubercle [10]. The anterior and posterior tubercles of the cervical vertebrae, "the two-humped camel," become more evident as you scan cranially to C6. The nerve root is identified as a hypoechoic round structure between the two tubercles [11]. Another method for identifying the correct cervical level is to trace the vertebral artery which lies

Table 10.1 Cervical radicular pain following ultrasound versus fluoroscopic guided injections

Comparison of verbal numeric pain scale			
	Baseline	2 weeks after injection	12 weeks after injection
Ultrasound-guided approach	6.15 ± 0.79	3.20 ± 0.51	2.62 ± 0.45
Fluoroscopy-guided approach	6.06 ± 0.82	3.17 ± 0.52	2.61 ± 0.42

D.A. Spinner, DO, RMSK
Department of Anesthesiology – Pain Medicine, Arnold Pain Management Center, Beth Israel Deaconess Medical Center, Harvard Medical School, Brookline, MA, USA
e-mail: dspinnerny@gmail.com

D.A. Spinner et al. (eds.), *Atlas of Ultrasound Guided Musculoskeletal Injections*, Musculoskeletal Medicine,
DOI 10.1007/978-1-4614-8936-8_10, © Springer Science+Business Media, LLC 2014

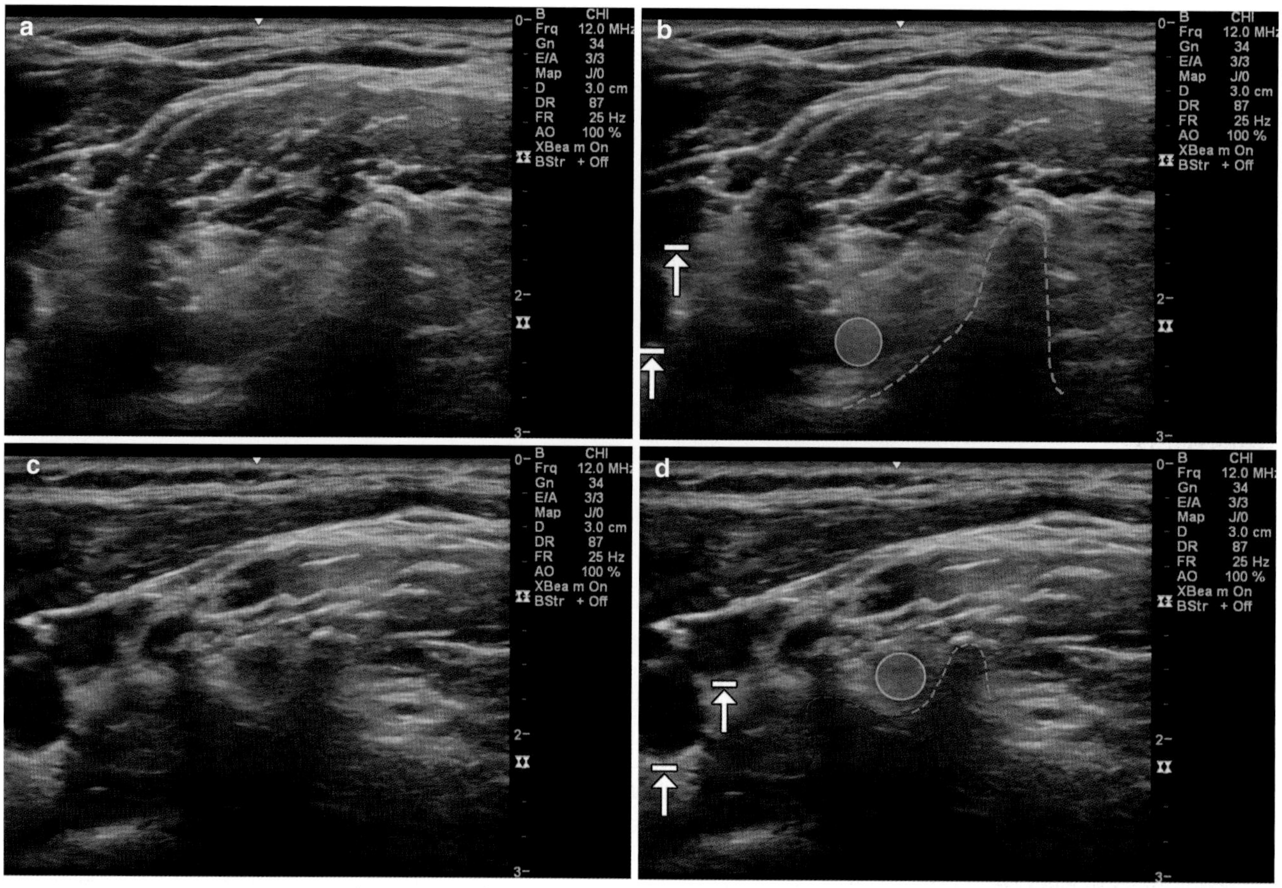

Fig. 10.1 (**a**) Transverse (axial) view over C7 with prominent posterior tubercle. (**b**) *Dashed orange line* outlines posterior tubercle, *yellow* indicates C7 spinal nerve, *arrows with stops* indicate carotid artery and internal jugular vein. (**c**) Transverse (axial) view over C6 with prominent anterior and posterior tubercles. (**d**) *Dashed orange line* outlines posterior tubercle, *dashed purple line* outlines anterior tubercle, *yellow* indicates C6 spinal nerve, *arrows with stops* indicate carotid artery and internal jugular vein

anterior to C7 and enters the C6 foramen 90 % of time. The remaining 10 % enter further cranially [12]. Be careful to keep the transducer perpendicular to the relevant cervical level as you travel to another level so you do not have the transducer angled downward at an unintended level. Use Doppler to identify the larger carotid artery, anterior and superficial to the anterior tubercle. Look for an anteriorly located vertebral artery. Lastly, try to identify any smaller feeder vessels in the foramen or in the way of the projected needle pathway (Fig. 10.1).

Injection Technique: In-Plane Axial Approach

Patient positioning: Lay the patient in the lateral decubitus position with the affected side facing upward with a pillow placed between the patient's legs and one under the arm to facilitate comfort. The patient can also lay supine with the head rotated and side bent away.

Probe positioning: Place the transducer transverse (short axis) over the C7 vertebrae, visualizing the rudimentary anterior tubercle and prominent posterior tubercle (Fig. 10.2a).

Markings: Identify the transverse process and tubercles of C7 as this differs from the other cervical vertebrae, marking the C7 level. If more than one level injection is planned, use a marker to identify the probe position at the desired vertebral levels and the needle entry site. Mark any vessels that are identified on Doppler to avoid inadvertent injury.

Needle position: Plan your needle path prior to insertion to avoid any feeding vessels or ones located in the posterior foramen. A blunt needle should be inserted from a posterior to anterior direction. The needle should be kept in-plane directed towards the desired nerve root.

Safety considerations: Care should be taken to avoid contact with a blood vessel or spinal nerve.

Pearls:

- The anterior spinal artery may receive some blood flow from the ascending and deep cervical arteries [1].
- Keep the transducer perpendicular as you scan to keep your desired vertebral level in site. Angling the transducer may cause you to view up or down a level.

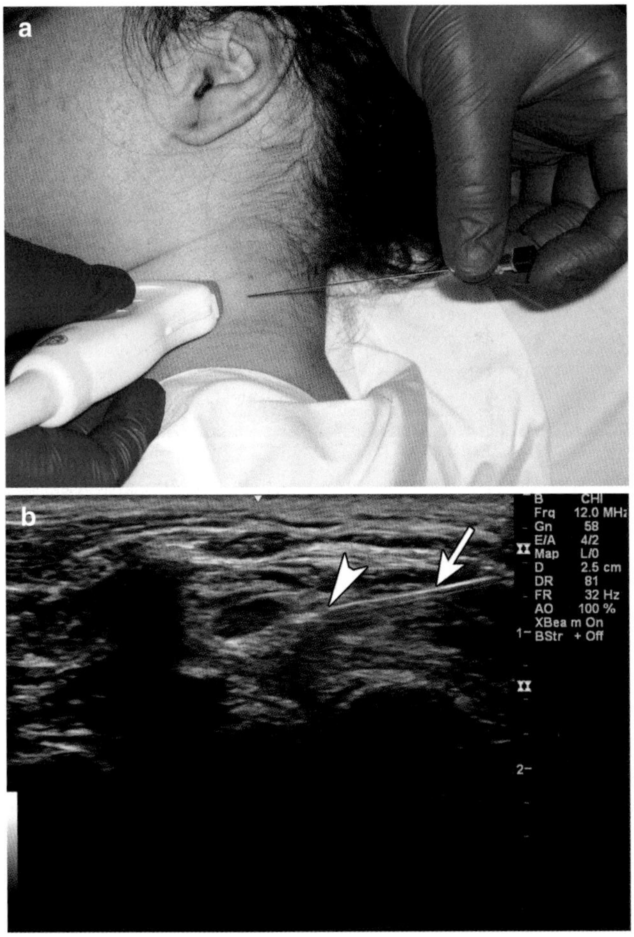

Fig. 10.2 (**a**) Example of transverse (axial) probe position over C6 level with in-plane needle position. (**b**) Example of in-plane axial injection towards to the C6 spinal nerve (probe angled slightly to position posterior tubercle out of the field of view to allow for easier needle trajectory), *arrowhead* indicates needle tip, *arrow* indicates needle

- Always inject from a posterior to anterior direction to avoid the internal jugular vein, vagus nerve, common carotid artery, and 80 % of anterior located radicular arteries in the cervical foramen.
- Doppler mode may help to identify feeding vascular structures in the posterior foramen.

Equipment needed:

- 6–12 MHz linear array transducer
- 22 or 25 gauge, blunt tip spinal needle
- Non-particulate steroid preparation
- 1–2 mL of local anesthetic or normal saline

Cervical Medial Branch Blocks (CMBB) and Third Occipital Nerve (TON)

Pain arising from the cervical zygapophysial (z-jt) aka facet joint is common and may present with aching or throbbing neck pain that radiates to the head (commonly C2–3) or shoulder or interscapular region (C5–6, C6–7) [13]. Patients may have pain and decreased range of motion with cervical side bending or rotation. The cervical z-jts are each innervated by two medial branches, and pain emanating from the joint is diagnosed by anesthetizing these nerves. Injection of the joints themselves is not as helpful diagnostically but may provide therapeutic benefit [14, 15]. Cervical medial branch block procedures are typically performed with fluoroscopic guidance but have the potential to miss the medial branch as there are variations in its course [16]. Ultrasound provides the opportunity to visualize the nerve towards the center of the articular pillars. The gold standard treatment for cervical z-jt pain is radiofrequency neurotomy, and the use of ultrasound guidance to perform the procedure has been described and may become a viable alternative to fluoroscopy [17, 18] (Table 10.2).

Table 10.2 Accuracy of ultrasound guided nerve blocks of the cervical zygapophysial joints [19]

Level	Accuracy (%)
Third occipital nerve	88
C4	94
C6	88
C7	41

Scanning Technique and Anatomy to Identify

The patient should lie in the lateral decubitus position. The transducer is placed longitudinally with the superior end on the mastoid process to obtain a coronal image. The articular pillars of the cervical vertebra (C2–7) are seen as hills, and the first trough between the hills of the C2–3 z-jt is identified by a characteristic depression. To confirm your level, the transverse process of C1 can be seen on the cephalad portion of the screen or turn on the Doppler to visualize the vertebral artery traversing anteriorly into the foramen of C2 [11]. The superficial medial branch of C3 differs from the other cervical medial branches in that it sits on top of the "hill" at the junction of the C2–3 z-jt and travels to become a cutaneous nerve. This is known as the third occipital nerve (TON). The TON can also be identified by placing the transducer over the mastoid process in the axial plane and moving it caudally until the transverse process of C1. Continuing caudally, the vertebral artery traverses into the foramen of C2 [20]. The TON is identified at the highest point of the convexity of the C2–3 joint [21]. The C4–8 cervical medial branches traverse dorsally over the articular pillars in the troughs between the hills and innervate the facet joint above and below [22]. They are found by the continuation of the longitudinal (coronal) scanning along the articular pillars. The medial branches appear as oval slightly hypoechoic structures in between the pillars (Fig. 10.3).

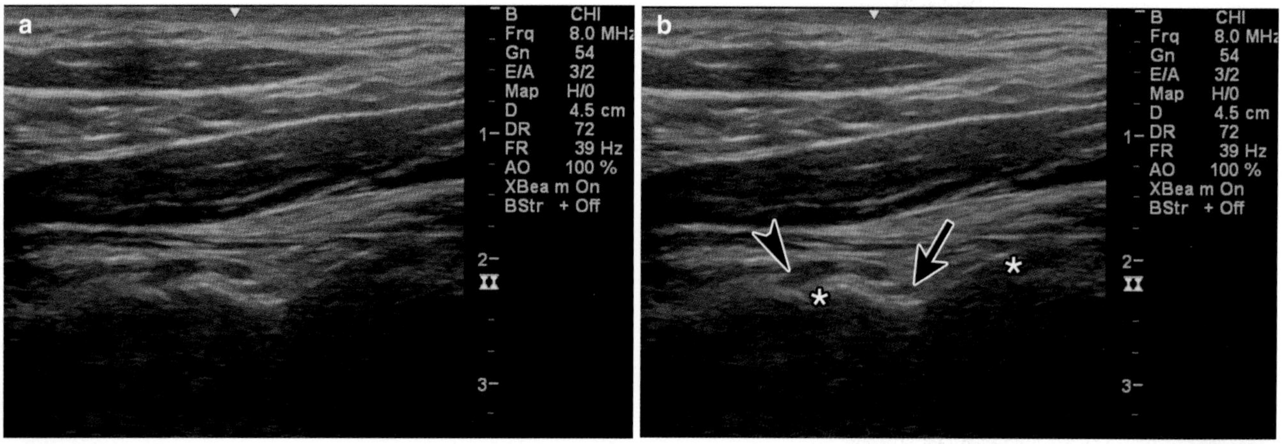

Fig. 10.3 (**a**) Coronal view of the cervical articular pillars. (**b**) *Black arrowhead* indicates TON, *black arrow* indicates C3 medial branch, *asterisk* indicates C2–3 and C3–4 z-jt

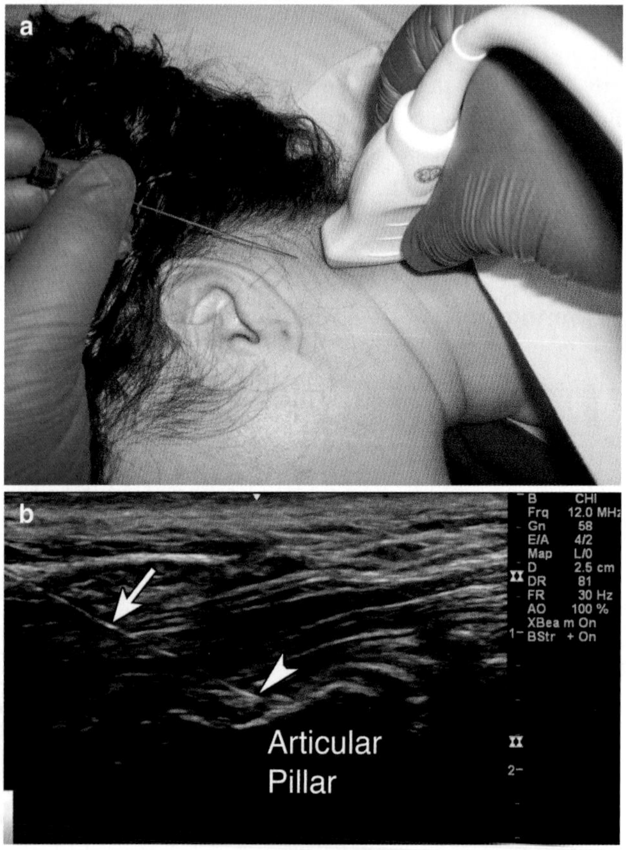

Fig. 10.4 (**a**) Example of coronal view over the cervical medial branches with in-plane needle position. (**b**) *Arrowhead* indicates needle tip adjacent to medial branch, *white arrow* indicates needle, articular pillar labeled

Injection Techniques: In-Plane Coronal Approach

Patient positioning: Lay the patient in the lateral decubitus position with pillows underneath the head, between the legs, and under the arm.

Probe positioning: Place the transducer coronally over the mastoid process and view the articular pillar, identifying the levels as you move caudally (Fig. 10.4a).

Markings: Identify and mark the desired cervical levels.

Needle position: The needle is inserted in-plane towards the medial branch if identified. If the nerve is not visualized, direct straight down between the articular pillars towards the deepest point, touching down on bone. For the TON, the needle is inserted in-plane towards the apex of the C2–3 joint.

Safety considerations: Keep the transducer and injection posterior to avoid the anterior vasculature.

Pearls for CMBB:

- Aim at the deepest point between the articular pillars.
- The medial branch may be difficult to visualize in an obese patient.
- The cervical medial branch becomes more difficult to identify as you proceed caudally.

Pearls for TON:

- Aim at the convexity of the C2–3 joint.
- The C2 level is also identified as having the first bifid spinous process [23]. The transducer can be placed axially over the spinous process of C2, and the lamina of C2 can be traced laterally until the C2–3 joint appears.

Equipment needed:

- High-frequency linear array transducer
- 22 or 25G 2.5–3.5″ spinal needle
- 0–1 mL of steroid preparation per level
- 0.5–1 mL local anesthetic per level

Cervical Zygapophysial Joint

The cervical z-jts are formed by the articulations of the superior and inferior articular pillars of adjacent vertebrae. Intra-articular injections can have diagnostic and therapeutic benefit [15, 24]. Cervical z-jt joint procedures are typically

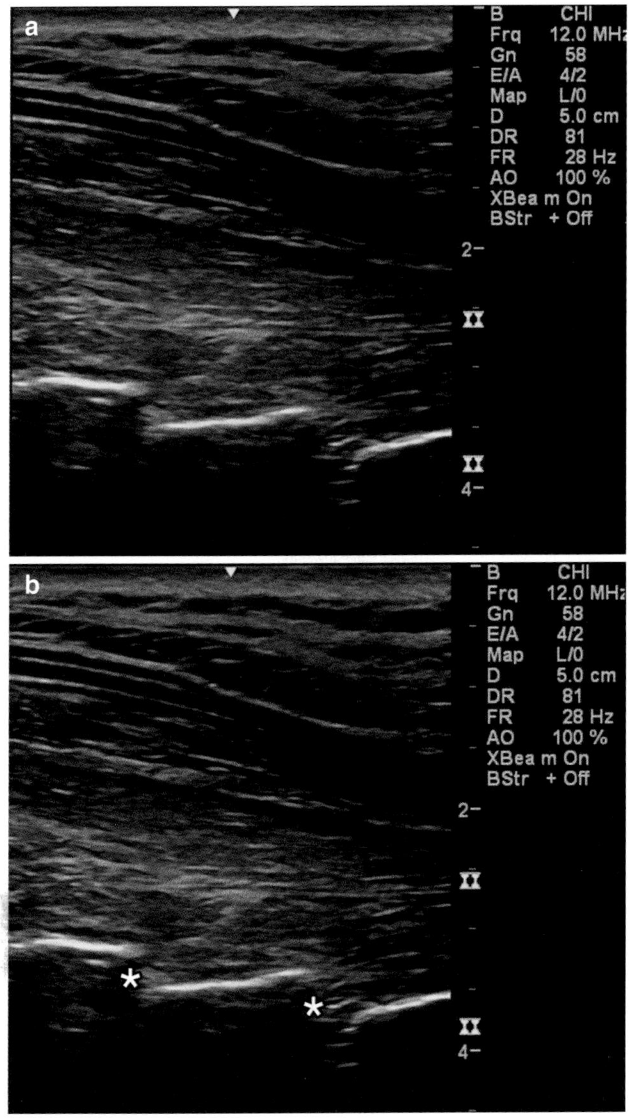

Fig. 10.5 (**a**) Sagittal view of the cervical facet joints. (**b**) *Asterisk* indicates cervical facet joints

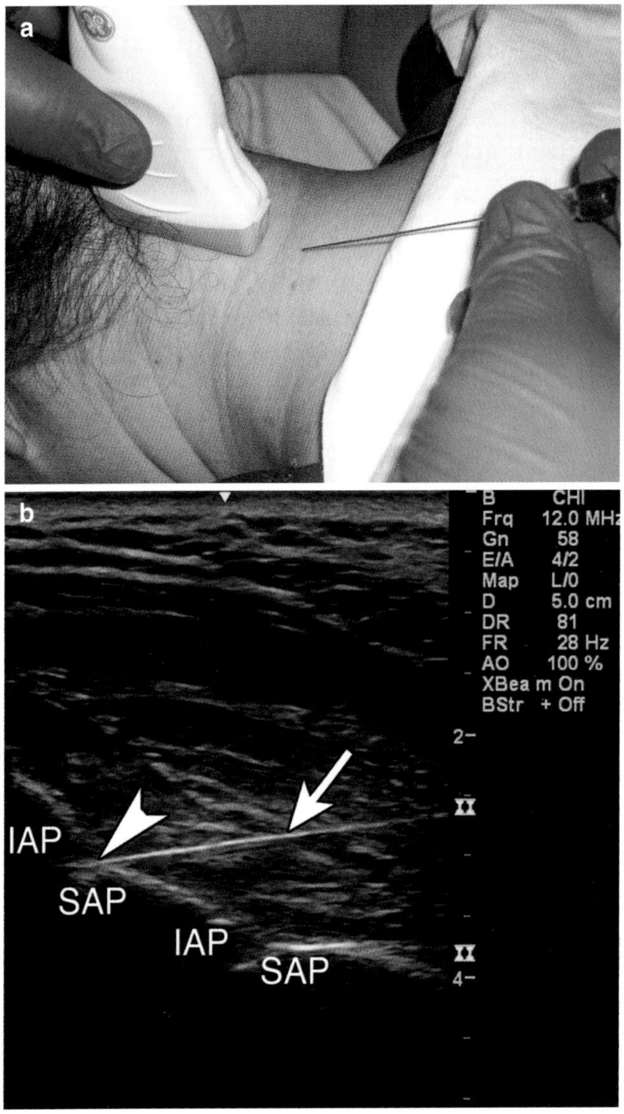

Fig. 10.6 (**a**) Example of sagittal probe position over cervical facet joint with in-plane injection technique. (**b**) *Arrowhead* indicates needle tip entering facet joint, *arrow* indicates needle, *IAP* inferior articular process, *SAP* superior articular process

performed with either fluoroscopic or CT guidance. Ultrasound-guided cervical facet joint injections have been shown to be faster than CT guidance, require fewer needle repositions, and have better pain scores at 1 month [25].

Scanning Technique and Anatomy to Identify

The patient should lie in the prone position. The transducer is placed midline in the sagittal plane (longitudinally) over the cervical spinous processes. The C2 level is identified as having the first bifid spinous process [13]. The cervical levels are counted as you move caudally by looking at the superficial midline hyperechoic spinous processes. Once you reach your desired level, moving the transducer laterally will bring a sawtooth image of the z-jt line into view. The z-jts become more vertical as you move caudally, becoming almost vertical in the thoracic spine [26, 27] (Fig. 10.5).

Injection Technique: In-Plane Sagittal Approach

Patient positioning: Lay the patient in the prone position with a pillow underneath the chest to allow for slight cervical flexion.

Probe positioning: Place the transducer in the sagittal plane over the cervical spinous processes and move laterally until the facet joints at the desired levels are in view (Fig. 10.6a).

Marking: Identify and mark the desire cervical levels.

Needle position: The needle is inserted in-plane from caudal to cephalad towards the facet joint.

Safety considerations: Keep the transducer and injection posterior to avoid the anterior vasculature.

Pearls:

- The cervical facets appear as shingles on a roof with the probe in the sagittal plane.
- Keeping the needle angle shallow will help to mimic the angle of the facet joint and ease the approach and needle placement for an intra-articular injection.
- The C2 vertebra has the first bifid spinous process.

Equipment needed:

- High-frequency linear transducer
- 25 gauge, 1.5″ needle
- 0.5–1 mL of steroid preparation per level
- 0.5–1 mL of local anesthetic per level

Stellate Ganglion

Stellate ganglion block (SGB) is an established treatment for sympathetically mediated pain conditions such as complex regional pain syndrome and Raynaud's disease [28]. The most widely practiced approach for this injection was originally described by Leriche [29], in which Chassaignac's tubercle, the anterior aspect of the C6 transverse process, is palpated and used as the needle target [30]. This approach is typically performed with or without fluoroscopy [31]. However, the stellate ganglion does not lie adjacent to this bony target but rather anteriorly in the prevertebral fascia [32, 33].

The stellate ganglion, or cervicothoracic ganglion, is the fusion of the inferior cervical ganglion and the first thoracic ganglion. The stellate ganglion lies posterior and lateral to the trachea, esophagus, and thyroid; medial to the common carotid artery and internal jugular vein; just lateral to the inferior thyroid artery and recurrent laryngeal nerve; and anterior to the vertebral artery and longus colli muscle [34]. The stellate ganglion is approximately 2.5 cm long, 1 cm wide, and 0.5 cm thick [35]. The fluoroscopic-guided approach cannot visualize any of these soft tissue structures. Ultrasound improves safety by allowing direct visualization of the related anatomical structures minimizing complications like recurrent laryngeal nerve palsy or inadvertent puncture of a major vessel with intravascular spread [36]. Ultrasound also helps to avoid retropharyngeal hematoma, which is reported to occur in 1/100,000 procedures; however, asymptomatic hematoma can be as high as 1/4 [37].

Scanning Technique and Anatomy to Identify

Place the patient in the supine position with the head in slight extension and rotated away from your desired side. Place the probe over the cricoid cartilage to obtain a transverse (axial) scan, and move laterally to identify the prominent anterior tubercle of C6. In this position, identify the carotid artery, internal jugular vein, cricoid cartilage, and longus colli muscle. Turn on the Doppler to look for the inferior thyroid artery and a vertebral artery that may not have moved posteriorly into the vertebral foramen yet [36]. To confirm your anatomical level, scan in the axial plane laterally over C7. C7 has a prominent posterior tubercle and a rudimentary anterior tubercle which differentiates it from C6 which has both anterior and posterior tubercles (Fig. 10.7).

Injection Technique: In-Plane Axial Approach

Patient positioning: Lay the patient supine with the neck in slight extension and slight rotation away.

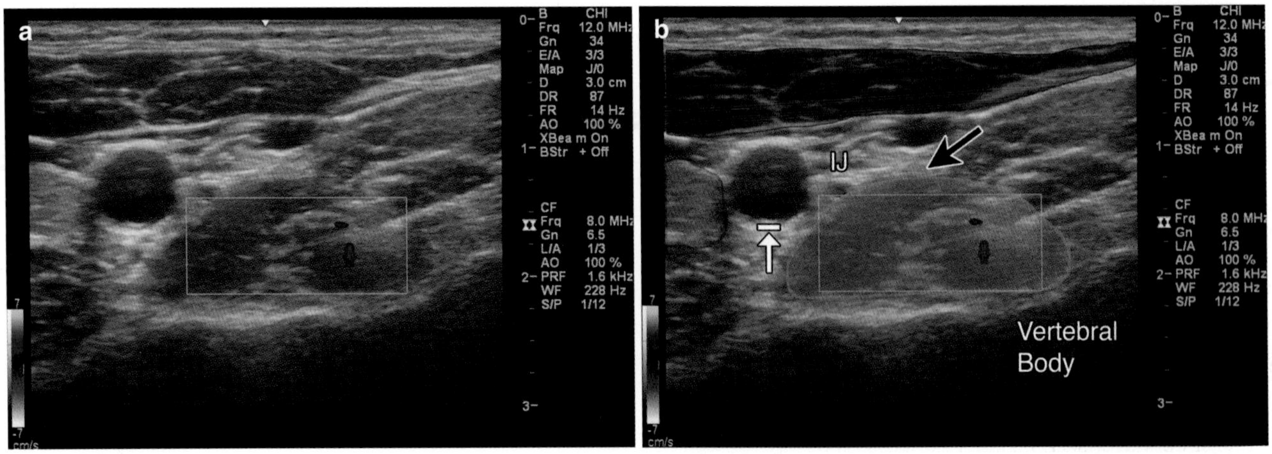

Fig. 10.7 (**a**) Transverse (axial) view of the stellate ganglion with Doppler. (**b**) *Magenta* indicates sternocleidomastoid, *purple* indicates anterior scalene, *orange* indicates longus colli, *black arrow* indicates location of stellate ganglion, *arrow with stop* indicates carotid artery, *IJ* internal jugular vein

Probe positioning: Start by placing the probe at C7 in the axial plane. As you scan cephalad, the anterior tubercle of C6 comes into view. Now at the level of C6, visualize the anterior tubercle of C6, longus colli muscle and prevertebral fascia, carotid artery, and thyroid gland (Fig. 10.8a).

Markings: There are a number of significant anatomical structures to mark and note in this region. Identify the esophagus, trachea, carotid artery, internal jugular vein, and inferior thyroidal artery.

Needle position: The needle is inserted in-plane from lateral to medial aiming at the prevertebral fascia just anterior to the longus colli muscle. Plan out the course of the needle to avoid puncturing important structures [8]. If the needle path can cause injury to these structures, adjust the probe position or insert the needle with a more oblique trajectory.

Safety considerations: Avoid the esophagus and trachea medially and the carotid artery, internal jugular vein, inferior thyroid, and vertebral arteries laterally. A phrenic nerve block can occur and cause diaphragmatic paresis [38].

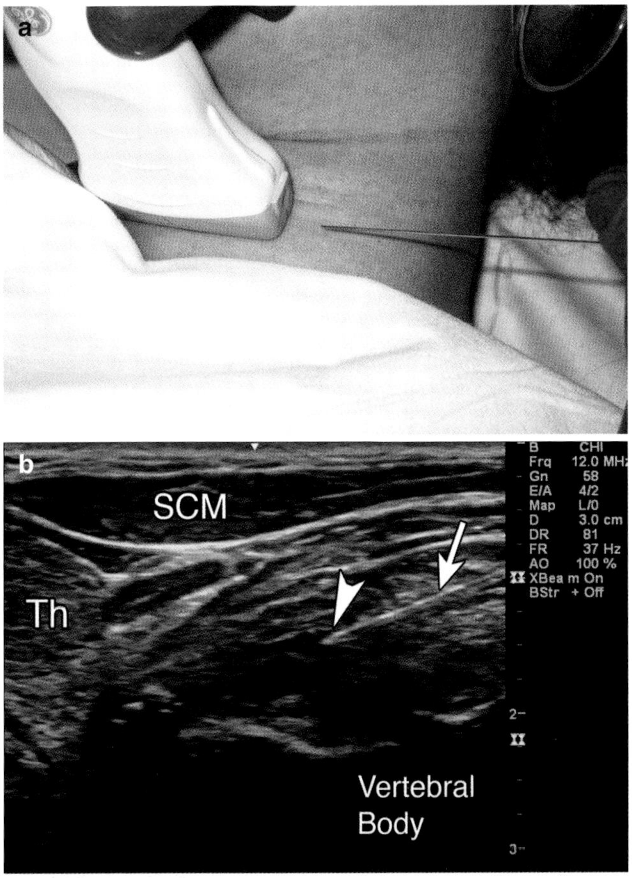

Fig. 10.8 (**a**) Example of axial probe position over stellate ganglion at level of C6 with in-plane injection technique. (**b**) *Arrowhead* indicates needle tip in the prevertebral fascia, *white arrow* indicates needle, *SCM* sternocleidomastoid, *Th* thyroid, vertebral body labeled

Pearls:

- The stellate ganglion lies medial to the scalene muscles.
- Stellate ganglion is formed by the fusion of the inferior cervical and first thoracic ganglion.
- A nerve stimulator can help to identify the phrenic nerve and avoid inadvertent diaphragmatic paresis [39].

Equipment needed:

- High-frequency linear array transducer
- 25G 3.5″ needle
- 1–3 mL short-acting anesthetic for local anesthesia
- 10–20 mL of long-acting anesthetic for the block

Greater Occipital Nerve

Greater occipital nerve (GON) block is used to treat occipital neuralgia and different headache conditions such as cluster, tension, cervicogenic, and migraine [39–42]. Occipital neuralgia is typically described as a painful paroxysmal stabbing pain in the distribution of the greater, lesser, and third occipital nerves [43]. Patients may exhibit tenderness over the affected nerve. The classical method of blind injection includes palpating just medial to the occipital artery at the level of the superior nuchal line [44]. Identification of the occipital artery by palpation can be difficult, however, and there can be variability in the course of both the occipital artery and GON. The GON arises from the C2 dorsal ramus and curves around the inferior aspect of the inferior oblique muscle (IOM) to then situate between the IOM and the semispinalis capitis (SSC) muscle [45]. There are a number of locations in which the GON can become irritated and entrapped including where the greater occipital nerve emerges from the C2 dorsal ramus between the atlas and the axis, where the nerve courses between the IOM and SSC muscles, and where the nerve pierces the belly of the SSC and at the nerve exit from the tendinous aponeurosis of the trapezius [46, 47] (Table 10.3).

Scanning Technique and Anatomy to Identify

The patient should lay prone on a table or cervical board with slight cervical flexion to expose the suboccipital region. Place the ultrasound probe transversely over the hyperechoic bony bifid C2 spinous process, and scan one level cephalad to C1. Identify the IOM just superficial to C1 and the SSC muscle superficial to that. The GON appears as a hypoechoic round or oval structure that lies within the plane of these two muscles before it pierces superficially through the SSC [48]. Use Doppler to visualize any branches of the occipital artery (Fig. 10.9).

Table 10.3 Accuracy of ultrasound guided GON injections

Study – GON	Author	Accuracy (%)
Ultrasound guided	Siegenthaler et al. [21]	100

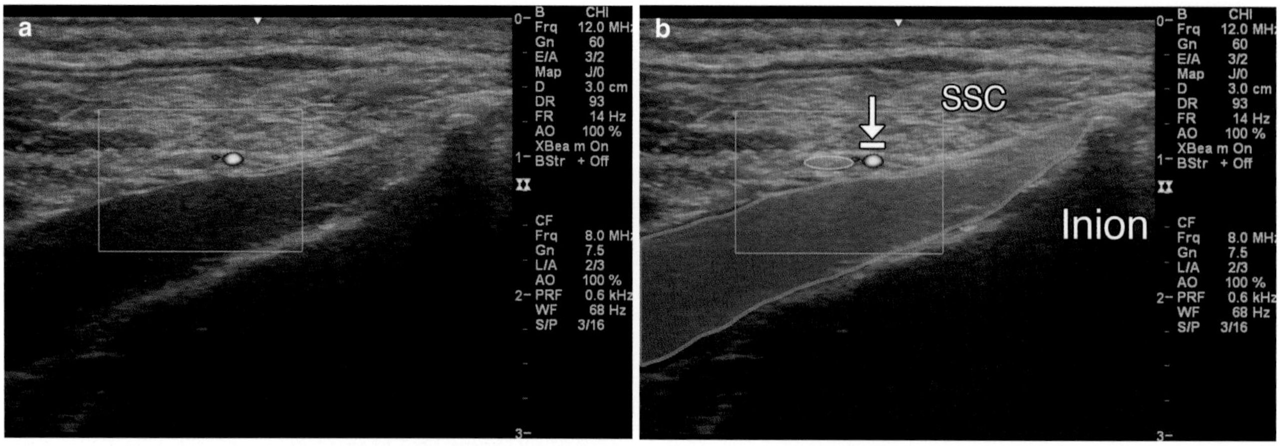

Fig. 10.9 (**a**) Axial view of the GON with Doppler. (**b**) *Orange* indicates IOM, SSC and inion labeled; *arrow with stop* indicates occipital artery; *yellow* indicates GON

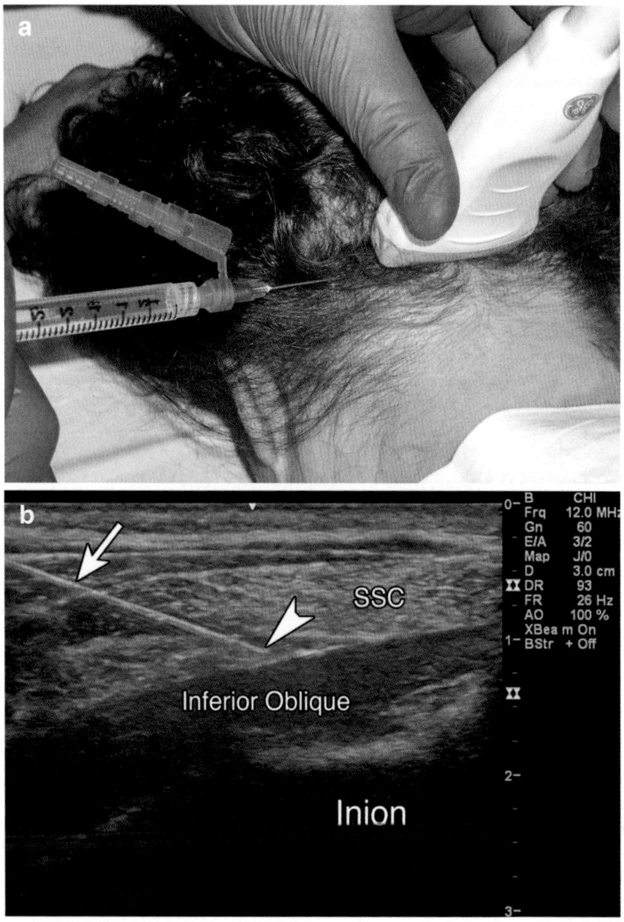

Fig. 10.10 (**a**) Example of axial probe position over GON with in-plane injection technique. (**b**) *Arrowhead* indicates needle tip adjacent to GON; *white arrow* indicates needle; SSC, inion, and inferior oblique labeled

Injection Technique: In-Plane Axial Approach [49]

Patient positioning: Lay the patient prone with the neck in slight flexion. A pillow can be placed under the chest.

Probe positioning: Start by placing the transducer transverse (axial) over the bifid spinous process of C2. The posterior arch of C1 will appear smooth. The inferior obliquus capitis muscle attaches to the spinous process of C2 and transverse process of C1. Follow the inferior obliquus capitis in-plane as it moves laterally and cranially. The GON sits in the fascial plane between the inferior obliquus capitis and semispinalis capitis muscle (Fig. 10.10a).

Markings: Use Doppler to identify any branches of the occipital artery to avoid inadvertent puncture.

Needle position: The needle is inserted in-plane from lateral to medial. Advance until the needle is close to the nerve sheath.

Safety considerations: Prior to placing the needle, Doppler may help to identify any vessels.

Pearls:

- The C2 spinous process is bifid which distinguishes it from the smooth posterior arch of C1.
- Placing the neck in slight flexion will help to clear room for the ultrasound probe.
- Rotate the probe slightly (lateral end more cranial than medial end) to help bring the inferior obliquus capitis muscle parallel to the probe.

Equipment needed:

- High-frequency linear array transducer
- 25G 1.5″ needle
- 0.5–1 mL of steroid preparation
- 1–3 mL local anesthetic

Lumbar Medial Branch Blocks and Zygapophysial Joint

Low back pain is very common and is often thought to arise from the zygapophysial or facet joints approximately 30 % of the time [50–52]. The z-jts joints are comprised of the superior and inferior articular processes (SAP and IAP) and are innervated by the medial branches of the dorsal rami of the level involved and level above [53]. Pain arising from these joints is typically localized to the low back but can radiate to the proximal lower extremities or buttocks. The pain is typically characterized as aching and dull. Loading the z-jt with oblique extension may reproduce the symptoms. History and physical exam are not the most reliable means of diagnosing z-jt-mediated pain; the gold standard is image-guided comparative anesthetic medial branch blocks [51]. Numerous studies have shown the accuracy of ultrasound-guided lumbar spine procedures, and newer evidence suggests that ultrasound-guided lumbar facet joint injections are just as effective as fluoroscopic-guided for improving pain and activities of daily living [19, 54–56] (Table 10.4).

Table 10.4 Accuracy of ultrasound guided lumbar medial branch blocks

Study – medial branch block	Author	Accuracy (%)
Ultrasound guidance with fluoroscopic confirmation	Greher et al. [55]	89
Ultrasound guidance with fluoroscopic confirmation	Shim et al. [56]	95
Ultrasound guidance with CT confirmation	Greher et al. [57]	94

Scanning Technique and Anatomy to Identify

The patient should lie prone resting comfortably. A pillow can be placed under the pelvis. The transducer is placed transversely (axial) over the upper crest of the sacrum. A superficial hyperechoic sacrum will be seen extending underneath the footprint of the probe. Keep the probe midline in the axial plane and scan cephalad. A small hypoechoic break will appear before the small superficial hyperechoic tip of the L5 spinous process. The lumbar vertebrae will have a distinctly different appearance from the sacrum. Just lateral to the midline, follow the spinous process down the lamina to the z-jt. Follow further laterally and deeper to identify the transverse process. Lumbar spine scanning can also be done starting longitudinally over the midline of the sacrum. The hyperechoic crest of S1, L5, and L4 can be seen separated by a laminar window. Staying midline and moving cephalad all the lumbar spinal levels can be identified. Sliding the probe laterally to a paramedian position will bring the z-jts in line (Fig. 10.11).

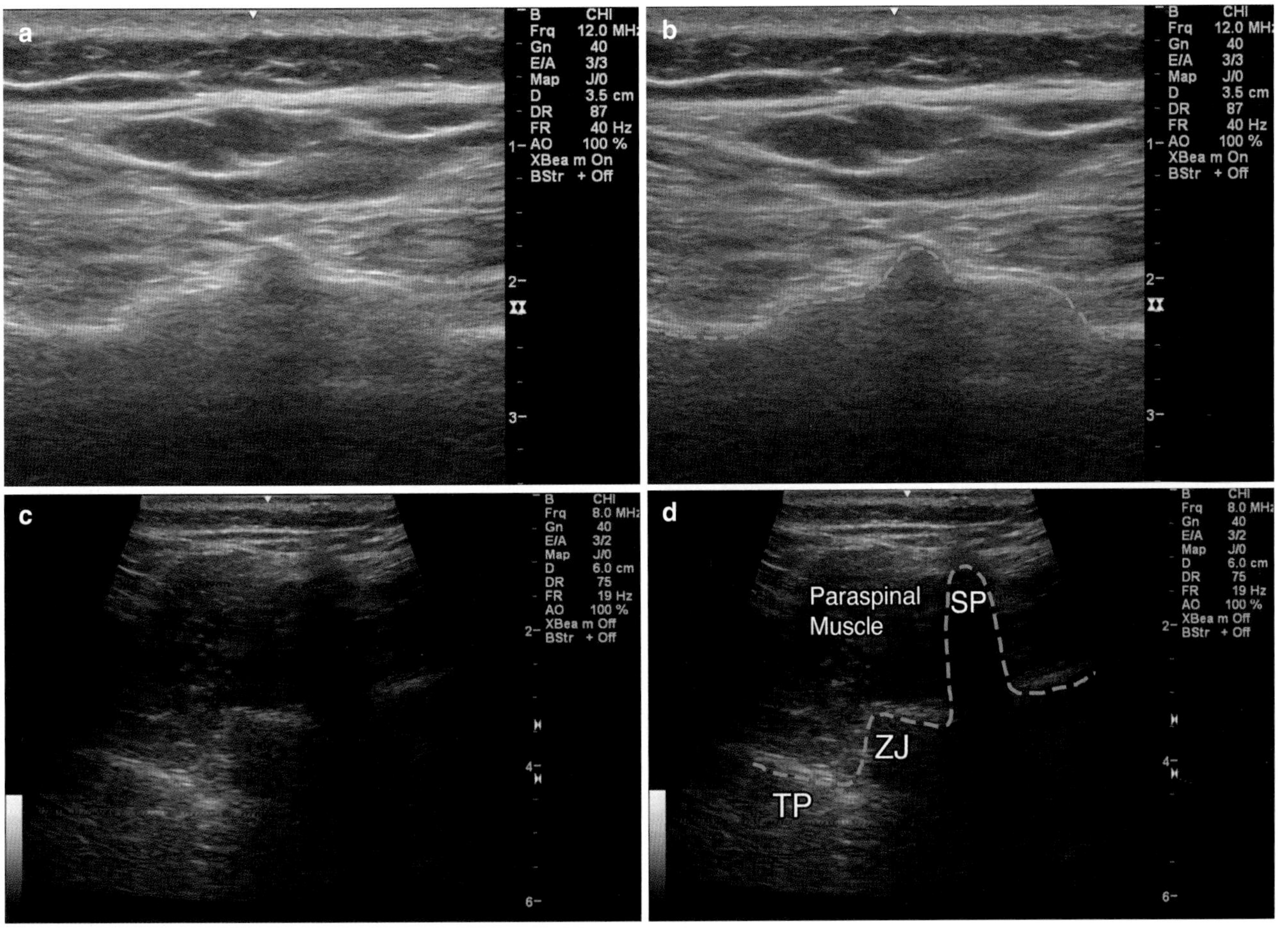

Fig. 10.11 (**a**) Axial view over sacrum. (**b**) *Dashed orange line* outlines dorsal sacrum. (**c**) Axial view over L5 vertebrae. (**d**) *Dashed orange line* outlines L5 posterior elements, *SP* spinous process, *ZJ* zygapophysial joint, *TP* transverse process, paraspinal muscle labeled

Injection Techniques: In-Plane Axial Approach

Patient positioning: Lay the patient prone with a pillow under the pelvis.

Probe positioning: Start by finding your desired level as above. Keep the probe in an axial view and identify the "triple crown" sign, transverse process deep, z-jt in the middle, and spinous process superficial, all in the same view. Center the probe over the z-jt (Fig. 10.12a).

Markings: Mark the spinal levels beginning at the sacrum as you scan cephalad. This can be done by scanning axially or sagittally from the midline using the sacrum as a landmark.

Needle position: The needle is inserted in-plane from lateral to medial towards the base of the SAP and the transverse process for the medial branches and towards the cleft formed by the IAP and SAP for the z-jt.

Safety considerations: Prior to placing the needle, Doppler may help to identify any vessels. If the needle is too caudal or cephalad, it may enter the epidural space.

Pearls:

- Fine-tuning or toggling the probe once it is in position over the facet joint in the axial plane will help to visualize the joint opening [58].
- After the target is reached, turn the probe sagittally to view the needle tip on the upper part of the transverse process to confirm it is in proper position for medial branch block.

Equipment needed:

- Curvilinear transducer or a wide-footprint linear transducer with a low frequency
- Spinal needle 22–25G 3.5–5
- 0.5–1 mL of steroid preparation per level
- 0.5–1 mL local anesthetic per level

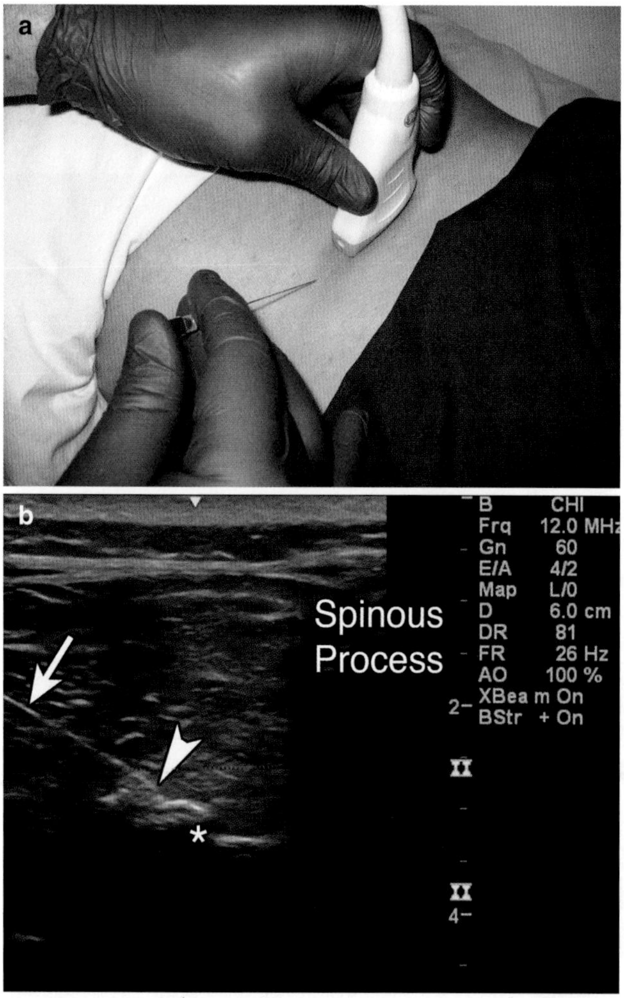

Fig. 10.12 (**a**) Example of axial probe position over L5 z-jt joint with in-plane injection technique. (**b**) *Arrowhead* indicates needle tip at z-jt, *arrow* indicates needle tip, *asterisk* indicates z-jt, spinous process labeled

Caudal

Caudal epidural injections are indicated for radicular pain due to lumbar spinal stenosis or disc herniations. Some physicians prefer the caudal approach because of the lower risk of intrathecal injection and inadvertent puncture, and some feel it is easier to perform in patients with a history of spinal surgery while still gaining access to the epidural space [23, 59, 60]. Caudal injections are typically performed with fluoroscopic guidance. Even with this image guidance, inadvertent needle placement can occur in up to 25.9 % of injections [61]. Ultrasound provides a great alternative to fluoroscopy. Blanchais et al. performed a feasibility study confirmed with epidurograms and found 96 % accurate needle placement [23]. Yoon et al. performed a study using color Doppler to assess for intravascular injections and found correct placement of medication in 52 of 53 patients [62]. Newer research has shown no statistical differences in pain or disability index between fluoroscopic or ultrasound-guided caudal injections [63] (Table 10.5).

Scanning Technique and Anatomy to Identify

The patient should lay prone in a comfortable position. Place the ultrasound probe transversely (axial) across the sacrum until two sacral cornua appear as two upside down U's. The sacrococcygeal ligament is seen as a hyperechoic line between the sacral cornua, centered along with a deep

Table 10.5 Accuracy of ultrasound guided caudal epidural injection

Study – caudal epidural space	Author	Accuracy (%)
Ultrasound guided	Blanchais et al. [64]	96

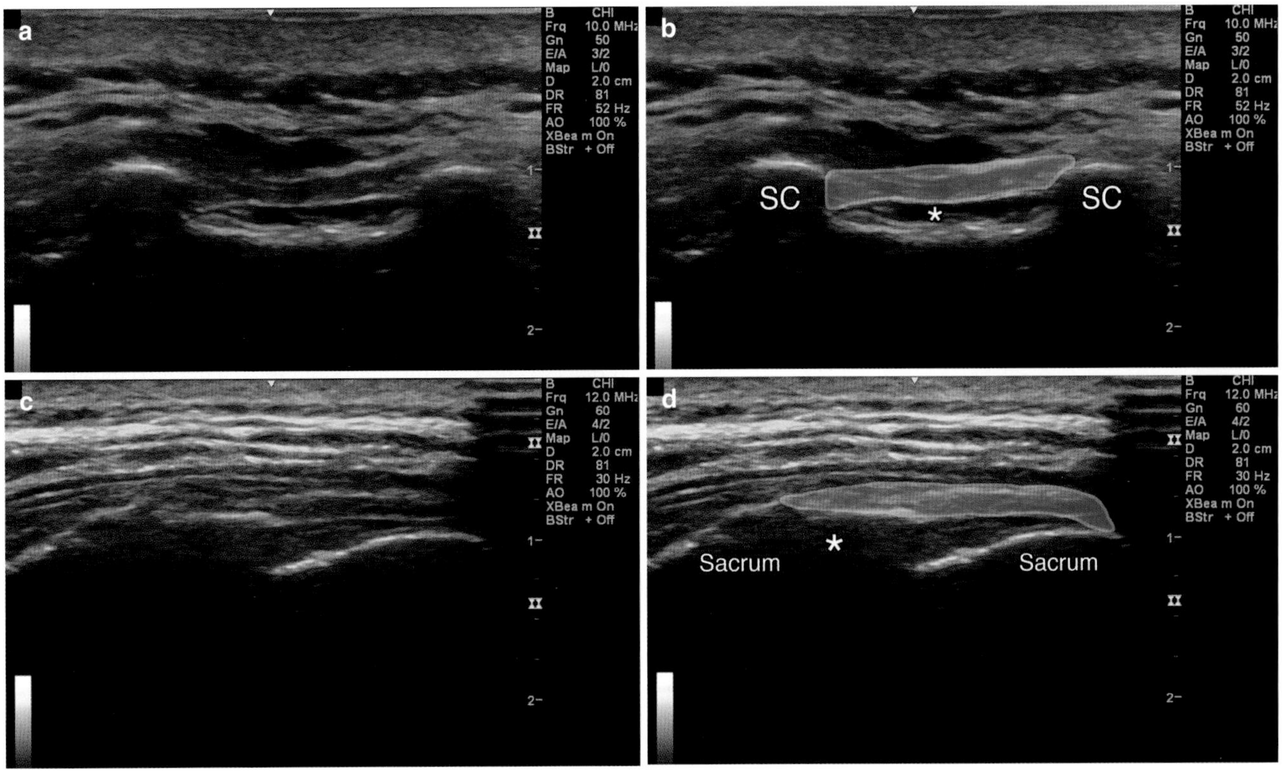

Fig. 10.13 (**a**) Axial view over sacral cornua. (**b**) *Green* indicates sacrococcygeal ligament, *SC* sacral cornua, *asterisk* indicates sacral hiatus. (**c**) Sagittal view of sacral hiatus. (**d**) Dorsal sacrum (*left*), *green* indicates sacrococcygeal ligament, *asterisk* indicates sacral hiatus

hyperechoic line representing the bony surface of the posterior side of the sacrum. The transducer is then rotated to obtain a longitudinal view of the sacral hiatus [23, 27, 65] (Fig. 10.13).

Injection Technique: In-Plane Sagittal Approach

Patient positioning: Lay the patient prone comfortably on table.

Probe positioning: Start by placing the transducer short axis (transverse) to the mid-sacrum and scan caudad until the sacral cornua appear. Rotate the probe 90° to give a sagittal and longitudinal picture, and center the sacral hiatus on the screen (Fig. 10.14a).

Markings: Mark the placement of the probe and needle entry site once the ideal position is found so that the area can be sterilized and found quickly again. You can also mark the distance between S2 and S4 so you know the distance to the thecal sac.

Needle position: The needle is inserted in-plane from caudal to cephalad aiming at the sacral hiatus. The needle should be inserted deep to the dorsal aspect of the sacrum. Some resistance by the sacrococcygeal ligament and a "pop" may be appreciated.

Safety considerations: Carefully aspirate to ensure no blood or cerebrospinal fluid.

Pearls:

- Once the needle advances through the sacrococcygeal ligament, begin aspiration and injection. Do not advance the needle too far as the dural sac typically ends at S2 and the needle cannot be visualized anterior to the dorsal bony aspect of the sacrum.
- Injection volume of 20 mL can reach S1 100 %, L5 89 %, L4 84 %, and L3 19 % of the time [23].

Equipment needed:

- High-frequency linear array transducer
- 22 or 25G 3.5″ spinal needle
- 2 mL of steroid preparation
- 0–4 mL local anesthetic
- 0–6 mL normal saline

Sacroiliac Joint

The SIJ is a diarthrodial joint with anterior and posterior innervation [66]. The complex nature of the ligamentous and muscular attachments from the SIJ to the hip make it a common pain generator [67]. Presenting symptoms may include low back and buttock pain as well as referred pain to the groin and thigh [30]. Physical exam maneuvers have

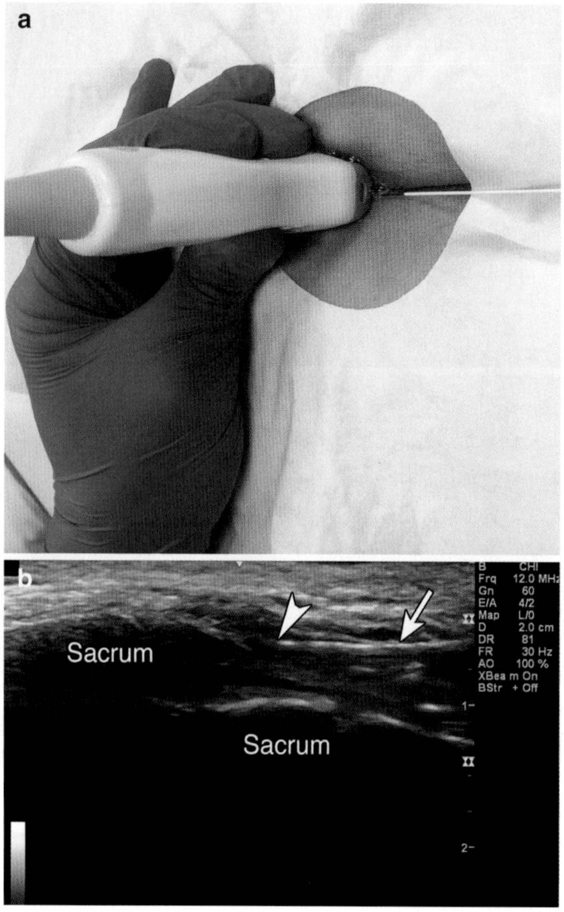

Fig. 10.14 (**a**) Example of sagittal probe position over sacrum with in-plane injection technique. (**b**) *Arrowhead* indicates needle tip traversing towards sacral hiatus, *arrow* indicates needle

Table 10.6 Accuracy of ultrasound guided SIJ injections

Study – SIJ injection ultrasound guided confirmed by fluoroscopy [36]	Accuracy (%)
First 30 injections	60
Second 30 injections	93.5
Last 20 injections	100

proven to have low sensitivity and specificity in diagnosing sacroiliitis, and SIJ injections have shown to serve both a diagnostic and therapeutic purpose [68–70]. Fluoroscopy is currently the gold standard for performing SIJ injections (Table 10.6).

Scanning Technique and Anatomy to Identify

The patient should lay prone. The transducer is placed transversely over the sacral hiatus and moved towards the affected side identifying the lateral edge of the sacrum. Continue cephalad until the ilium comes into view and the cleft between the sacrum and ilium are identified [30, 71]. Alternatively, identify the PSIS laterally and the sacrum medially, and move the probe inferiorly until the cleft of the joint space comes into view (Fig. 10.15).

Injection Technique: In-Plane Axial Approach

Patient positioning: Lay the patient in the prone position with a pillow under the pelvis.

Probe positioning: Start by placing the transducer short axis (transverse) to the sacrum at the level of the sacral hiatus. Move the probe lateral and cephalad until the cleft between the sacrum and ilium is centered on the screen. The probe should be positioned 1 cm above the lower end of the joint (Fig. 10.16a) [72].

Markings: No significant vascular or neural structures need to be marked.

Needle position: The needle should be inserted in-plane from medial to lateral parallel to the transducer for optimal needle visualization.

Safety considerations: Prior to placing the needle, Doppler may help to identify any vessels. Take care in osteoporotic individuals to not advance the needle through bone.

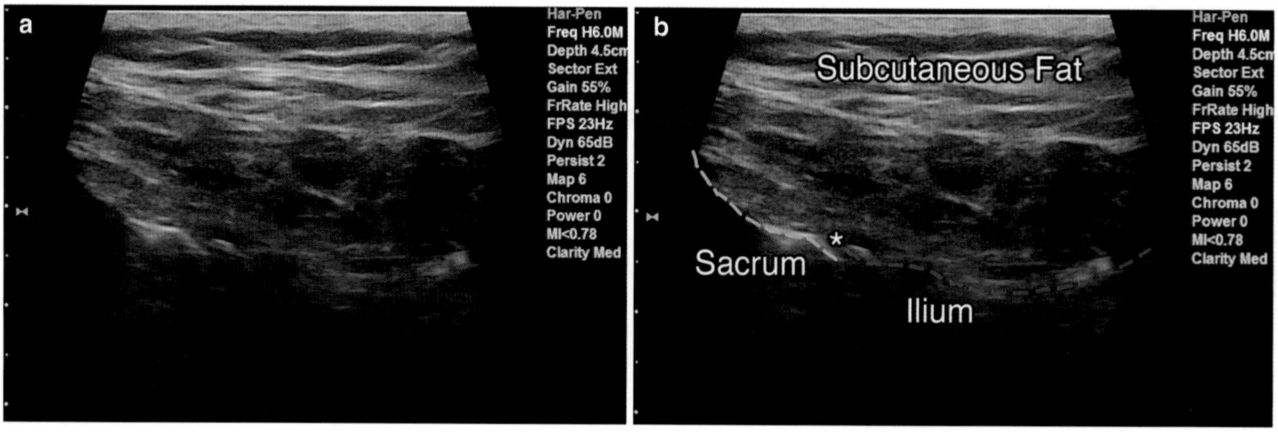

Fig. 10.15 (**a**) Axial view of the SIJ. (**b**) *Dashed orange line* outlines sacrum, *dashed purple line* outlines ilium, *asterisk* indicates joint space, subcutaneous fat labeled

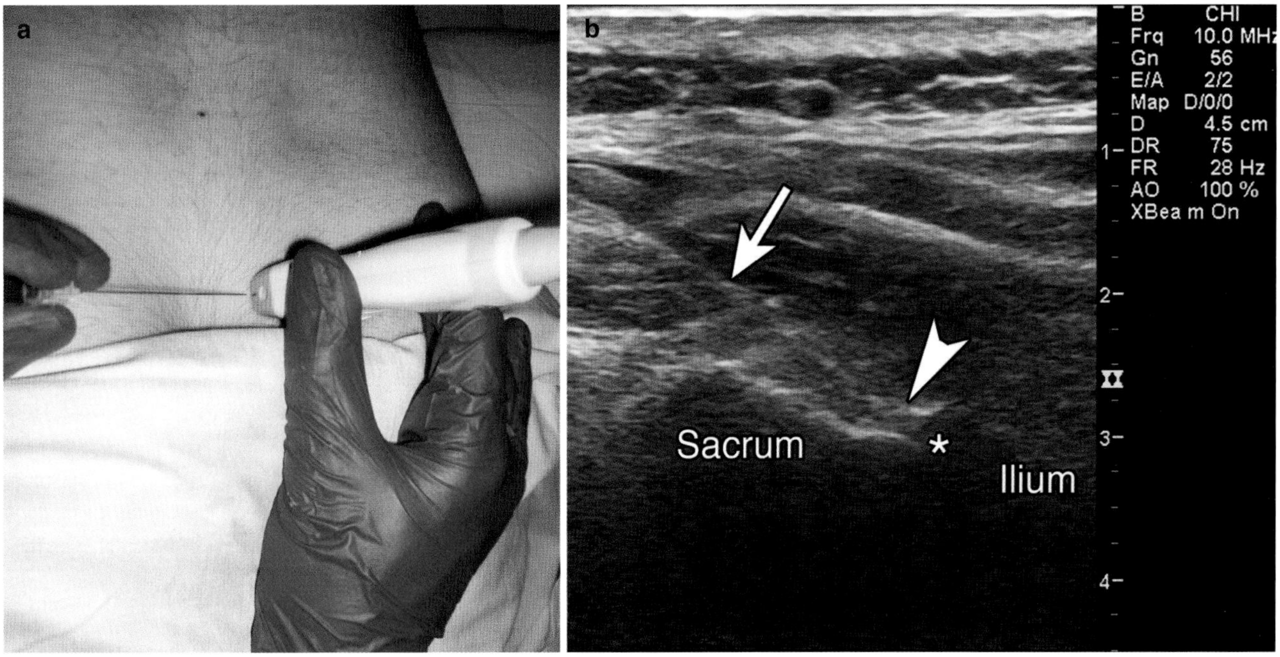

Fig. 10.16 (**a**) Example of axial probe position over SIJ with in-plane injection technique. (**b**) *Arrowhead* indicates needle tip entering SIJ, arrow indicates needle, *asterisk* indicates joint space, sacrum and ilium labeled

Pearls:

- The injection can be performed in the lower third of the SIJ which is synovial, while the upper portion is fibrous and not a true joint [36, 73, 74].
- Target the most inferior portion of joint.
- Push the needle through the posterior ligament, and feel a pop to help confirm joint entry rather than a periarticular injection.

Equipment needed:

- Curvilinear or linear array 6–10 mHz transducer
- 22G 3.5″ spinal needle
- 1–2 mL of steroid preparation
- 1–2 mL local anesthetic

References

1. Bush K, Hiller S. Outcome of cervical radiculopathy treated with periradicular/epidural corticosteroid injections: a prospective study with independent clinical review. Eur Spine J. 1996;5:319–25.
2. Jee H, Lee JH, Kim J, et al. Ultrasound-guided selective nerve root block versus fluoroscopy-guided transforaminal block for the treatment of radicular pain in the lower cervical spine: a randomize, blinded, controlled study. Skeletal Radiol. 2013;42: 69–78.
3. Narouze SN. Ultrasound-guided interventional procedures in pain management: evidence-based medicine. Reg Anesth Pain Med. 2010;35:55–8.
4. Huntoon MA. Anatomy of the cervical intervetebral foramina: vulnerable arteries and ischemic neurologic injuries after transforaminal epidural injections. Pain. 2005;117:104–11.
5. Hoeft MA, Rathmell JP, Monsey RD, Fonda BJ. Cervical transforaminal injection and the radicular artery: variation in anatomical location within the cervical intervertebral foramina. Reg Anesth Pain Med. 2006;31:270–4.
6. Narouze S, Vydyanathan A, Kapural L, Sessler DI, Mekhail N. Ultrasound-guided cervical selective nerve root block: a fluoroscopy-controlled feasibility study. Reg Anesth Pain Med. 2009;34:343–8.
7. Pobiel RS, Schellhas KP, Eklund JA, et al. Selective cervical nerve root blockade: prospective study of immediate and longer term complications. Am J Neuroradiol. 2009;30:507–11.
8. Wallace MA, Fukui MB, Williams RL, Ku A, et al. Complications of cervical selective nerve root blocks performed with fluoroscopic guidance. Am J Roentgenol. 2007;188:1218–21.
9. Brouwers PJ, Kottink EJ, Simon MA, Prevo TL. A cervical anterior spinal artery syndrome after diagnostic blockade of the right C6-nerve root. Pain. 2001;91:397–9.
10. Martinoli C, Bianchi S, Santacroee E, Pugliese F, Graif M, Derchi LE. Brachial plexus sonography: a technique for assessing the root level. AJR Am J Roentgenol. 2002;179:699–702.
11. Narouze S, Vydyanathan A. Ultrasound-guided cervical transforaminal injection and selective nerve root block. Tech Reg Anesth Pain Manag. 2009;13:137–41.
12. Matula C, Trattnig S, Tshabitscher M, Day JD, Koos WT. The course of the prevertebral segment of the vertebral artery: anatomy and clinical significance. Surg Neurol. 1997;48:125–31.
13. Dwyer A, Aprill C, Bogduk N. Cervical zygapophyseal joint pain patterns. I: a study in normal volunteers. Spine. 1990;15(6): 453–7.
14. Barnsley L, Bogduk N. Medial branch blocks are specific for the diagnosis of cervical zygapophyseal joint pain. Reg Anesth. 1993;18:343–50.
15. Boswell MV, Colson JD, Sehgal N, et al. A systematic review of therapeutic facet joint interventions in chronic spinal pain. Pain Physician. 2007;10:229–53.
16. Siegenthaler A, Schliessbach J, Curatolo M, Eichenberger U. Ultrasound anatomy of the nerves supplying the cervical zygapophyseal joints: an exploratory study. Reg Anesth Pain Med. 2011;36: 606–10.
17. Lee SH, Kang CH, Lee SH, et al. Ultrasound-guided radiofrequency neurotomy in cervical spine: sonoanatomic study of a new technique in cadavers. Clin Radiol. 2008;63:1205–12.

18. Lord SM, Barnsley L, Wallis BJ, et al. Percutaneous radiofrequency neurotomy for chronic cervical zygapophyseal-joint pain. N Engl J Med. 1996;5:1721–6.
19. Siegenthaler A, Mlekusch S, Trelle S. Accuracy of ultrasound-guided nerve blocks of the cervical zygapophyseal joints. Anesthesiology. 2012;117:347–52.
20. Eichenberger U, Greher M, Kapral S, et al. Sonographic visualization and ultrasound-guided block of the third occipital nerve: prospective for a new method to diagnose C2-3 zygapophysial joint pain. Anesthesiology. 2006;104:303–8.
21. Siegenthaler A, Narouze S, Eichenberger U. Ultrasound-guided third occipital nerve and cervical medial branch nerve blocks. Tech Reg Anesth Pain Manag. 2009;13:128–32.
22. Galiano K, Obwegeser AA, Bale R, et al. Ultrasound-guided and CT-navigation-assisted periradicular and facet joint injections in the lumber and cervical spine: a new teaching tool to recognize the sonoanatomic pattern. Reg Anesth Pain Med. 2007;32:254–7.
23. Narouze S, Peng PW. Ultrasound-guided interventional procedures in pain medicine: a review of anatomy, sonoanatomy, and procedures. Part II: axial structures. Reg Anesth Pain Med. 2010;35:386–96.
24. Sehgal N, Shah RV, McKenzie-Brown AM, et al. Diagnostic utility of facet (zygapophysial) joint injections in chronic spinal pain: a systematic review of evidence. Pain Physician. 2005;8:211–24.
25. Obernauer J, Galiano K, Gruber H, et al. Ultrasound-guided versus computed tomography- controlled facet joint injections in the middle and lower cervical spine: a prospective randomized clinical trial. Med Ultrason. 2013;15:10–5.
26. Pal GP, Routal RV, Saggu SK. The orientation of the articular facets of the zygopophyseal joints at the cervical and upper thoracic region. J Anat. 2001;198:431–41.
27. Yoganandan N, Knowles SA, Maiman DJ, Pintar FA. Anatomic study of the morphology of human cervical facet joints. Spine. 2003;28:2317–23.
28. Aeschbach A, Mekhail NA. Common nerve blocks in chronic pain management. Anesthesiol Clin North America. 2000;18:429–59.
29. Leriche R, Fontaine R. L'anesthesie isolee du ganglion etoile. Sa technique, ses indications, ses resultats. Presse Med. 1934;41:849–50.
30. Janik JE, Hoeft MA, Ajar AH. Variable osteology of the sixth cervical vertebra in relation to stellate ganglion block. Reg Anesth Pain Med. 2008;33:102–8.
31. Abdi S, Zhou Y, Patel N, Saini B, Nelson J. A new and easy technique to block the stellate ganglion. Pain Physician. 2004;7:327–31.
32. Kiray A, Arman C, Naderi S, Guveneer M, Korman E. Surgical anatomy of the cervical sympathetic trunk. Clin Anat. 2005;18:179–85.
33. Civelek E, Kiris T, Hepgul K, Canbolat A, Ersoy G, Cansever T. Anterolateral approach to the cervical spine: major anatomical structures and landmarks. J Neurosurg Spine. 2007;7:669–78.
34. Hogan Q, Erickson SJ. Magnetic resonance imaging of the stellate ganglion: normal appearance. Am J Roentgenol. 1992;158:655–9.
35. Narouze S, Vydyanathan A, Patel N. Ultrasound-guided stellate ganglion block successfully prevented esophageal puncture. Pain Physician. 2007;10:747–52.
36. Peng P, Narouze S. Ultrasound-guided interventional procedures in pain medicine: a review of anatomy, sonoanatomy, and procedures: part 1: nonaxial structures. Reg Anesth Pain Med. 2009;34(5):458–74.
37. Kapral S, Krafft P, Gosch M, Fleischmann D. Ultrasound imaging for stellate ganglion block: direct visualization of puncture site and local anesthetic spread. Reg Anesth. 1995;20:323–8.
38. Ojeda A, Sala-Blanch X, Moreno LA, et al. Ultrasound-guided stellate ganglion block what about the phrenic nerve? Reg Anesth Pain Med. 2013;38(2):167.
39. Vincent MB, Luna RA, Scandiuzzi D, Novis SA. Greater occipital nerve blockade in cervicogenic headache. Arq Neuropsiquiatr. 1998;56:720–5.
40. Naja ZM, El-Rajab M, Al-Tannir MA, Ziade FM, Tawfik OM. Occipital nerve blockade for cervicogenic headache: a double-blind randomized controlled clinical trial. Pain Pract. 2006;6:89–95.
41. Bovim G, Sand T. Cervicogenic headache, migraine without aura and tension-type headache. Diagnostic blockade of greater occipital and supra-orbital nerves. Pain. 1992;51:43–8.
42. Shim JH, Ko SY, Bang MR, et al. Ultrasound-guided greater occipital nerve block for patients with occipital headache and short term follow up. Korean J Anesthesiol. 2011;61(1):50–4.
43. Headache Classification Subcommittee of the International Headache Society. The international classification of headache disorders. 2nd ed. Cephalalgia. 2004;24(Suppl 1):9–160.
44. Greher M, Moriggl B, Curatolo M, Kirchmair L, Eichenberger U. Sonographic visualization and ultrasound-guided blockade of the greater occipital nerve: a comparison of two selective techniques confirmed by anatomical dissection. Br J Anaesth. 2010;104:637–42.
45. Mosser SW, Guyuron B, Janis JE, Rohrich RJ. The anatomy of the greater occipital nerve: implications for the etiology of migraine headaches. Plast Reconstr Surg. 2004;113:693–7.
46. Loukas M, El-Sedfy A, Tubbs RS, et al. Identification of greater occipital nerve landmarks for the treatment of occipital neuralgia. Folia Morphol (Warsz). 2006;65:299–304.
47. Natsis K, Baraliakos X, Appell HJ, et al. The course of the greater occipital nerve in the suboccipital region: a proposal for setting landmarks for local anesthesia in patients with occipital neuralgia. Clin Anat. 2006;19:332–6.
48. Cho J, Haun DW, Kettner NW. Sonographic evaluation of the greater occipital nerve in unilateral occipital neuralgia. J Ultrasound Med. 2012;31:37–42.
49. Greher M, Moriggl B, Curatolo M, et al. Sonographic visualization and ultrasound-guided blockade of the greater occipital nerve: a comparison of two selective techniques confirmed by anatomical dissection. Br J Anesth. 2010;104(5):637–42.
50. Boswell MV, Colson JD, Spillane WF. Therapeutic facet joint interventions in chronic spinal pain: a systematic review of effectiveness and complications. Pain Physician. 2005;8:101–14.
51. Manchikanti L, et al. Cervical medial branch blocks for chronic cervical facet joint pain: a randomized, double-blind, controlled trial with one-year follow-up. Spine. 2008;33:1813–20.
52. Manchikanti L, Boswell MV, Singh V, Pampati V, Damron KS, Beyer CD. Prevalence of facet joint pain in chronic spinal pain of cervical, thoracic, and lumbar regions. BMC Musculoskelet Disord. 2004;5:15.
53. Boswell MV, Shah RV, Everett CR, et al. Interventional techniques in the management of chronic spinal pain: evidence-based practice guidelines. Pain Physician. 2005;8:1–47.
54. Yun DH, Kim HS, Yoo SD, et al. Efficacy of ultrasonography-guided injections in patients with facet syndrome of the low lumbar spine. Ann Rehabil Med. 2012;36:66–71.
55. Greher M, Scharbert G, Kamolz LP, et al. Ultrasound-guided lumbar facet nerve block: a sonoanatomic study of a new methodologic approach. Anesthesiology. 2004;100:1242–8.
56. Shim JK, Moon JC, Yoon KB, et al. Ultrasound-guided lumbar medial-branch block: a clinical study with fluoroscopy control. Reg Anesth Pain Med. 2006;31:451–4.
57. Greher M, Kirchmair L, Enna B, et al. Ultrasound-guided lumbar facet nerve block: accuracy of a new technique confirmed by computed tomography. Anesthesiology. 2004;101:1195–200.
58. Gofeld M. Ultrasound-guided zygapophysial nerve and joint injection. Reg Anesth Pain Man. 2009;13:150–3.
59. Tsui BC, Tarkkila P, Gupta S, et al. Confirmation of caudal needle placement using nerve stimulation. Anesthesiology. 1999;91:374–8.
60. Botwin KP, Gruber RD, Bouchlas CG, et al. Complications of fluoroscopically guided caudal epidural injections. Am J Phys Med Rehabil. 2001;80:416–24.

61. Stitz MY, Sommer HM. Accuracy of blind versus fluoroscopically guided caudal epidural injection. Spine. 1999;24:1371–6.
62. Yoon JS, Sim KH, Kim SJ, et al. The feasibility of color doppler ultrasonography for caudal epidural steroid injection. Pain. 2005;118:210–4.
63. Park Y, Lee JH, Park KD, et al. Ultrasound-guided vs. fluoroscopy guided caudal epidural steroid injection for the treatment of unilateral lower lumbar radicular pain: a prospective, randomized, single-blind clinical study. Am J Phys Med Rehabil. 2013;92(6): 1–12.
64. Blanchais A, Le Goff B, Guillot P, et al. Feasibility and safety of ultrasound-guided caudal epidural glucocorticoid injections. Joint Bone Spine. 2010;77:440–4.
65. Chen CP, Wong AM, Hsu CC, et al. Ultrasound as a screening tool for proceeding with caudal epidural injections. Arch Phys Med Rehabil. 2010;91:358–63.
66. Vydyanathan A, Narouze S. Ultrasound-guided caudal and sacroiliac joint injections. Tech Reg Anesth Pain Manag. 2009;13:157–60.
67. Deer TR. An overview of interventional spinal techniques. Semin Pain Med. 2004;2:154–66.
68. Van der Wurff P, Buijs EJ, Groen GJ. A multitest regimen of pain provocation tests as an aid to reduce unnecessary minimally invasive sacroiliac joint procedures. Arch Phys Med Rehabil. 2006;87(1):10–4.
69. Berthelot J, Labat J, Le Goff B, et al. Provocative sacroiliac joint maneuvers and sacroiliac joint block are unreliable for diagnosing sacroiliac joint pain. Joint Bone Spine. 2006;73(1):17–23.
70. Manchikanti L, Staats P, Singh V, et al. Evidence-based practice guidelines for the interventional techniques in the management of chronic spinal pain. Pain Physician. 2003;6:3–81.
71. Harmon D, O'Sullivan M. Ultrasound-guided sacroiliac joint injection technique. Pain Physician. 2008;11:543–7.
72. Pekkafali MZ, Kiralp MZ, Basekim CC, et al. Sacroiliac joint injections performed with sonographic guidance. J Ultrasound Med. 2003;22:553–9.
73. Maldijian C, Mesgarzadeh M, Tehranzadeh J. Diagnostic and therapeutic features of facet and sacroiliac joint injection: anatomy, pathophysiology, and technique. Radiol Clin North Am. 1998;36:497–508.
74. Calvillo O, Skaribas I, Turnipseed J. Anatomy and pathophysiology of the sacroiliac joint. Curr Rev Pain. 2000;4:356–61.

Appendix

Sample Ultrasound Procedure Notes

Name	DOB	Medical Record Number
David	5/14/1948	660000

Providers	
Physician performing procedure	Name, M.D./D.O.
Assistant	Resident/fellow/PA/NP
Referring provider	Name, M.D./D.O.
Facility identification:	Examination date:

Procedure: {RIGHT/LEFT/BILATERAL} **Location injection with ultrasound guidance**

Findings:

Procedure note:
Thank you, Dr. (referring provider) for allowing me to participate in the care of your patient. Please do not hesitate to contact me with questions or concerns.

D.A. Spinner et al. (eds.), *Atlas of Ultrasound Guided Musculoskeletal Injections*, Musculoskeletal Medicine, DOI 10.1007/978-1-4614-8936-8, © Springer Science+Business Media, LLC 2014

Name	DOB	Medical Record Number
Alpha	5/14/1948	660000

Providers	
Physician performing procedure	Name, M.D./D.O.
Assistant	Resident/fellow/PA/NP
Referring provider	Name, M.D./D.O.
Facility identification:	Examination date:

Procedure: {RIGHT/LEFT/BILATERAL} **Subacromial/subdeltoid bursa (SASDB) corticosteroid injection with ultrasound guidance**

Findings: An ultrasound evaluation was performed of the {RIGHT/LEFT/BILATERAL} SASDB using a 12 MHz linear array transducer. The supraspinatus was visualized with the SASDB just superficial sliding under the acromion. There was a small amount of fluid and bunching of the bursa seen with dynamic testing.

Procedure note: After risks, benefits, and alternative treatment options and prognosis were discussed, the patient signed the informed consent. The {RIGHT/LEFT/BILATERAL} SASDB was evaluated under ultrasound using a 12 MHz linear array transducer. The findings are described above. The {RIGHT/LEFT/BILATERAL} subacromial region was then prepped with betadine and a sterile probe cover applied. The probe was positioned in the coronal plane parallel to the long axis of the supraspinatus. A wheal of 2 mL of 1 % lidocaine was injected as local anesthetic. A 25G 1.5″ needle was then inserted about 2–3 cm from the lateral end of the probe and directed towards the SASDB using an in-plane approach under direct ultrasound visualization. After negative aspiration, 6 mL total was then placed consisting of 40 mg Kenalog and 5 mL 1 % lidocaine without resistance. Excellent flow and fluid distention was noted in the bursal space confirming placement. There was no bleeding or complications. Post-procedure impingement maneuvers yielded no residual pain. Post-procedure care instructions were given, including applying ice with 15-min intervals up to three times daily for the next 48 h as needed. The patient is to follow up with us in 2 weeks for reevaluation and was instructed to contact us with any questions or concerns. The patient tolerated the procedure well.

Thank you, Dr. (referring provider) for allowing me to participate in the care of your patient. Please do not hesitate to contact me with questions or concerns.

Name	DOB	Medical Record Number
Alpha	5/14/1948	660000

Providers	
Physician performing procedure	Name, M.D./D.O.
Assistant	Resident/fellow/PA/NP
Referring provider	Name, M.D./D.O.
Facility identification:	Examination date:

Procedure: {RIGHT/LEFT/BILATERAL} **Lateral epicondyle percutaneous needle tenotomy with ultrasound guidance**

Findings: An ultrasound evaluation of the {RIGHT/LEFT/BILATERAL} common extensor tendons (CET) was performed with a 12 MHz linear array transducer. The CET appeared to have mild heterogeneity, focal hypoechoic areas, tendon thickening, mild cortical irregularity, and a few punctate calcifications consistent with tendinosis.

Procedure note: After risks, benefits, and alternatives were discussed, the patient signed informed consent. The {RIGHT/LEFT/BILATERAL} lateral elbow region was evaluated under ultrasound using a 12 MHz linear array transducer. The findings are described above. The {RIGHT/LEFT/BILATERAL} CET was then prepped with betadine and a sterile probe cover applied. Using an in-plane, long-axis, distal-to-proximal approach, the area was infiltrated with a 25 gauge needle. Gentle percutaneous tenotomy was performed with 3.0 mL 1 % lidocaine without epinephrine under direct ultrasound visualization. There was no bleeding or complication noted. Post-procedure care instructions were given, including applying ice for 15-min intervals up to three times daily for the next 48 h as needed. The patient is to follow up with us in 2 weeks for reevaluation and was instructed to contact us with any questions or concerns. The patient tolerated the procedure well.

Thank you, Dr. (referring provider) for allowing me to participate in the care of your patient. Please do not hesitate to contact me with questions or concerns.

Name	DOB	Medical Record Number
Alpha	5/14/1948	660000

Providers	
Physician performing procedure	Name, M.D./D.O.
Assistant	Resident/fellow/PA/NP
Referring provider	Name, M.D./D.O.
Facility identification:	Examination date:

Procedure: {RIGHT/LEFT/BILATERAL} **Carpal tunnel corticosteroid injection with ultrasound guidance**

Findings: An ultrasound evaluation was performed of the {RIGHT/LEFT/BILATERAL} carpal tunnel using a 12 MHz linear array transducer. The median nerve appeared enlarged, swollen, and flattened in the carpal tunnel, measuring # in diameter and #cm^2 in cross-sectional area. The flexor retinaculum appeared normal/thickened. The radial and ulnar arteries as well as the ulnar nerve were identified.

Procedure note: After risks, benefits, and alternative treatment options and prognosis were discussed, the patient signed the informed consent. The {RIGHT/LEFT/BILATERAL} carpal tunnel was evaluated under ultrasound using a 12–10 MHz linear array transducer. The findings are described above. The {RIGHT/LEFT/BILATERAL} ulnar-sided distal wrist region was then prepped with betadine and a sterile probe cover applied. The probe was positioned in the axial plane along the distal wrist crease. A 25G 1.5″ needle was then inserted about 1–2 cm from the ulnar side of the probe above/below the ulnar artery and nerve and directed towards the median nerve using an in-plane ulnar-sided approach under direct ultrasound visualization. 2 mL total was then placed consisting of 20 mg Kenalog and 1.5 mL 1 % lidocaine adjacent to the median nerve. Excellent flow of fluid was noted above/below the median nerve. The patient had increased numbness in D1-3 confirming median nerve block. There was no bleeding or complication noted. The patient tolerated the procedure well and was instructed to apply ice for 15-min intervals PRN.

Thank you, Dr. (referring provider) for allowing me to participate in the care of your patient. Please do not hesitate to contact me with questions or concerns.

Name	DOB	Medical Record Number
Alpha	5/14/1948	660000

Providers	
Physician performing procedure	Name, M.D./D.O.
Assistant	Resident/fellow/PA/NP
Referring provider	Name, M.D./D.O.
Facility identification:	Examination date:

Procedure: {RIGHT/LEFT/BILATERAL} **Greater trochanteric bursa corticosteroid injection with ultrasound guidance**

Findings: An ultrasound evaluation was performed of the {RIGHT/LEFT/BILATERAL} lateral hip using a 5–10 MHz linear or curved array transducer. The gluteus minimus and medius muscles were visualized inserting onto the anterior and posterolateral facets respectively. Both tendons appeared thickened with cortical irregularity at their insertion zones, heterogeneous in appearance without focal tears, consistent with mild tendinosis. There was a small amount of fluid identified in the subgluteus maximus (greater trochanteric) bursa.

Procedure note: After risks, benefits, and alternative treatment options and prognosis were discussed, the patient signed the informed consent. The {RIGHT/LEFT/BILATERAL} trochanteric bursa region was evaluated under ultrasound using a 10 MHz linear array transducer. The findings are described above. The lateral hip region was then marked, prepped with betadine, and draped. A sterile probe cover was applied. The probe was positioned in a coronal oblique plane parallel to the long axis of the gluteus medius tendon. A wheal of 2 mL of 1 % lidocaine was injected as local anesthetic. A [22/25] G 3″ spinal needle was then introduced using an in-plane approach. After negative aspiration, 5 mL total was then placed consisting of 40 mg Kenalog and 4 mL 1 % lidocaine was then placed under direct ultrasound visualization and without resistance. Fluid distention was appreciated on ultrasound confirming placement. There was no bleeding or complications. Post-procedure palpation yielded no residual tenderness. Post-procedure care instructions were given, including applying ice for 15-min intervals up to three times daily for the next 48 h as needed. The patient is to follow up with us in 2 weeks for reevaluation and was instructed to contact us with any questions or concerns. The patient tolerated the procedure well.

Thank you, Dr. (referring provider) for allowing me to participate in the care of your patient. Please do not hesitate to contact me with questions or concerns.

Name	DOB	Medical Record Number
Alpha	5/14/1948	660000

Providers	
Physician performing procedure	Name, M.D./D.O.
Assistant	Resident/fellow/PA/NP
Referring provider	Name, M.D./D.O.
Facility identification:	Examination date:
Viscosupplementation injection with ultrasound guidance	
Joint	Knee, shoulder, hip
Side	Right, left, bilateral
Substance	Hyalgan
Lot number	12345
Expiration date	12/31/2015

Findings: An ultrasound evaluation was performed of the {RIGHT/LEFT/BILATERAL} knee using a 12 MHz linear array transducer. There was a {SMALL, MED, LARGE} effusion noted. The quadriceps tendon appeared normal.

Procedure note: The {RIGHT/LEFT/BILATERAL} knee was examined using ultrasound, with the findings as noted above. After risks, benefits, and alternatives were discussed, the patient signed the informed consent. The {RIGHT/LEFT/BILATERAL} knee joint was evaluated under ultrasound using a 12 MHz linear array transducer. The {RIGHT/LEFT/BILATERAL} superolateral knee region was then prepped with betadine and a sterile probe cover applied. A wheal overlying the target of 1 mL of 1 % lidocaine was injected as local anesthetic. A 25G 1.5″ needle was then inserted into the suprapatellar joint recess using an in-plane approach under direct ultrasound visualization. Hyalgan 2 mL was then injected into the joint's suprapatellar recess under direct ultrasound visualization. Excellent flow of fluid was noted in the joint space. There was no bleeding or complications. The patient tolerated the procedure well.

Thank you, Dr. (referring provider) for allowing me to participate in the care of your patient. Please do not hesitate to contact me with questions or concerns.

Name	DOB	Medical Record Number
Alpha	5/14/1948	660000

Providers	
Physician performing procedure	Name, M.D./D.O.
Assistant	Resident/fellow/PA/NP
Referring provider	Name, M.D./D.O.
Facility identification:	Examination date:

Procedure: {RIGHT/LEFT/BILATERAL} **Plantar fascia corticosteroid injection with ultrasound guidance**

Findings: An ultrasound of the {RIGHT/LEFT/BILATERAL} foot was performed with a 12 MHz linear array transducer. There was thickening, hypoechogenicity, and cortical irregularity at the calcaneus consistent with plantar fasciitis.

Procedure note: After risks, benefits, and alternative treatment options and prognosis were discussed, the patient signed the informed consent. The {RIGHT/LEFT/BILATERAL} foot was evaluated under ultrasound using a 12 MHz linear array transducer. The findings are described above. The {RIGHT/LEFT/BILATERAL} medial hindfoot was then prepped with betadine and a sterile probe cover applied. A wheal of 2 mL of 1 % lidocaine was injected as local anesthetic. A 25G 1.5″ needle was then inserted about 2–3 cm from the medial end of the probe using a medial-to-lateral in-plane short-axis approach under direct ultrasound visualization with location confirmation by long-axis out-of-plane visualization. After negative aspiration, 4 mL total was then placed in multiple locations superficial and deep consisting to the fascia consisting of 20 mg Kenalog and 3.5 mL 1 % lidocaine. Excellent flow of fluid was noted around the plantar fascia. There was no bleeding or complications. Patient reported 100 % immediate pain relief following the procedure. Post-procedure palpation yielded no residual tenderness. Post-procedure care instructions were given, including applying ice for 15-min intervals up to three times daily for the next 48 h as needed. The patient is to follow up with us in 2 weeks for reevaluation and was instructed to contact us with any questions or concerns. The patient tolerated the procedure well.

Thank you, Dr. (referring provider) for allowing me to participate in the care of your patient. Please do not hesitate to contact me with questions or concerns.

Name	DOB	Medical Record Number
Alpha	5/14/1948	660000

Providers	
Physician performing procedure	Name, M.D./D.O.
Assistant	Resident/Fellow/PA/NP
Referring provider	Name, M.D./D.O.
Facility identification:	Examination date:

Procedure: {RIGHT/LEFT/BILATERAL} **Trigger point injection with ultrasound guidance**

Findings: An ultrasound of the {RIGHT/LEFT/BILATERAL} rhomboid muscle was performed with a 12 MHz linear array transducer. Viewing longitudinally, the layers noted include subcutaneous tissues, trapezius, rhomboid, ribs, pleura, and lungs. There were focal, hypoechoic regions within the rhomboid muscle combined with probe pressure confirm the trigger point and the pain referral pattern described.

Procedure note: After risks, benefits, and alternative treatment options and prognosis were discussed, the patient signed the informed consent. The {RIGHT/LEFT/BILATERAL} rhomboid muscle was evaluated under ultrasound using a 12 MHz linear array transducer. Ultrasound was medically indicated due to the thin layer of the rhomboid muscle and its close proximity to the pleura and lungs. The findings are described above. Using color Doppler, no vasculature was identified within the needle path. The upper back region was then prepped with alcohol. The probe was positioned perpendicular to the long axis of the rhomboid muscle. A wheal of 2 mL of 1 % lidocaine was injected as local anesthetic. A 25G 1.5″ needle was then inserted about 1–2 cm from the caudal end of the probe and directed towards the muscle using an in-plane approach under direct ultrasound visualization. The needle was guided to the muscle keeping superficial to the costal margin to avoid lung puncture. After negative aspiration, 5 cc of 1 % lidocaine was then injected into the area following a dry needling technique. There was no bleeding or complications. Post-procedure palpation showed decreased tenderness over the trigger point without pain referral. Post-procedure care instructions were given, including applying ice for 15-min intervals up to three times daily for the next 48 h as needed. The patient is to follow up with us in 2 weeks for reevaluation and was instructed to contact us with any questions or concerns. The patient tolerated the procedure well.

Thank you, Dr. (referring provider) for allowing me to participate in the care of your patient. Please do not hesitate to contact me with questions or concerns.

Name	DOB	Medical Record Number
Alpha	5/14/1948	660000

Providers	
Physician performing procedure	Name, M.D./D.O.
Assistant	Resident/fellow/PA/NP
Referring provider	Name, M.D./D.O.
Facility identification:	Examination date:

Procedure: {RIGHT/LEFT/BILATERAL} **Botulinum toxin injection with EMG and ultrasound guidance**

Muscles	Biceps	Brachialis	Brachioradialis	Pronator teres	FCU
# of locations	2	1	1	1	1
Total dose (units)	75	25	40	30	30
Total dose: 200 units in 2 mL preservative free saline					
Lot #			Expiration date:		

Diagnosis: Spasticity

Procedure note: After risks, benefits, and alternative treatment options and prognosis were discussed, the patient signed the informed consent. The muscles listed above were prepped with alcohol. An injectable 3″ monopolar needle was inserted into the above muscles using an in-plane approach under direct ultrasound visualization. Live ultrasound guidance using a 10 MHz linear array transducer was used to avoid neurovascular structures of the arm and forearm. The limb was passively ranged and large MUAP activity was generated with passive stretch confirming correct location. After negative aspiration, the above botulinum toxin was placed in the various locations. The patient tolerated the procedure well without complication. Post-procedure care instructions were given, including applying ice for 15-min intervals up to three times daily for the next 48 h as needed. The patient is to follow up with us in 3–4 weeks for reevaluation and was instructed to contact us with any questions or concerns.

Thank you, Dr. (referring provider) for allowing me to participate in the care of your patient. Please do not hesitate to contact me with questions or concerns.

Name	DOB	Medical Record Number
Alpha	5/14/1948	660000

Providers	
Physician performing procedure	Name, M.D./D.O.
Assistant	Resident/Fellow/PA/NP
Referring provider	Name, M.D./D.O.
Facility identification:	Examination date:

Procedure: {RIGHT/LEFT/BILATERAL} **Sacroiliac joint (SIJ) injection with ultrasound guidance**

Findings: No effusion was noted.

Procedure: After risks, benefits, and alternative treatment options and prognosis were discussed, the patient signed the informed consent. The risks include but are not limited to infection, allergic reaction, nerve damage, paralysis, epidural hematoma, syncope, headache, respiratory or cardiac arrest, and scar formation. The {RIGHT/LEFT/BILATERAL} SIJ was evaluated under ultrasound using a 10 MHz linear array transducer. The findings are described above. The SIJ region was then prepped with betadine and a sterile probe cover applied. A 10 MHz linear array transducer was used to identify the {RIGHT/LEFT} PSIS in the axial plane. The transducer was moved inferiorly until the inferior sacroiliac joint margin could be identified. The skin was anesthetized with 3 mL of 1 % Lidocaine without Epinephrine. A 22G 3″ spinal needle was then inserted obliquely in a medial-to-lateral in-plane fashion into the SIJ under direct ultrasound visualization. After negative aspiration, a total of 3.0 mL consisting of 1.0 mL of Depo-Medrol (80 mg/mL), with the remainder of 0.25 % Marcaine without Epinephrine was then injected into the SI joint, with excellent intra-articular flow noted, and no extravasation of injectate. There was no bleeding or complications. Patient reported 100 % immediate pain relief following the procedure. Post-procedure care instructions were given, including applying ice for 15-min intervals up to three times daily for the next 48 h as needed. The patient is to follow up with us in 2 weeks for reevaluation and was instructed to contact us with any questions or concerns. The patient tolerated the procedure well.

Thank you, Dr. (referring provider) for allowing me to participate in the care of your patient. Please do not hesitate to contact me with questions or concerns.

Index

A
Abductor pollicis longus (APL), 31–33, 39
Achilles tendon, 75–78
Acromioclavicular (AC) joint, 10, 11, 119
Acromion, 9–11, 14–16, 91
Active trigger point, 89
Adductor brevis, 47, 48, 105
Adductor longus, 47, 48, 105
Adductor magnus, 47, 48, 105
Anechoic, 4, 10, 14, 26, 66, 69, 71, 111
Anisotropy, 3, 4, 9, 15, 29, 30, 38, 46, 63, 66, 77
Ankle inversion, 109–112
Anterior superior iliac spine (ASIS), 43, 49–53, 106
Anterior talofibular ligament (ATFL), 73–75
Anterior tibiotalar ligament, 72, 73
Anterior tubercle, 93, 123, 124, 128, 129
APL. *See* Abductor pollicis longus (APL)
ASIS. *See* Anterior superior iliac spine (ASIS)
ATFL. *See* Anterior talofibular ligament (ATFL)
Atlas of Ultrasound Guided Musculoskeletal Injections
Attenuated, 1

B
Baker's cyst, 57, 66–67
Biceps brachii tendon, 7
Bicipital groove, 7–10
Botulinum toxin (BTX), 1, 90, 94, 95, 101–104, 106, 107, 111–117, 119

C
Calcaneocuboid joint, 77–79
Calcaneofibular ligament (CFL), 73, 74
Calcaneus, 70–79, 84, 85
Carotid artery, 93–95, 124, 125, 128, 129
Carpal tunnel syndrome (CTS), 29–31
Carpometacarpal (CMC) joint, 33–35, 39–41
Cartilage uncovering sign, 4
Caudal, 12, 63, 128, 132, 133
Cervical dystonia, 101–104, 112–113
Cervical medial branch block (CMBB), 125–126
Cervical radiculitis, 123
Cervical spinal nerve, 123–125
Cervical vertebrae, 123, 124
CFL. *See* Calcaneofibular ligament (CFL)
Chemodenervation, 101–119
Chopart joint, 77
Chronic aspiration, 113–119
Circumflex humeral artery, 7, 8
Clavicle, 7, 9, 10, 91–93, 95
Clenched fist, 102–106
Color Doppler, 3, 92, 94–97, 132
Common extensor tendon (CET), 22–24
Common flexor tendon (CFT), 17–20
Complex regional pain syndrome, 128
Compression neuropathy, 24, 29
Crouched gait, 105–109
CTS. *See* Carpal tunnel syndrome (CTS)

D
Deep fibular nerve, 69, 70, 110, 111
Deflection, 1–2, 111
Deltoid ligament, 71–73
Deltoid muscle, 14, 16
DeQuervain's disease, 31
Distal radioulnar joint (DRUJ), 31, 32
Dystonia, 101

E
Electrical stimulation, 1, 101
Electromyography (EMG), 89, 95, 101, 106–109, 111–113
Equinovarus, 105, 109–112
Extensor hallucis longus, 69, 70
Extensor pollicis brevis (EPB), 31–33, 39
External oblique, 52

F
FCU. *See* Flexor carpi ulnaris (FCU)
FDP. *See* Flexor digitorum profundus (FDP)
Femoral head, 43–45, 50, 51
Femur, 57–59, 63–65, 106
Fibula, 62, 63, 69, 74, 75, 82–84, 109–111
Fibular tendon sheath, 82–84
First annular (A1) pulley, 37
First extensor compartment, 31–34
First metatarsophalangeal joint (MTP), 80–82
Flexor carpi radialis (FCR), 30, 34, 35, 102–107
Flexor carpi ulnaris (FCU), 20, 102, 104–107
Flexor digitorum, 37, 71, 72
Flexor digitorum longus, 85, 86, 105, 109, 110
Flexor digitorum profundus (FDP), 29, 37–39, 102–107
Flexor digitorum superficialis (FDS), 29, 37, 38, 101, 102, 104–107
Flexor hallucis longus, 71, 72, 85, 86
Flexor pollicis longus, 29, 30, 37, 102, 104–106
Flexor retinaculum, 29–31, 85, 86
Flexor superficialis muscle, 30
Focal zone, 3
Forearm flexor spasticity, 102–106
Frequency, 3, 44, 106, 108, 111, 112, 116, 117

D.A. Spinner et al. (eds.), *Atlas of Ultrasound Guided Musculoskeletal Injections*, Musculoskeletal Medicine,
DOI 10.1007/978-1-4614-8936-8, © Springer Science+Business Media, LLC 2014

G

Gain, 3, 51, 59
Ganglion cyst, 35–37
Gastrocnemius, 66, 67, 105, 109–111
Gel standoff, 5, 10, 11, 18, 32, 36, 38–40, 60, 61, 70, 71, 73, 78, 79, 81, 82, 87
Gerdy's tubercle, 65
Geyser sign, 4
Glenohumeral (GH) joint, 7, 11–14
Glenoid labrum, 12, 14
Gluteus medius, 45, 46, 65
Golfer's elbow, 17
Gracilis, 47, 61, 105
Greater occipital nerve (GON), 129–130
Greater trochanteric bursa, 45
Greater trochanteric pain syndrome (GTPS), 45–46
Greater tuberosity, 8, 9

H

Heel-toe, 3, 4, 6, 44
High frequency linear array transducer, 2, 9, 10, 12, 18, 20, 22, 24, 26, 27, 30, 31, 33, 35, 37, 39, 41, 46, 48, 50, 58, 59, 62–66, 71, 72, 74, 76, 77, 80, 82, 85–87, 93, 94, 96, 97, 119, 126, 129, 130, 133
Hip adductor tendinopathy, 46
Hip adductor tendinosis, 46–48
Hip joint, 43–45, 50, 51
Hip joint capsule, 44, 51
Hockey stick transducer, 3
Humeral head, 7, 12, 14
Hyperechoic, 4, 6, 7, 10, 14, 17–21, 26, 27, 29, 30, 34, 35, 37, 38, 43, 45, 49, 59, 61–63, 65, 66, 69, 80, 85, 90, 91, 93, 108, 127, 129, 131–133
Hypoechoic, 4, 6, 14, 17–21, 23, 25, 26, 29, 37, 47, 54, 57, 59, 65, 66, 80, 84, 90, 91, 108, 118, 123, 125, 129, 131

I

Iliacus, 49, 50, 105, 106
Iliofemoral ligament, 43, 44
Iliohypogastric nerve, 52, 53
Ilioinguinal nerve, 52–53
Iliopsoas, 44, 45, 47, 101, 105
Iliopsoas bursitis, 50–51
Iliopsoas spasticity, 106–109
Iliopsoas tendinopathy, 50–51
Iliotibial band friction syndrome, 64
Iliotibial band syndrome (ITBS), 64–66
Inferior oblique muscle (IOM), 129, 130
Infraspinatus muscle, 7, 11–14, 92
In-plane, 2, 4, 6–16, 18–27, 29–40, 43–54, 57–67, 70–87, 92–98, 104–112, 118, 124–130, 132–135
Interdigital neuroma, 80, 81
Internal jugular vein, 93–95, 124, 125, 128, 129
Internal oblique, 52
IOM. *See* Inferior oblique muscle (IOM)
Isoechoic, 4
ITBS. *See* Iliotibial band syndrome (ITBS)

J

Jumper's knee, 59

K

Kager's fat pad, 75, 77
Kirschner turn (K-turn), 6, 59, 85
Knee osteoarthritis, 57–59
K-turn. *See* Kirschner turn (K-turn)

L

Latent trigger point, 89
Lateral epicondylosis, 22–24
Lateral femoral cutaneous nerve, 49–50
Lateral ligament complex, 23, 24, 69, 73–75
Lesser tuberosity, 7, 8
Levator scapulae (LS), 91, 96–97, 104, 112, 113
Lister's tubercle, 31, 32
Long axis, 2, 9, 18, 20, 23–24, 35–37, 39, 45, 48, 59, 62, 66
Low frequency curvilinear transducer, 44
LS. *See* Levator scapulae (LS)
Lumbar medial branch block, 130–132

M

Medial collateral ligament (MCL), 61, 62
Medial epicondylosis (ME), 17–18
Medial malleolus, 71–73, 78, 82, 85–87, 109
Median nerve, 2, 4, 29–31, 36
Meralgia paresthetica, 49
Metacarpophalangeal joint, 37, 39
Midtarsal joint, 77–80
Morton's neuroma, 80–81
Myofascial pain syndrome (MPS), 89–90

N

Neuromuscular, 101–119

O

Obturator nerve, 46–48
Occipital neuralgia, 129
Olecranon bursitis, 26–27
Out-of-plane, 2, 5, 18, 23, 24, 30–31, 33–35, 37–40, 62–63, 71–72, 80–81, 83, 85, 86, 118–119

P

Paratenon, 76–77
Parotid gland, 113, 118, 119
Patella, 57–60
Patellar tendinopathy, 59
Patellar tendinosis, 59
Peroneal tendon sheath, 74, 82
Peroneus brevis, 82
Peroneus longus, 82
Pes anserine bursitis, 59–62
Phrenic nerve, 91, 93, 94, 129
Physical medicine and rehabilitation, 1
Piriformis, 53–54
Plantar fascia, 84–85
Plantar nerves, 71, 72, 85, 86
Pleura, 4, 93, 98
Popliteal cysts, 66
Popliteus, 57, 63–64

Popliteus muscle tendon unit (PMTU), 63, 64
Posterior interosseous nerve, 24–26
Posterior interosseous nerve syndrome, 24
Posterior scalene, 93, 112
Posterior tibial nerve, 85, 86
Posterior tubercle, 96, 123–125, 128
Power Doppler, 3, 7, 17, 76–78, 81, 86
Prefemoral fat pad, 57, 58
Pronator quadratus, 102, 105
Pronator teres, 102, 104–106
Proximal humerus, 7
Psoas, 49, 50, 52, 105–108

Q
Quadriceps, 57, 58, 105

R
Radial collateral ligament, 23
Radial nerve, 24, 25, 33, 106
Radial tunnel syndrome, 24
Reflection, 2, 4
Refraction, 2
Retrocalcaneal bursa, 75–76
Rhomboid muscle, 91, 92, 97–98

S
Sacral cornua, 132, 133
Sacrococcygeal ligament, 132, 133
Sacroiliac joint, 133–135
Salivary glands, 113–119
Sartorius, 44, 49, 50, 61
SASDB. *See* Subacromial/subdeltoid bursa (SASDB)
Scalene muscle, 93, 139
Scalenus anterior, 93–94, 113
Scaphoid, 29, 34–36
Scaphotrapeziotrapezoid (STT) joint, 33–35
Scatter, 2
SCM. *See* Sternocleidomastoid muscle (SCM)
Semimembranosus-gastrocnemius bursa, 66
Semispinalis capitis (SSC), 104, 129, 130
Semitendinosus, 61, 105
Short axis, 2, 8, 18, 21, 23–26, 29, 31–33, 36, 37, 59, 61, 63, 66, 82, 83, 123, 124, 133, 134
Sialorrhea, 103, 113–119
Spasticity, 1, 47, 101, 102, 108
Spinal accessory nerve (SAN), 91, 92, 96
Spine, 11, 12, 91, 92, 97, 123–135
Spinoglenoid notch, 12, 14
Spring ligament, 77, 78
Starry sky, 4
Stellate ganglion, 128–129
Stenosing tenosynovitis, 37
Sternocleidomastoid muscle (SCM), 93–96, 112, 113, 129
Subacromial/subdeltoid bursa (SASDB), 7, 8, 14–16
Subluxation, 20, 82
Submandibular gland, 113, 114, 118, 119
Submedius bursa, 45
Subminimus bursa, 45
Subscapularis muscle, 8, 9
Subscapularis tendon, 7
Subtalar joint, 70–72
Supinator syndrome, 24
Suprapatellar fat pad, 57, 58
Suprapatellar joint space, 57
Suprascapular artery, 11, 12, 14, 91
Suprascapular ligament, 11, 12
Suprascapular nerve, 4, 11, 12
Suprascapular nerve block, 11–12
Suprascapular notch, 11, 12, 91
Supraspinatus muscle, 11, 12, 15, 91, 92
Sustentaculum tali, 71, 72, 77

T
Talar dome, 69, 70
Talonavicular joint, 78, 79
Talus, 69–75, 78, 79
Tarsal tunnel, 71, 72
Tarsal tunnel syndrome, 85–87
Tendinopathy, 6, 22, 43, 45, 89
Tennis elbow, 22
Tenosynovitis, 7, 29, 31, 37, 82
Third occipital nerve (TON), 125–126, 129
Thumb in palm, 102–106
Tibia, 61–63, 65, 69, 71, 76, 86, 87, 109–111
Tibialis anterior, 69, 70, 109–111
Tibialis posterior, 71, 72, 85, 86, 101, 105, 109–112
Tibiofibular joint, 57, 62–63
Tibiotalar joint, 69–71
Time gain compensation (TGC), 3
Toggling, 4, 30, 132
Torticolllis, 102, 112, 113
Transducer, 1–10, 12, 14, 16, 18–27, 29–39, 41, 43–54, 58, 59, 61–66, 69–78, 80–87, 90, 91, 93–97, 104, 106, 108, 110–112, 118, 119, 123–135
Transverse abdominis, 52
Transverse carpal ligament, 29
Transverse humeral ligament, 7, 8
Transverse tarsal joint, 77–80
Trapezium, 29, 34, 35, 39, 40
Trapezius muscle, 11, 90–93, 97, 112
Trapezoid, 49
Trigger finger, 37–39
Trigger point, 1, 37, 89–98, 112
Triple crown sign, 108, 132

U
Ulnar collateral ligament, 17–20, 23
Ulnar nerve, 18, 20–22, 27, 29, 30, 106, 107
Ulnar neuritis, 20

V
Vagus nerve, 93, 95, 125
Volar plate, 37

W
Walk off, 5, 14

Z
Zygapophysial facet joint, 130

Printed in the United States of America